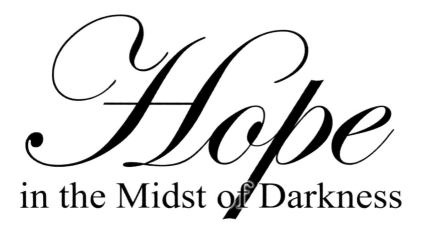

Hope
in the Midst of Darkness

A breast cancer survivor's journey

Nancy Horton

HOPE IN THE MIDST OF DARKNESS: A BREAST CANCER SURVIVOR'S STORY

ISBN-13: 978-1-77069-194-0

Printed in Canada.

Word Alive Press
131 Cordite Road, Winnipeg, MB R3W 1S1
www.wordalivepress.ca

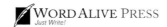

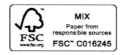

Library and Archives Canada Cataloguing in Publication

Horton, Nancy Jane
    Hope in the midst of darkness / Nancy Horton.

ISBN 978-1-77069-194-0

    1. Horton, Nancy Jane--Health. 2. Breast--Cancer--Patients--Canada--Biography. 3. Mothers--Canada--Biography. 4. Breast--Cancer--Patients--Religious life. 5. Breast--Cancer--Religious aspects--Christianity. 6. Breast--Cancer--Psychological aspects. I. Title.

BV4910.33.H67 2010   248.8'6196994490092   C2010-907713-X

The advice herein is not intended to replace the services of trained health professionals, or be a substitute for medical advice. You are advised to consult with your health care professional with regard to matters relating to your health, and in particular regarding matters that may require diagnosis or medical attention.

Front cover photo taken by Tim Girard (www.impressionistics.ifp3.com).

Back cover photo taken by Vicki Cain.

Acknowledgements

My deepest appreciation to...

God for giving and sustaining my life.

Rob. Thank you for being the man of integrity that you are. For loving me and standing by me through everything. You are truly a wonderful husband, father and friend.

Our three boys, Ben, Carter and Spencer. You inspire me to live, play and laugh. Your smiles, infectious laughter and warm hugs make each day worth living. Thank you for your understanding and allowing me the time to write this book. I'm proud of you!

Mom and Dad. Thank you for giving me your blessing so that I can openly share the pain of our past to allow others to experience healing. I love you.

A special thanks to my editor Jackie, and my great team of proof readers Cindy, Mom and Wanda for a job well done and Tim Girard for the photo on the front cover.

To my family, friends, church and even the strangers that prayed and offered support; each one of you made walking this journey much easier than you'll ever know! I love you all and will always remember your kindness! So, it is with my deepest affection, that I dedicate this book to each and every one of you.

Lastly, it is with great honour that I must acknowledge the greats such as Joyce Meyer, Beth Moore and Gloria Copeland. It is the teachings of these godly women that I've learned from and speak through. God has used you to strengthen and anchor my soul, to the point of continued existence on this earth. May God continue to richly bless you through your faithful service to the King!

Contents

Acknowledgements   v

One – The Onset of Darkness   1

Two – You're Beautiful! (Even After a Mastectomy)   12

Three – Chemotherapy   37

Four – Herceptin   78

Five – Radiation   82

Six – Why Me?   87

Seven – Fear   107

Eight – Reconstruction   144

Nine – Inner Healing   162

Ten – Don't Give Up!   216

Eleven – Managing Stress   234

Twelve – Entering Your Promised Land   272

Thirteen – God's Will to Heal!   316

Fourteen – Jesus Our Great Shepherd!   345

Chapter One
The Onset of Darkness

What's it about a physical that makes it so uninviting? If I took a survey, I'm sure people would all agree that it's not the smiling faces at the reception desk! I'm certain it's the annual humiliation of the poking and prodding of body parts we all wish could stay hidden, those places now affected by gravity that worsen with time!

December 2, 2004, seemed like any other ordinary snowy day. I hustled our two oldest boys out the door to ensure they wouldn't be late for school. A physical was the last thing I anticipated, as I stood watching my husband Rob turn the page of our country calendar. Surprise! Oh, I was surprised all right! Time sure flies when you're having fun!

It seemed like just yesterday when I was in my doctor's office discussing the constant dull ache I'd experienced in my right breast for over a year. Along with the ache, a thick mustard–orange discharge crusted in my undergarment. Yeah, okay, I might as well be frank, my bra. This is big stuff we are talking about here... or in my case, big issue, little stuff! I experienced quite a few problems with clogged ducts and had mastitis on the right side with each boy while nursing, especially when it came time to wean. Mastitis is inflammation of the breast, usually caused by a bacterial infection due to a break or crack in the skin, or when milk becomes stagnant because the breast is unable to be emptied.[1] A year had passed since my doctor diagnosed my problem as nothing! To my knowledge, there wasn't any family history of breast cancer; I wasn't overweight, I didn't drink or smoke, and because I nursed each child for almost a year I was told it was nothing to worry about and was left with no further examination.

This is not a ploy to take shots at my doctor; people need to pay attention to their bodies and be aware of symptoms so they don't run into trouble as I did. When our bodies are doing weird things, we need to investigate the problem until we get an answer, especially one that we are comfortable with, even if it means getting a second opinion. Don't worry about hurting your doctor's feelings. This is your health we're talking about! Unfortunately, the medical system is overloaded and we need to become well-informed so we can act as our own advocates.

I was a busy wife and mother, burning the candle at both ends for too long, trying to ensure that life was perfect for everyone around me. So much so, that I neglected to look after myself. After discussing the new problem of an inverted nipple, my doctor decided I needed further testing. She assured me it was probably nothing other than fibroid tissue and scheduled me for a mammogram one week later.

Several nights after my physical, I had a very vivid dream of missing my right breast. In the same dream, I stood by a doctor's chart and was restored on both sides. Hey, I looked pretty good, a much perkier version than before! When I awoke, an unfamiliar Scripture stirred in my mind. I quickly referred to my Bible to verify its authenticity. It read, *Lord, even though I have trouble all around me, you will keep me alive.* (Psalm 139:7; NCV)

Alive! Alive is good! A knot tightened in my stomach. Reaching across into my pine night table, I retrieved my "God's Promise" book. I flipped it open directly to the comfort section. I began to pray, "Lord, please give me two Scriptures to confirm what I think you're trying to tell me." The two Scriptures He gave me were: "*So do not fear, for I am with you; do not be dismayed, for I am your God. I will strengthen you and help you; I will uphold you with my righteous right hand... For I am the Lord, your God, who takes hold of your right hand and says to you, Do not fear; I will help you."* (Isaiah 41:10, 13) and *"Fear not, for I have redeemed you; I have summoned you by name; you are mine. When you pass through the waters, I will be with you; and when you pass through the rivers, they will not sweep over you. When you walk through the fire, you will not be burned; the flames will not set you ablaze. For I am the Lord, your God, the Holy One of Israel, your Saviour."* (Isaiah 43:1b–3a)

Yes, this was something I was definitely going to have to go through. Then a peace came that surpasses all understanding as I prayed (Philippians 4:6). That week, I had my mammogram, a series of squish-and-squash tests that detect abnormalities, at our local hospital. Much to my surprise, it didn't hurt nearly as bad as rumours had led me to believe. Then again, they say "No brain, no pain." Hopefully that wasn't it!

Days later, my doctor called to notify me that I was being sent for a biopsy because there was a questionable area on the mammogram. Because of the approaching Christmas holiday, the breast clinic was unable to fit me in until January 10th. Our family went about life, performing our usual daily routines.

One day, as I stood washing my lunch dishes at the kitchen sink, I felt as if an explosion went off inside my right breast. It was a sudden sharp, tearing sensation that went throughout the tissue and then immediately dissipated. I had a strong gut feeling it wasn't a good sign, not to mention the indication that came from my dream. Regardless, I formed a good distraction by organizing and entertaining for both my husband's and my family's Christmas dinners at our home.

January 10th soon arrived, and Rob and I were on our way to Ottawa for my biopsy. My Mom overslept and arrived three-quarters of an hour late to watch the boys. I quietly prayed as Rob raced as fast as the wet, slippery roads would allow. It was snowing quite hard, but we managed to be only twenty minutes late. Rob dropped me off near the front of the hospital to gain time and I ran across the lawn in running shoes, through a foot of snow, while he parked. I was relieved when the receptionist said she could still fit me in.

After I slipped into a thin, pastel blue gown, the nurse explained the procedure and then had me lie face down on a table. She carefully positioned me with my breast poking through a hole. She washed my skin with an iodine solution and clamped my breast in an instrument that reminded me of a vice grip. As I lay completely still, a radiologist took several x-rays from different angles, to help locate the particular areas needing biopsy. The technologist then froze my breast with several needles and proceeded, seconds later, making a small incision in my skin. A metal core cylinder was then inserted into the incision. By using the x-rays to guide his way, the technologist was able to manoeuvre the core cylinder to each specific area. Each time the cylinder was set in place, a long needle projected out and into the tissue to remove flesh samples, then retracted back into the cylinder. I believe they removed ten or eleven samples. Then another x-ray was taken to ensure that the abnormal calcifications seen on the x-rays had been properly sampled. As they placed Steri-tape on the incision, the nurse informed me that the results of the biopsy were expected back in five days.

While searching the Internet to educate myself on types of breast cancer, I discovered that I had all of the symptoms listed: lumps, inverted nipple, skin irritation, pain, and discharge from the nipple. The dimpling of the skin can be located anywhere on the breast.[2] Additional symptoms, swelling, redness, and hot to touch, were listed for a different type of breast cancer called Inflammatory.[3] Also, eighty-five percent of women who are diagnosed with breast cancer have no family history of breast cancer.[4] Did I ever want to kick myself in the rear end! Self–examination was something I neither practiced nor felt comfortable with. The attitude I carried was why bother learning about such things when they won't likely ever happen to you? I figured, "I'm young, thirty–six years old! I eat well." Or so I thought, until recently. We'll get into that one later. Girls, we need to be our own advocates and get educated!

Five days of waiting turned into nine, and after playing phone tag for a while with receptionists, my G.P. received the results and had her nurse contact me. I was to meet her at the hospital the next morning before she started her obstetrics clinic. I knew it! It had to be bad news; why else would she have had her nurse call and insist I meet with her? Otherwise, she would have given the results over the phone.

I convinced my husband to come to my appointment because I was sure of the results. He, on the other hand, didn't think it was anything. I'm not certain if it was a case of denial or just optimistic thinking. I had told Rob about my dream and the Scriptures God had given me. He felt that I was putting too much weight on my dream; at that point, he didn't under–stand God talking to someone through Scripture. In the past, God gave me several dreams that came into fruition and I believed this to be no differ–ent.

After a short wait in the small, crowded waiting room, the nurse called Rob and me into the examination room and encouraged us to sit down. My doctor promptly entered the room and slowly closed the door. It seemed like eternity as she slowly leaned back against a small, white cabinet in the corner, and in quiet hesitation, searched for the right words. There was no need. The solemn expression of her thin, pale face said it all.

"It's not good, is it?" I voiced.

"No, she replied. "You have breast cancer, Nancy."

The words hit my husband like a ton of bricks. Glancing quickly over at Rob to see his reaction, my heart felt sick for him. His mother had suffered from cancer for approximately 23 years. She lost her battle to cancer in 2000, and now this. He slumped forward in his chair with both hands over his mouth. What was he thinking?

It's no big deal; I'll have my breast removed and have reconstruction. I was never too crazy about them anyway. It shouldn't be a big deal. I can handle this, I thought to myself, until I heard. "You're young and strong, Nancy. They will hit you with everything they've got. Surgery, chemo, and radiation," the doctor said confidently.

Wait a minute! Chemo! My bluish green eyes welled up with tears. I never even thought about that! The rest was pretty much a blur... I remember jumping off the table and Rob wrapping his left arm around my waist as we quietly walked out of her office. God's strength gripped us as we walked through the waiting room, full of smiling faces, cooing babies and young expectant mothers rubbing their tummies. My family doctor booked me in to see the surgeon for a consultation appointment two days later and I had surgery six days after that. Now, if that isn't God's favour nothing is!

On the truck ride home after receiving the news, Rob filled with anger. "Were things going too well for the Horton family? Finally, when things were starting to really come together and we were finally getting ahead, now God does this to us!" he exclaimed.

"No, Rob, God didn't do this to us. God loves us and wants what's best. I don't have all the answers right now, but please don't blame God." Silence filled the truck.

Rob is this amazingly sweet, burly redhead who is strong and kind hearted. He held me in his muscular arms as I sat in a fetal position on our couch. I remembered back to the time we were joyfully planning our wedding, when Rob received the call that his mother had stomach cancer. I wondered if he felt the same way. We were both in shock, even though God had shown me beforehand what was now taking place. Shock is a great defence mechanism God designed to help our bodies to cope in time of crisis! We made all the necessary phone calls to family and a few close friends.

An hour had passed, and I decided I needed to go to my "Mom's Time Out" group that meets bi-weekly on Wednesday mornings for Bible study. The ladies are from all different denominations, all very special and unique. I had asked for prayer a few weeks previously and felt it would be easier to share the news all at once. As I walked into the cool basement room of the old Wesleyan Church, I could hear Rebecca, our leader, finishing the discussion on the other side of the door. I entered quietly to be sure not to disturb them and sunk my numb body down into the first open chair next to the door. Rebecca stopped flat in mid-sentence, glanced up with her hopeful brown eyes and asked, "Was the news good?" I shook my head no. My heart began to race.

Eyes streamed with tears as my dear friends gathered around me in loving prayer and prayed as the Spirit led them. They prayed for my healing, for strength, for my family's needs to be met, and most of all for my husband and children to draw close to the Lord and to feel His comfort. Reb prayed Isaiah 43, without knowing that was the exact Scripture God had given me. God is so good to confirm things and to give us assurance in the uncertain times of our lives. The next day, I attended "Coffee Break" Bible study, where Spencer and I went religiously on Thursdays. My sister Debbie, who also attended, had coaxed me to ask for prayer the previous week. I hadn't planned on telling anyone else because of my pride. Obviously, God had another plan. When prayer request time came, I spoke up and explained the situation. When it was time for us to go to our classes everyone just sat there. Full of compassion and love, these beautiful women formed a circle around me and prayed. God again confirmed the Scriptures He initially gave me. The Lord also reminded me to... *"Be still and know that He is God."* as it states in Psalm 46:10. It's at times like this that we need to let God be God and put our lives in His hands. He is more capable than what we give or allow Him credit for.

I burst into tears, wondering what terrible thing I had done. I loved the Lord, went to church regularly, and spent regular time in the Word and in prayer daily! What? What did I do? These questions kept ringing in my ears. I will share what the Lord revealed about these questions in a later chapter. Cindy, my group leader and friend, spoke God's love into me and reminded me that nothing can separate us from His perfect love.

At bedtime, we gathered our boys, ages four, eight and ten, in Ben's room to read bedtimes stories. Normally, our routine would be to read individually to them and have quiet, sharing time. Experience has found it's the best time for them to open up. Then came the hard part! How do you explain to three little boys about a serious situation without filling them with fear? They would hear us talking and it was only fair to involve them in what was going on. My heart was filled with compassion as I gazed into their innocent faces and shared the unfortunate state and how it was going to affect our lives for the next year. Three shades of beautiful, blue eyes watered as they stared with serious intent. Their chins began to quiver as they realized the severity of the circumstances.

We shared that Mommy was very sick and needed to have one, possibly two surgeries as well as medication that would most likely make her sick to her tummy, lose her hair, and perhaps make her too weak to play at times. We cried and prayed, asking God to heal Mommy and protect our family. My heart wrenched as the boys sobbed themselves to sleep, embraced in each other's arms. I used this situation as a tool, to teach them to talk to God and to trust Him. The Word says, *"The Lord is faithful to all His promises and loving towards all He has made"* (Psalms 145:13b). God is a God of His Word and He will do what He says (Hebrews 10:23).

Carter, my middle son, was sent into a crying fit every time hair loss was mentioned. He would inquire repeatedly, hoping the outcome had changed. He loved my straight, blond hair more than I did, I think. On a few past occasions, he would ask me to put my hair into pigtails to play. I finally asked the Lord for wisdom in how to deal with this situation, after his third outburst of tears. I don't know why we don't save ourselves the trouble and ask right away! Wisdom spoke right out of my mouth before it even registered. "You mean to tell me, you won't love mommy with her big, fat, bald head?" I said. Carter laughed and laughed. Bubbles of joy rolled up from the depths of our bellies and from that moment on, he was fine. The Word says,

"A cheerful heart is good medicine." (Proverbs 17:22)

And it's true! After I lost my hair, Carter always gave my shiny bald head a kiss and a rub while passing by or during snuggle time. He'd accepted, and loved me just the same, and knew in his heart that one day I would again wear my hair in pigtails while we played!

Amazingly, the night of my diagnosis I dozed off serenely just as if it were any other night. When 3:00 a.m. hit, I awoke from a deep sleep, weeping uncontrollably. My subconscious mind had finally registered the gut-wrenching reality I was about to experience. I had endured much hardship and heartache in my past, but nothing had ever caused such excruciating pain as this! I cried out, "Lord, please comfort me!" Immediately I felt a warm presence and great peace cover me—I honestly, physically, felt

God's arms of love wrap around me, loving me, comforting me. I rolled over onto my stomach and immediately drifted away into a restful sleep.

The following night, I encountered God in exactly the same way as I had the previous night. Any misconception I had about God being angry with me fell away. All the lies I believed about having to earn God's love dissipated.

"The Lord is gracious and compassionate, slow to anger and rich in love. The Lord is good to all; he has compassion on all he has made." (Psalm 145:8, 9)

God's love is a gift, and gifts are free! We don't need to strive to attain it; it is ours to receive. The only thing we need to do is be willing to accept it. Things I had been taught as a young girl and had read in the Bible about God's character were becoming truth to me. God's Word promises that He will never leave us nor forsake us (Hebrews 13:5) and I finally understood what that meant. God revealed His gentle, kind spirit to me and met with me in the most incredible, intimate way. He is not distant or uninterested and He is right there waiting for you to reach out to Him also.

"Taste and see that the Lord is good; blessed is the man who takes refuge in him." (Psalm 34:8)

Something to Think About!

Our earthly authority sets a standard within our minds of how we interpret God to be.[5] When such people fail to show us the proper love and respect, whether by treating us harshly, through abandonment, unjust ridicule, abuse or neglect, we form mistrust issues with God. As you read this book, God will reveal Himself to you for who He truly is, and remove the walls that hinder healing and wholeness for your body, mind, and soul.

Dear God,

I need You in my life! I ask that You would reveal Yourself to me in an amazing way. I want to experience Your presence. Help me to trust You with my life. Lavish me in Your amazing love and bless me with the Spirit of wisdom and revelation, so that I can come to know You (Ephesians 1:17). Open my heart and mind that I might see and understand how much You really do care and bring healing to my body, mind and soul. In Jesus' name I pray. Amen.

---

[1] "Mastitis-Causes, Symptoms, Treatment, Diagnosis-Conditions." *Med Broadcast*. 04 January 2005 (www.medbroadcast.com/condition_info_details.asp).

[2] "Breast Cancer Symptoms and Information on Breast Cancer." *National Breast Cancer Foundation* (Early Detection). 04 January 2005 (http://www.nationalbreastcancer.org/early_detection/index.html).

[3] "Breast Cancer Symptoms Signs of Breast Cancer Early Detection." *National Breast Cancer Foundation* (Signs and symptoms). 04 January 2005 (http://www.nationalbreastcancer.org/signs_and_symptoms/index.html).

[4] "Breast Cancer Symptoms Signs of Breast Cancer Early Detection." *National Breast Cancer Foundation* (Signs and symptoms). 04 January 2005 (http://www.nationalbreastcancer.org/signs_and_symptoms/index.html).

[5] Jones, AJ. *Finding Father: The Father Heart Series/ 6-Disc Set*; (Toronto, ON: Catalyst Home International, 2006), (www.catalysthome.org).

Chapter Two
You're Beautiful!
(Even After a Mastectomy)

I praise you because I am fearfully and wonderfully made;
your works are wonderful, I know that full well.

Psalm 139:14

As a teenager, like many other girls, I constantly stared into the mirror picking out the imperfections about myself, wishing I could change particular things. Whether discontented with my straight, stringy hair, the bump on my nose or my body structure, I compared myself to others' qualities and rejected my own. I even carried it into my adult life, thinking that it was physical attractiveness that made one valuable. I pressured myself, trying to add up to the magazine super models and Hollywood stars. Reality is, they spend hours on makeup and hair and wipe out blemishes with photography touch ups. We need to give God credit and ourselves a break!

I even wished my body was perfect, thinking that would make my husband love me more. It's silly to think I actually thought that way, knowing love is based on far more than just fuzzy feelings and animal attraction. It's not lust! Love is respecting someone for who they are, seeing their inner beauty rather than their outward appearance. Love is caring so deeply your heart aches when they're hurting. Love is standing by them regardless of their faults and wanting to add joy to their day whenever possible.

You see, love is a choice we make concerning how we are going to act toward others. It's not about doing those things that bring satisfaction to our fleshly desires. It's about keeping others' best interests in mind when making choices. We need to be mindful to bless others, especially during those times when they're not treating us the way we think they should. Love is not based on emotions; it's a choice we make!

My Mastectomy

Ten days after my diagnosis, my mastectomy was performed at our local hospital. My breast was sent to pathology to investigate whether the cancer was invasive (moved outside the duct walls). In the meantime, I was sent for an abdominal ultrasound to check my liver, kidneys, and bladder and I had a bone scan for metastasis. Thankfully, the results of the scans were clear, but unfortunately eleven days later, I received the biopsy report that confirmed it was invasive (completely throughout my breast). I would have to receive surgery again to remove approximately 10–12 lymph nodes from under my right arm.

Eight days later, on a Tuesday morning, I was back under aesthetic. They removed 18 lymph nodes. The following Thursday, during my post-op appointment, the drain under my arm had clogged because of a blood clot, and the fluid was running down my side. My surgeon decided to remove the drain. By Friday night, I had what looked like a golf ball stuffed underneath the skin of my armpit. I went to emergency and the doctor, on call, drained my underarm with a needle and syringe to prevent lymphodema.

Lymphodema is a permanent condition of swelling in the arm, and sometimes in the surrounding area, due to fluid build–up because the fluid is unable to drain back out. It is the function of the auxiliary lymph nodes to carry bodily fluid in and out of the arm. This becomes more difficult with strenuous activities such as exercising or lifting or when there is any type of trauma. In the next week, I made five trips to see my family doctor to have the area drained because of recurring swelling. During the last visit, the doctor was successful in removing three large syringes full of fluid. By that time, I was extremely tender and feeling like a pincushion, but very thankful my arm wasn't swollen!

The biopsy results showed one out of the 18 lymph nodes had cancer cells within. Thank God, they were able to catch it before it had spread any further. Health professionals also gave me special exercises and massages to do to help prevent lymphodema. They encouraged me to no longer carry anything with that arm, whether it is groceries or a hand bag. I now needed to wear rubber gloves while doing dishes, gardening, and housework, to avoid cuts or abrasions. I could no longer do simple tasks like clipping my cuticles.

Having a mastectomy didn't even cross my mind as being difficult because I was a very optimistic person and only thought positively about the day when I would receive reconstruction. The doctors and plastic surgeon would take the left side and kindly match it with the right. This time I had a choice of size and could even be perky, a word I never thought I would use to describe myself! I felt in control and viewed the situation as just a big bump in the road. This was going to be absolutely "no problem" or so I thought, until the day I approached my husband thinking I should be a good wife and take care of his manly needs, regardless of how tired I felt! I discovered he had absolutely no desire to be intimate with me. It wasn't a matter of him not being in the mood. Men are visual; that's the way God wired them.

In my heart I felt crushed; the woman he once knew was gone. I may have been missing a breast, but I was still the same person on the inside, a very vulnerable one, who had the same desires as everyone else to be loved and accepted regardless of their imperfections. He was no longer attracted to me sexually, even though it was not my breasts that attracted him to me in the first place. He wept and held me in his arms as he reassured me that he still loved me and would always be there for me. He so wanted to be a good husband. I respected his honesty and always will.

Knowing these things gave me some comfort but didn't take the pain of rejection away. Part of me just wanted to die at that point. I made Rob promise me that if I died he wouldn't remarry anyone unless she had a close relationship with the Lord because I needed the boys to be brought up in faith and with the knowledge of God's truth. He told me to stop talking foolishly because I wasn't going anywhere.

I had two choices here, I could accept the rejection and choose to believe that I was worthless, or I could believe what the Bible says about me. Knowing that my Heavenly Father's love never fails and that my value rests in who I am in Christ, not in what I look like or in what I can or cannot do, brought me all the comfort anyone would ever need (see Ephesians 1:3–8).

For those who have accepted Jesus as their Lord and Saviour, we are "in Christ" and seen as "righteous" in God's eyes. He sees us through Jesus because of the perfect blood sacrifice Jesus made on the cross for our sins. We are then, heirs with Christ and have value in Him because we are adopted as God's children. We are always accepted by God regardless of the rejection we may experience from others.

I had to pray and trust that God would work about a change in Rob's heart. Two days later, my oldest brother called to see how I was. He couldn't get me off his mind. That's a God thing! We discussed the problem and it was great to hear the situation from a male's perspective. We prayed in agreement that whatever difficulty Rob was having, he would work through it quickly.

The next night, Rob approached me. Whatever caused his hesitation with intimacy was gone. He wanted us to be together as a real couple. I challenged him, making sure he was certain with his decision. I didn't want to subject myself to any more emotional pain. He assured me, and the rest is history. God not only restored our relationship completely, He made it better! In fact, Rob has put that so far out of his mind that he barely remembers struggling with this issue!

In difficult times, it can be emotionally hard for our husbands as well. It's important to remember to give them the space they need to digest and process everything in their minds, to cope and continue on. It's not only about us! Their world has been shaken too! They have fears and insecurities just like we do, even though they may not voice them. If we are sensitive to their needs, love will melt down the walls. The same can be said for our friends. Just because we are coping well, doesn't mean it's easy for them. Try to be patient! You will reap the benefit from it sooner or later.

When You're Hurting!

It's always on the days that you're hurting, or trusting God to bring about change, that the enemy will send people your way to say things that discourage you, knock your faith or set you up to speak or think negatively. These people mean well, and don't realize they're part in Satan's scheme. He's sneaky and works by putting thoughts, negative thoughts or lies in people's minds (see Ephesians 2:2).

People would sincerely come and ask me how I was. After I had optimistically shared some light details they'd reply, "Really it's no big deal, it's not like you had big breasts, you really can't tell anyway" or "You've had your kids, your breasts have served their purpose."

I tell you, it is a big deal when your femininity is being attacked and you're fighting to keep your marriage and life together. We are surrounded by sensuality everywhere we go. Unfortunately, it's not only the men and women who are being saturated by it, our children are as well. We're seeing young girls walking around half dressed on the streets, models with their breasts and tummies exposed on the covers of magazines or television commercials and programs that are inundated with these images. Most people have gotten so used to it that we've become desensitized. For me, it was like a slap in the face constantly reminding me of the loss I had suffered.

Others' Hurtful Comments

When others made hurtful comments, I had to make a conscious choice not to take offense, and love them anyway. Offense is the bait Satan uses to pull us into sin.[1] We often feel justified because of the way we have been treated, and we allow pride, bitterness, anger and resentment to stand in our way of freedom. This tends to blind us from seeing our faults. One day, we will stand before the judgment seat of Christ to give account for our actions, which includes our reaction to situations. It won't matter, at that point, who did what to stir you up, only how you chose to respond.

"For our struggle is not against flesh and blood, but against the rulers, against the authorities, against the powers of this dark world and against the spiritual forces of evil in the heavenly realms." (Ephesians 6:12)

People aren't the real enemy. They're the vessels which Satan uses, at times, to get to us. We need to guard our hearts with faith, hope and love, believing the best. Who really knows what they were thinking anyway? Maybe they were trying to place a wall of excuses up to cope, or they were expressing how they think they would feel. Perhaps they just didn't know what to say, because they were nervous or uncomfortable, and it was the first thing that came to their mind! From my experience, I feel it would be wise for the person who doesn't know what to say to say nothing or "I'm sorry, I just don't know what to say." Rather than fill the air with awkward words that may offend, especially when they've never been in that person's shoes. It's really not our place to give advice unless we're asked anyway. A listening ear soothes the soul more than words could ever say. I have several friends who did exactly that. It brought me so much comfort knowing that they sincerely cared for me. The fact that I was in their hearts and thoughts was enough.

Sometimes, our "pat-on-the-back" comments may actually be insults. We always react out of our own wounding; things said or done that may trigger a rise within me may not have any effect on you at all. There will be times we may offend others unintentionally. When this happens, it's important to see the sincerity of heart behind one's actions or words towards you, rather than to judge. We have all said wrong things, there's no way of getting around that. There are always three sides to every story, ours, theirs and God's. Only God knows the whole picture and that is why we shouldn't judge. Many offenses are a result of misunderstandings.

Taking time to respectfully and openly discuss concerns with others involved will often reveal truth and bring healing. We all need to walk in God's love with one another, being gracious and merciful, to gain inner peace.

There may be times when others are intentionally hurtful. Words or the lack of them have the ability to wound, mend or heal. What should we do in this situation? By nature, our first reaction is to lash out, or place a wall of protection around ourselves. Does that really solve anything? Our flesh might feel gratified for a moment, but this can cause serious repercussions and create additional issues to deal with.

Job, a righteous man of God, endured a season of great suffering. His friends drew close, but instead of bringing him comfort, they judged him, proclaiming that he must have sinned, to cause such an infliction. Job could have become angry, but instead he prayed for them as instructed by God. In the process, Job was healed. The Lord tells us to leave room for God's wrath and allow Him to be our vindicator. This is the very thing that sets us free and opens the door of blessing. God will work in their heart and deal with them appropriately if you give Him the situation. When we pray for those who hurt us, we invoke a blessing in God's time. I don't know about you, but I would much rather be blessed than cursed.

"Do not repay evil with evil or insult with insult, but with blessing, because to this you were called so that you may inherit a blessing." (1 Peter 3:9)

God Winks

Have you ever had a moment where you felt you couldn't go on the way things were because life seemed hopeless? Previously, I talked about how the enemy attempts to discourage us, and beat our faith down, but there is an upside! God is always watching over us and has an army of angels that follow His commands (Psalm 103; Psalm 91:11). God is just as able to put good thoughts and ideas into people's minds. He brings people alongside us at just the right moment to encourage, pray, and give a smile or hug. Whatever it is we need, He knows! These things are actually from God to us (James 1:16–17). Isn't it great to have a God who loves us so much that He is always watching over us, providing what we need. He doesn't change. We can count on Him. He is faithful!

Finding a Positive View

"You are a beautiful woman, a complete package, put together by many feminine qualities, not just one."

Over time, I have learned to be content in all things. I have chosen to have a positive mindset and to be grateful for all blessings in my life. I had to say to myself, "I may not have a breast, but thank God I'm alive to see the sparkle in my boys' eyes as they smile, and to feel my husband's embrace." I may have suffered a great amount of pain but I have become a confident, stronger person who has gained great wisdom and understanding through these life's challenges.

Are there certain aspects within your life you need to reframe with a positive twist? Just because you might be missing a few body parts doesn't make you any less of a woman. A man isn't any less of a man if he's missing his left testicle, is he? I think not! That may sound crude, but you need to clearly see my point. Breasts don't solely identify a female's gender.

We automatically think of the physical characteristic but there are many facets to femininity and beauty. Women have countless qualities to share. They can be affectionate, romantic, tender, devoted, comforting, heroic, gentle, sensitive and compassionate. The range is widely diverse. "You" are a beautiful woman, a complete package, put together by many qualities, not just one.

We can hold certain female traits and not others. Many women are nurturers. For some, this attribute arrives with their bundle of joy. Yet others find it difficult to muster up, even one ounce. Our upbringing can shape or diminish this characteristic. I have girl-friends whose parents dressed them in frilly dresses and gave them dolls to play with. Their mothers fussed over their hair, always making sure their daughters' braids and pony tails were kept just so. As they grew older, they were taught how to cook, bake, apply makeup properly and act like a lady. On the contrary, I also have friends whose parents wished their girls were boys, gave them boy names and taught them how to throw a football. This has made it difficult for them to embrace femininity, causing pain and rejection. Our circumstances determine much of our personality and behaviour.

We can hold certain female eminences and not others. In grade school I knew an extremely bright girl who, although dainty in stature, had dark body hair covering her arms and legs. Other women have deep, husky voices, behave like tomboys or lack femininity in the way they carry themselves. Nevertheless, this doesn't decrease their value as women. On the inside, they're loving, sensitive and considerate. We all have different qualities!

Do the best with what you have! There are other ways you can make yourself feel good. Applying a little make-up, wearing your favourite color (pink makes me feel feminine), experimenting with an attractive new hairstyle or buying yourself a new outfit can give you a needed boost to feel more beautiful. There's waxing for unwanted body hair. Take etiquette lessons if you feel the need. The possibilities are endless. Have a massage, go on a trip or take some time for yourself!

Give Yourself a Boost

- Apply a little make-up
- Wear pink to help you feel more feminine
- Try a new hairstyle
- Shower daily
- Exercise

- Treat yourself to a new outfit

- Get a prosthesis or reconstruction

- Wax away unwanted body hair

Warning: Many cosmetics and beauty products may contain carcinogens (can-cer causing ingredients).[2] For information regarding safe products go to www.safecosmetics.org.[3] Health Stores will also carry shampoos, conditioners, body lotions, hair colors and other products that do not contain harmful chemicals.

Society's Mindset

We have allowed society to frame our minds about what beautiful is. Everyone has a different idea or perception about what beautiful should be. Dove, along with National Geographic, did an international study in 2007, to compare the diverse practices of cultures revealing their beliefs about what makes women beautiful. The Japanese consider straight hair and a clear complexion to exemplify a woman's beauty. They go to great lengths to straighten their hair with chemicals and heat. Until the 1930's, China practiced foot binding to inhibit the growth of the young girl's feet because they considered small feet to be more feminine. The Kayak tribe, near the border of Burma and Thailand, believe an elongated neck makes women attractive and elevates her status. They place brass rings around the necks of the girls, starting at the age of five and increase the number of rings as they age, to give their necks a giraffe like appearance. Can you imagine having up to an extra twenty-two pounds of weight on your shoulders everywhere you go? In southern Ethiopia, they cut scars into a girl's stomach and they're not to marry until they have received the last of their scars. The Maori people of New Zealand tattoo their lips and chins blue. In Mauritania, the larger a woman is the more desirable she is. Against the government's wishes, parents force feed the young girls and some are given black market drugs used to fatten livestock. We all know too well that in North America skinny is in![4]

No matter where people live, they will go to the extreme to fit in with society's idea of beautiful. It's crazy! And many times unhealthy! Chemicals, starving, purging, cutting, force feeding; that's not natural!

We shouldn't allow society to shape or dictate to us what 'beautiful' is any longer. It has given us a very narrow view and it has become extremely unhealthy. There are many forms of beauty. Let's open our eyes to see ourselves from God's perspective. After all, He is our Creator. Enjoy being who He created you to be.

God's Mindset

"God saw all that he had made, and it was very good." (Genesis 1:31a)

When God created you, He was pleased. He considered what He made to be good. Only you can choose to believe that for yourself. God is not always fond of your choices but that doesn't change the fact that He loves you and always will.

It's important to feel secure in who you are as a person, accepting who God created you to be as an individual, and not feel inferior to others because they may hold certain gifts and talents, even attaining looks you wish were yours. I think it's important to be the best you can be and enjoy your individuality. You will never feel fulfilled if you are always trying to be like others. You have your own experiences and personality that make you interesting and special. As you walk in your own gifting and abilities, and allow others to be the individuals God created them to be, it will make the world a more interesting place. Besides, if God wanted us all to be the same, He would have created us that way!

Our Differences

Outside the window where I'm writing is a pair of cardinals eating the fruit off the crab–apple tree we planted the spring after Ben was born. This reminds me of the conversation I once heard Joyce Meyer have with John C. Maxwell on "Enjoying Everyday Life." It made me contemplate how our uniqueness should be something we treasure. John invited the audience to imagine what the world would be like if God had only created one species of bird. I think nature would seem boring, don't you think? Cardinals capture a beauty of their own, with brilliant red feathers and crested heads, but the thought of solely having them alone makes me feel sad. Picture a humming bird as it hovers over a vibrant red honey suckle, drawing nectar with its long bill. It seems almost motionless, yet moves its wings 80 times per second. They are absolutely fascinating to watch. God has created each person unique and beautiful as well. That's why He gave each of us our own D.N.A. and finger prints, to be one of a kind. You were meant to be different too. Embrace it. It's good a thing!

Think about insects for a moment. What would life be like if there were only houseflies and mosquitoes? You probably view these bugs as pests, a mere nuisance, but even these have a special place in our ecosystem. Life without the bumblebees would be tragic. It goes much deeper than not having any sweet, sticky honey for your toast! If that were the case, pollination wouldn't happen. Think of the repercussions of such a thing and how it would affect our world. Do you see how imperative diversity is? Like the bumblebee, we each have a special part and destiny in life. We need each other to operate in our different strengths and abilities to survive and grow. Be thankful for your differences and respect others for theirs.

Are you suffering from a poor self–image? Many struggle with this stronghold without even having a mastectomy. A stronghold is anything that has a tight grip on you. Poor self–image can affect someone's confidence and hinder a person from enjoying even the simplest things in life. Many women refuse to wear shorts on a scorching hot day because they would rather sweat buckets than have someone see their varicose veins. How many women lose out on family fun because they don't want anyone to see them in a bathing suit at the beach because they think they have fat thighs? These people need to be thankful they have legs to walk, run and stand on! Things in life aren't always ideal so we need to constantly put things in perspective.

Do you tend to compare yourself to others, including the media and advertising, and then gauge your self–worth according to what you believe others think you should be like, rather than what you are? This isn't healthy. Even people that haven't had a mastectomy have imperfections. Make a mental choice to accept yourself and work with what you have. Instead of concentrating on the things you don't like about yourself, focus on the good!

Finding Purpose

Everyone has a purpose in this life. Sometimes it takes a life–changing experience to cause a person to re–evaluate this. God has placed specific desires within our hearts for a reason. What are you passionate about? Is there something positive you can bring out of the negative situations you face to help others? Let your pain become someone else's healing ointment. If you're not sure what your purpose is, I suggest reading *The Purpose Driven Life* by Rick Warren.

When time began, *God* already knew you and had plans for your life. He set in place certain giftings that you would operate out of and one day, use for good. Satan knows this! He is familiar with all your strengths and abilities as well as your weaknesses. He roams around watching and waiting for just the right second to attack. He wants to stop you from enjoying your life and especially from making a difference in this world.

Please take a moment to jot down your strengths on a piece of paper. This tends to be more difficult to do than writing your weaknesses. At times we focus on the negative so much that we forget to see the positive. Each one of us is special and unique with specific gifts, talents, strengths and weaknesses and there is a special purpose and meaning for each one of our lives! We each need to do our part and stop thinking our element is less or more important than others. It is time to come together in unity and in love for the sake of all! Remember, you are an important member of life's team!

Developing Your Inner Beauty

There is something to be said about the beauty that emanates from the inner depths. Lovely attributes that shine forth from one's character, for the world to see, naturally drawing others. There's no striving. Their personality radiates an amazing love for life and unspeakable joy and peace with the world. They are able to face themselves and mankind with honesty and integrity because they have first learned to love themselves and now are able to love others in return. Inner beauty starts within the heart and then emanates out through one's attitude and spirit.

Although God made everything beautiful, it isn't the exterior He is concerned with. Man looks at the outer appearance but the Lord is concerned about the condition that our hearts are in (1 Samuel 16:7). It's what's on the inside that counts! God examines our hearts to determine our character and motives. Do you need an internal check-up? We, as people, get so caught up in our outward appearance that we sometimes forget what's really important!

Jesus is what makes someone beautiful on the inside. He takes our mistakes and our filth and washes us clean, fills us with His goodness and gives us purpose and meaning in exchange. God loves us so much that He's continually working within our hearts to bring change for self-improvement and allowing us contentment where we are, each step of the way.

"Let not yours be the [merely] external adorning with [elaborate] interweaving and knotting of the hair, the wearing of jewelry, or changes of clothes; But let it be the inward adorning and beauty of the hidden person of the heart, with the incorruptible and unfading charm of a gentle and peaceful spirit, which [is not anxious or wrought up, but] is very precious in the sight of God." (1 Peter 3:3, 4; Amplified)

I again, gleaned understanding from Joyce Meyer from the above passage from watching "Enjoying Everyday Life." The word "merely" is used in this passage to point out that we should not only concern our-selves with outward beauty. I truly believe God does not frown upon those who fix themselves up to look beautiful. He created you beautiful and desires you to look that way. After all, we are God's children and royalty wear fine things, don't they? God has a golden crown waiting for us in eternity so I don't see any reason why we can't enjoy wearing a lit-tle fancy stuff now.

In the above Scripture Paul was addressing a concern within the Ephesian church, at that particular time in history, for those who con-centrated on these aspects alone. Vanity was a great problem among them. He wanted the women to stand out differently from the Romans by giving attention to what held greater worth and significance. So how can we apply this Scripture to our own lives in this day and age? Pride and beauty can easily become an obsession as it was a stronghold for the

Ephesians. Just don't let it be your main focus! It is the beauty of our inner man that is of great value; the quiet gentle spirit. These are the qualities we should focus on. Moreover, outer beauty is fleeting, while inside beauty is a quality you control by choice.[5]

We all have good and bad in our hearts. It is our sinful desires that can get us into trouble. The key is to overcome our sinfulness with righteousness. I love the ancient tale the wise Old Cherokee taught his grandson to impart morals. The story is called "Good Wolf, Bad Wolf." It goes like this:

"One evening an Old Cherokee told his grandson about a battle raging inside mankind. He said, "My son, inside each one of our hearts is a battle between a good wolf and bad wolf. The evil one is angry, envious, hateful, jealous, fearful, sorrowful, greedy, arrogant, pitiful, resentful, inferior, deceitful, and every other negative characteristic. The other is good. It is full of love, joy, peace, hope, humility, kindness, empathy, generosity, truth, compassion, faith and every good trait."

After a few moments of contemplation the boy asked, "Which wolf wins?"

The grandfather replied, "The one you feed!"[6]

There truly is an inner war that rages for our souls. Our behaviour and attitudes feed the wolf of choice. The bad wolf is always hungry and is never satisfied but, with God's help, we can fight the battle. Starving the bad wolf by making consistent right choices will allow the good wolf to overcome and the desired qualities of true beauty to radiate out from within as your character reflects the fruits of the good spirit. This beauty can last forever providing we continue to feed the right wolf, the good wolf!

"But now you must rid yourselves of all such things as these: anger, rage, malice, slander, and filthy language from your lips. Do not lie to each other, since you have

taken off your old self with its practices and have put on the new self with its practices and have put on the new self, which is being renewed in knowledge in the image of its Creator." (Colossians 3:8, 9, 10)

This Scripture seems to go hand in hand with that wise Old Cherokee tale. How can we possibly rid ourselves of evil traits that seem so naturally ingrained within our souls? If we have difficulty with such weaknesses, we must deal with the roots of these issues. Repetitive actions create habits, right? Since our habits created the problem, our habits can be overcome by forming new ones. We must first make a decision to put such behaviour to rest. As we purposely choose to stop the less desirable behaviour, we must also settle in our minds to put on the new-self (new behaviour).

Similar to getting dressed, we must choose to clothe ourselves with compassion, kindness, humility, gentleness and patience; bearing with one another and forgiving one another. As we utilize these life principles, our inner strength grows stronger and it becomes easier over time to deny our fleshly reactions. As we bind each of these qualities together with love, God promises that it will bring perfect harmony to our lives (see Colossians 3:8–10, 12–14). It's amazing how God's kingdom works! When keeping our lives pure, by doing what is righteous in the eyes of the Lord, we can and will triumph over the negative forces of this world. It may seem uncomfortable for our flesh, but when we refuse to give in God promises we will reap a blessing.

"*Do not be overcome by evil, but overcome evil with good.*" (Romans 12:21)

Accepting Ourselves

The world is full of gorgeous people who can't seem to see or appreciate their value. Why is this so difficult for women? We seem to have such deep-rooted body issues. We worry so much about how others view us.

We rely on the opinions of others to gauge how we feel about ourselves. The truth is, people can compliment us all they want, but until we accept and love ourselves, we aren't able to receive the good from what they're saying! It's like there is a wall there, a physical barrier that stops the positive from penetrating.

As I've talked to different women, I am shocked to see how many struggle with insecurity. We try to get our identity from our jobs and relationships when we need to become dependent in God and find our identity in Him. Many women feel insecure, yet they hide it. I hid it. We wear masks pretending everything is okay in our world, yet it really isn't. Why do so many women feel this way? Society has trained women to believe they have to look a certain way, weigh a certain amount and perform with excellence in all aspects to be of any worth. When we don't meet these specific standard requirements, set by the world, we struggle with inadequacy, guilt and condemnation. Beauty is based on much more than external appearance and outward performance. True beauty occurs when you are able to drop all pretences, gain inner peace by accepting yourself for who you truly are and enjoy the freedom that comes with it. Do you feel free to be yourself?

I believe the attack on our femininity stems right back to the beginning of creation were God created the most beautiful angel Lucifer.[7]

This is what the Sovereign Lord says:

"You were the model of perfection, full of wisdom and perfect in beauty. You were in Eden, the garden of God; every precious stone adorned you: ruby, topaz and emerald, chrysolite, onyx and jasper, sapphire, turquoise and beryl. Your settings and mountings were made of gold: on the day you were created they were prepared." (Ezekiel 28:12b–14)

This passage is talking about when God created and anointed Lucifer to be a guardian angel. The most beautiful stones and gems were of no comparison to his mesmerizing beauty. It was this beauty that filled him with pride and caused his downfall. Out of pride, rebellion and jealousy, he wanted to take over God's throne (Ezekiel 28:17). God threw him and a third of the angels who were his followers down from Heaven (Revelation 12:4). Satan became God's rival and enemy. He is jealous of God and all He has made that is beautiful and has been trying to destroy God's creation ever since. [8]

Satan is the one that comes to steal, kill and destroy (John 10:10). God stands for everything that is good, Satan for evil, and both desire your soul.

God created the garden as a beautiful paradise and placed Adam and Eve there to walk and talk with God. God created good things and wanted to share it with us. When Adam and Eve disobeyed God and were removed from the garden, enmity was placed between the serpent (Satan) and the woman. God created Eve as the picture of beauty, with all the curves... the mother of all the living. Women were created to represent God's nurturing side and it was through the woman's womb the Saviour of the earth was born. Jesus, God in flesh, the One born to crush and defeat the enemy. [9]

We imagine Satan as dark and evil, yet he disguises himself as an angel of light to deceive. All through history, there has been one attack after another on women. [10] They have had to fight to be recognized as valued human beings so they could gain the privilege to vote, to become doctors and lawyers, as well as to attain equal rights in the work place.

Women have also struggled with equality within the church as a result of the Word being taken out of context. Paul addressed letters written by the Corinthian church on issues that were relative to that time and place. Scholars feel that in his letters he first repeated the questions before he answered them. This is where it has caused confusion. If you refer back to these Scriptures with this in mind, it makes complete sense. This particular church was having difficulty keeping ordinance because many of the women were newly converted Christians, from a background of pagan worship. Hollering out was a common practice of that belief system. Old habits sometimes die hard and needed to be addressed. This is why the women were placed in a different section of the church and asked to keep quiet. They were clearly causing disruption. [11]

If you read the whole Bible you will read of several different women (Miriam, Tabitha, Euodia, Priscilla, Junia, Deborah etc.) who were prophets, apostles and coworkers for the Lord's work. And Jesus had a number of women who supported Him in ministry (Exodus 15:20; Judges 4&5; 2 Kings; 2 Chronicles 34:22; Acts 9:36; Acts 21:8; Phil 4:2; Romans 16:1, 3,7).

Satan is determined to destroy everything and anything beautiful God has created.[12] There has even been an attack on women's femininity from the start. I guess he figured if he couldn't destroy women, he would attack them one way or another.

God wanted men to have Lordship over their wives and children, as a means of ordinance, to act as the head of the home and to provide protection, not to cause dysfunction. Regrettably, many men have dominated and oppressed women from the beginning of time out of selfishness and pride. This is a perversion of what God intended. He meant it to be an act of love and service. God intended the unity of man and woman to be a relationship of give and take, not one of domination and control.

The outcome has caused a feminist movement to rise up, as an act of self-preservation, kicking women into survival overdrive and creating a new female version that is tough like men. These women are independent and out of balance because they are trying to rule and overtake the place of men (men's role).

God created man and women to come together, in unity, carrying their masculine and feminine traits to complement and strengthen one another. In the Garden of Eden, God saw that Adam needed a companion and helpmate, not someone to control, manipulate or devalue, but a female companion that was very much needed, esteemed and treasured! God took one of Adam's ribs from his side to create Eve. This was a representation that she was made equal, and fully part of him. In 1 Peter 3:7; NKJV we read, *"Husbands, likewise, dwell with them with understanding, giving honour to the wife, as to the weaker vessel."* Women are actually to be honoured. They are to be seen as a weaker vessel because they are more delicate, not because they are less valuable as a person.

When reading the New Testament, you will see that Jesus gave more value to the women than the men did. Jesus only ever preformed the acts of the Father. Therefore, we should look to His example, rather than to men. Old culture gave women few rights and saw them as property and of little value. This is a mindset we still fight today. We can be grateful to those who have fought so hard to win the fight to freedom. The right to be seen as equal, that to which we are!

Seeing Your Value

Liking yourself is a process that starts in your mind. If you have been in the habit of self-loathing it will take time to turn these thoughts around. It is possible, one thought at a time.

Mephibosheth was the son of Jonathon, the grandson of King Saul. Although he was a royal heir, he carried a low opinion of himself. He was crippled in both his feet, at a young age, and saw himself as worthless.

"Mephibosheth bowed down and said, 'What is your servant, that you should notice a dead dog like me?'" (2 Samuel 9:8)

Jonathon, Mephibosheth's father, loved David as himself and made a covenant with him (1 Samuel 18:1–3). David eventually became King and after the death of Jonathon, searched for family, for Jonathon's sake, to whom he could show kindness. This is when Mephibosheth was brought before him and he uttered the words that weighed so heavily upon his heart. Because of David's covenant with (Mephibosheth's father) Jonathon, David restored all the land to him, that had belonged to his grandfather, he had Saul's servants work the land for him, and he allowed Mephibosheth to eat at his table (2 Samuel 9:1–13).

When we accept Jesus as our Lord and Saviour, we have a new covenant with God because of Jesus' sacrifice on the cross. It is through the new covenant that we can receive forgiveness for our sins and be accepted into the family of God. We become heirs of God in Heaven, for Jesus' sake. I pray you find your rightful place of acceptance in Christ. We do not need to see ourselves as Mephibosheth did. He saw himself as a lowly dog and yet the king esteemed him. He gained a rightful place at the King's table every day. We are welcome to dine with The King of all Kings, anytime, for the same reason. Like Mephibosheth, we tend to focus on what we consider wrong with us, our dislikes, rather than the qualities of strength and the things we have to be thankful for. Having a positive outlook about your qualities is the first key to unlocking the door, to loving and accepting yourself.

Loving Yourself

Part of loving yourself means looking after yourself. There is nothing selfish about taking time for your own needs. As the demands of life, such as work, family and other obligations, press continuously, it's easy to get tired and worn out if you are not depositing something beneficial back into your own life. When we do, we are able to better meet the needs of those we love. We will be doing them a favour by giving them a healthier, happier you. If we don't have any energy, how will we be of any help to those we love? Therefore, we need to rejuvenate our lives by giv-ing to ourselves. As women, we tend to put ourselves last. It's our nature. Perhaps this attitude has been ingrained in us from our past. The prob-lem is, when you put everyone else first all the time, you don't have the time or energy left for you and eventually you can slip into a resentful mindset. I get a chuckle out of the saying, "If mama's happy, everyone's happy!" It's the truth. We can set the atmosphere for our entire house-hold, by our mood! If you were to describe the aroma in your house, would it be that of a freshly baked chocolate chip cookie or burnt toast? Let's do everyone a favour and be good to ourselves. Listed below are some helpful hints to improve your everyday life.

Helpful Hints

- Eat properly
- Get enough sleep
- Exercise
- Get a yearly physical
- Visit your dentist for regular check–ups
- Feed your mind with good things
- Speak and think positive thoughts about yourself
- Learn to laugh at yourself and your mistakes
- Practice Forgiveness
- Accept yourself for who you are, so you can love others in return

[1] Bevere, John. *The Bait of Satan* (Lake Mary, Florida: Charisma House, A Strange Company, 2004).

[2] Colbert, Don, MD. *The Seven Pillars of Health* (Lake Mary, Florida: Siloam, 2007), p. 161.

[3] Ibid.

[4] Killeen, Peter. Hommel, Robin (Co-Executive Producers). (2008). The Oprah Show. Baltimore: Harpo Productions.

[5] Meyer, Joyce. *The Confident Woman* (Avenue of the Americas, New York, NY: Warner Faith, Hatch Book Group, USA, 2006).

[6] Osteen, Joel. *Becoming a Better You Journal: A Guide To Improving Your Life Every Day* (New York: Free Press, Published by Simon & Schuster, 2008), p. 93.

[7] Eldredge, John & Stasi. *Captivating* (Nashville, Tennessee: Thomas Nelson, Inc., 2005).

[8] Ibid.

[9] Eldredge, John & Stasi. Captivating (Nashville, Tennessee: Thomas Nelson, Inc., 2005).

[10] Ibid.

[11] Ibid.

[12] Eldredge, John & Stasi. *Captivating* (Nashville, Tennessee: Thomas Nelson, Inc., 2005).

Chapter Three
Chemotherapy

Give thanks in all circumstances,
for this is God's will for you in Christ Jesus.

1 Thessalonians 5:18

I was to start Chemo six to eight weeks after surgery, but because of the heavy waiting list, my chemo treatment was delayed to nine weeks after my second surgery. I agreed to have the tumour sent away to Germany to be tested for a protein called Her2. There was a trial being performed on this type of cancer, which was proving to be quite effective. I received a call from my medical oncologist wanting me to wait another week to allow more time for the results to return before making my decision on which type of chemo to receive. I felt I had waited long enough and decided to proceed with F.E.C. This chemo is a combination of three drugs, which is red in color and nick-named "The Red Devil." A total of six treatments were to be given every three weeks.

On March 31, I had a port-a-cath inserted into my chest on the left side. This is a round plastic device that has a titanium ball covered with rubber in the center and a tube that comes out the side, which leads straight into the left ventricle of the heart. It allows the nurses to administer drugs or draw blood repeatedly without collapsing your veins from trauma to your arm. F.E.C. also tends to streak your veins black.

On April 11, the night before my first chemotherapy treatment, I had a very vivid dream. I sat looking at a children's Bible at the kitchen table in the house where I grew up, with the new owner. She wore a white and red plaid tea towel on her head while repeating, "I just don't know, there is something different about the situation with Nancy." I left the table and quietly climbed up the long, oak staircase to my old bedroom. Curious, I slowly opened the door; it was dark and cold. A canopy bed, draped with dark heavy linen, sat on the east wall. A glimmer of sunlight beamed through a small window above the headboard across the dark bedding. As I climbed up onto the end of the bed, a soft pink knitted blanket appeared. I curled up into a ball and nestled in the blanket, feeling feminine, peaceful and safe. I heard my mother's voice say, "I'm sure Nancy will be okay. I just know it!"

I prayed and asked the Lord what He wanted to say to me regarding the dream. This is what I felt Him say to my heart: "Rest in Me my child. Use My wisdom, read My Word and rest. It's comfortable, familiar and warm in My arms. Rest in Me. Rest in Me. You'll be okay. Read Hebrews 4 and Isaiah 43, remember the flames will not burn or hurt you!"

Hebrews 4 talks about the rest we have in God when we put our trust in Him. This is something we attain by putting our faith in Him about our circumstances. He has given us all the promise of finding rest in Him but we must be obedient to what He tells us to enjoy this peace. If people harden their hearts and choose disobedience, they'll never enter this place (vs.7b). God finished His work at the beginning of creation. There's no need to strive, let Him act on your behalf. When facing a valley in life as cold and dark as cancer, it can be scary. The Lord wants to be our comforter and light. He wants us to find rest in Him. He wants to be our safe place. Will you trust Him with your life?

On April 12, I received my first chemo in Ottawa at the General Hospital. The Lord blessed me with a new friend Christine, who had just completed treatment herself. Chris accompanied me and brought great comfort and support. I appreciated the fact that she had already walked this familiar road. I met her through one of my many wonderful neighbours Leslie, who, like Chris, also extended remarkable compassion. As I looked across the room, I felt very thankful. A man directly in front of me had a tumour the size of a large grapefruit that engulfed his face and throat. Regardless of how bad a situation may seem, we should always count our blessings because there is always someone far worse off than us.

The chemo unit was set up in a large circle with patients on the outside wall facing the center and patients in the inner circle facing outward, with the nurse's station directly in the middle of the room. It smelled of strong medicine and the air had a chill from the air conditioner, unlike warm hospital rooms. The nurses were dressed in an array of colourful uniforms with plastic blue smocks over and wore double gloves on their hands to protect themselves from coming into contact with the powerful drugs. The disease didn't discriminate, for patients from all ethnic backgrounds and races were affected. I recall one of the nurses mentioning they administer chemo to approximately 100 patients a day.

The chemo took three and a half hours to administer. I felt peculiar as the toxic medication raced through my veins. A strange taste filled my mouth as they administered the first drug. The nurse gave me ice to suck on, to numb the insides of my mouth to prevent mouth sores. The second, and the last, drug cocktail mix sent my head into a swirl. After returning home, I ate some supper and made the boys' lunches for school the next day. Rob and my mom encouraged me to sit down, even though I felt fine.

At approximately six o'clock, four hours after my treatment, I started violently projectile vomiting every few minutes non-stop. Shortly after midnight, relief finally came. My private nurse arrived to give me an ejection in my right hip to stop the vomiting. She came consecutively every three hours after that, until the vomiting had subsided. I had moved to the room of one of the boys for the night, because I didn't want to keep Rob awake with the sound effects (he had to work in the morning).

Everything within me felt like I was going to die, as my body shook with chills. I repeatedly quoted to myself the verse "*I can do all things through Christ who strengthens me.*" Thankfully, it gave me the strength to pull through. I was sick for 14 hours steady. My stomach settled somewhat over the next three days.

I really wasn't sure how I was going to do this for six months. My eyes were extremely sensitive to the light, so I spent the next week sitting or lying down with my eyes closed. It took everything in me to think and speak. I had *never* taken drugs before (illegal narcotics), but I imagined this experience was how someone felt after an overdosed high. It was not a pretty sight, or so I've been told!

Chemo can be fatal and is a toxic poison. It can cause leukemia, heart failure or damage, as well as osteoporosis, and force your body into early menopause.[1] My blood pressure had dropped severely low and I had sharp stabbing pains in my heart. The nurse was concerned that I was having a heart attack due to the chemo. After a trip to our local hospital, the doctors on call concluded that the pain was from muscle spasms in the chest wall. The other symptoms resulted from a bad reaction to the anti-nausea drug, Stemitil. It took one week for the effects of the medication to wear off. When it did, I really appreciated feeling good! People often take their health for granted. For my second chemo treatment, my medical oncologist changed the anti-nausea drugs to Maxeran and Zofran, and Dexidron for pain. She also decided to put me on three days' hydration so I would not lose weight.

The acid from my stomach began to eat away at my esophagus, making my throat raw and sore. The doctor performed regular blood tests every three weeks, before each chemo treatment, to ensure that my platelets and white blood cells were up at a good level. Chemo destroys the healthy cells along with the bad ones. Everyone needs white blood cells to fight off infection and disease. This is why many patients (usually really old or young) have died during treatment. After catching a simple cold, which can then turn into pneumonia, it becomes fatal as their bodies are unable to fight the germs.

I had a dream that I was in an unlocked, dilapidated house and sensed in my spirit that someone was trying to steal something that belonged to me. Something I needed to treasure and guard. When I awoke, the Lord gave me the sense that the house was my body, the treasured possession was my health and that something needed to change.

My niece, Kimberly, arrived on the Tuesday (for four days) to help out with the boys, while I received my chemo. Unfortunately, my white blood cell count was very low. The doctor postponed my treatment and prescribed more rest. Because I didn't want the circumstances to burden my family, I was doing too much and wore myself out in the process. Kim got a taste of busy family life and decided she was going to wait a long time before having children. She was a terrific help. After several days, my blood was retested and I was able to receive my treatment on the Friday, one day before Kim went home. This turn of events turned out to be a blessing because, from that day forward, I always received my Chemo just before the weekend when Rob was home with the children. By Monday, I was back to my old self.

One night, I dreamt I was a princess living in a castle situated in a valley. My father also lived in a nearby castle on top of a grand hill. As I sat in the corner, my father told me to stay away from foods containing sugar, caffeine, corn, and anything deep fried, like chips. The enemy un-expectedly slipped in and attacked my castle. At first, I didn't fight back. My father, with his army, came to help me. Each one of us held a sword and shield with a cross emblem, provided by my father. Together, we began to defeat each adversary.

This is what it meant: I am royalty, a daughter of the King (God). Even though we're in a valley, our Heavenly Father is nearby to help fight our battles. He gives us direction to protect us. The enemy will use entic-ing things like food against us to cause sickness and attack our bodies (castle). I need to watch what I eat, so the enemy can't use this to attack my body (castle). The cross and sword (the Word) are mighty weapons that defeat the enemy. They're ours to use. Don't let the enemy defeat you, fight back with the armour God has given you.

Twenty–four hours after each chemo treatment, I needed to receive an injection into my stomach, called Neulasta, to help induce my body to create white blood cells. Thank God, the treatment was covered by my husband's health plan because it cost $2,622.00 for each injection. There was a similar treatment, provided by the government at no cost to patients who don't have coverage, but the down side is that it causes constant ar-thritic aches and pains rather than for only a day or two, and the injections are daily. There was a short period of uncertainty about what was going to happen, which caused me quite a bit of stress. Rob was so kind and com-passionate; he was determined to obtain the superior treatment for me, regardless of the cost. I hated the thought of adding additional financial burden onto our family. The truth of the matter was that I really didn't feel like I was worth it, at that time. We'll get into that can of worms later.

God reminded me of the power in His Word (Bible). I needed to pray and speak that into my situation, lining my words up with the will of God. The Word of God speaks, and is alive and full of power (Hebrews 4:12).

"As the rain and the snow come down from heaven, and do not return to it without watering the earth and making it bud and flourish, so that it yields seed for the sower and bread for the eater, so is my word that goes out from my mouth: It will not return to me empty, but will accomplish what I desire and achieve the purpose for which I sent it." (Isaiah 55:10–11)

God's Word is powerful and has the ability to deliver a person from any dark situation that may threaten to overcome them. When He sends His Word things happen, lives are changed! Proverbs 4:20–22 says, *"My son, pay attention to what I say; listen closely to my words. Do not let them out of your sight, keep them within your heart; for they are life to those that find them and health to a man's whole body."* The Hebrew translation for the word "health" in the above verse is "medicine." The Word of God acts as medicine in our bodies and brings health to all our flesh. For this to happen, we need to partake in a daily dose of His healing Word, for it to be most effective. If someone is sick, and the physician prescribes medication, the medicine won't do its job properly if it isn't taken according to the directions. How many people have had a sickness return because they only took their medication for a few days and the remainder sat on a shelf in the medicine cabinet? It's the same idea with God's Word! Our Bible won't be of any benefit, collecting dust on a shelf. We need to partake of it regularly, in healthy doses. As you do, it will empower your body, mind and spirit with healing energy.[2]

During each subsequent chemo treatment, I prayed Isaiah 41 as well as Psalm 41:3, which talks about the Lord sustaining you on your sick bed and healing all infirmities. Each time, I improved immensely and threw up less! The acid reflux also disappeared. Because chemo attacks all the fast growing cells, it can cause thinning of the lining of your stomach and make it more sensitive, which can make it difficult to eat. I had no problem in this area, which is awesome because I enjoy my food.

A doctor and several nurses told me to eat whatever I wanted during treatment. They don't like to take that comfort away from chemo patients. Because I knew the importance of only putting good things in my mouth, I watched, very carefully, what I ate. During treatment, there were patients who sat stuffing themselves with fried food, chips and pop. Their choices made me cringe! Why not give yourself the best chance you can?

Seeking Comfort

"Praise be to the God and Father of our Lord Jesus Christ, the Father of compassion and the God of all comfort, who comforts us in all our troubles, so that we can comfort those in any trouble with the comfort we ourselves have received from God." (2 Corinthians 1:3, 4)

As humans, we all desire to be comfortable and when things aren't copasetic around us, we automatically tend to look for external sources to make us feel better. People are inclined to avoid or numb pain with substances or things, sometimes without even realizing it. Have you ever wondered why some people are constantly drowning themselves in fantasy novels, soap operas, or any kind of television in general? To get away from reality, that's why. It goes far beyond just having a favourite author or program. Drugs and alcohol are abused for the same reasons.

People crave certain comfort foods like candy bars, sweets, French fries and ice cream because it makes them feel good.[3] The fact is our brains release a feel-good hormone when we consume them, but these foods can actually do our bodies more harm than good.[4] These snack foods turn directly into sugar in our bodies, which pulls our immune system down and causes cancer cells to produce rapidly because they literally feed off sugar.[5] Foods that are deep fried not only contain fats that cause cancer cells but also form carcinogens while deep fried under immensely high temperatures.[6]

Shopping is another form of escapism that millions of people turn to, digging huge holes of debt for themselves, trying to bring some sort of contentment. Unfortunately, comfort, from any source other than God, only produces temporary results and draws people into a cycle of addiction.[7]

"Now this is what the Lord Almighty says: 'Give careful thought to your ways.' You have planted much, but have harvested little. You eat, but never have enough. You drink, but never have your fill. You put on clothes, but are not warm. You earn wages, only to put them in a purse with holes in it. This is what the Lord Almighty says: 'Give careful thought to your ways." (Haggai 1:5–7)

God reminds us to take a good look at how we turn to things to bring us comfort, how we give them precedence and yet we still remain dissatisfied and empty. We often expect others to meet our need for comfort. The loving support of family and friends is a gift in times of hardship but they are not meant to be our all in all. Essentially, we need to rely on God. He is the only true source of lasting comfort. Have you been looking for comfort in the wrong places? If you reach out and ask God to meet your need, He will empower you with the needed strength and grace to continue on.

Dear God,

I confess that I have been looking for comfort from worldly sources and not from You. Please forgive me and remove any feelings of guilt and condemnation that are weighing me down. Help me recognize when I fall into this trap and help me look to You to be my true source of comfort. Break the cycle of addiction off my life and fill me with Your everlasting peace. Empower those people in whom

You choose to bring comfort, and may I recognize Your hand in my circumstances that I may give You the praise and glory. In Jesus' name I pray. Amen.

After each chemo treatment, I spent three consecutive days lying in bed. When the boys and Rob weren't visiting me in my room, I passed the time reading healing Scriptures, praying and thanking God for all the blessings in my life. Staying positive stilled the fear, gave me peace and kept me hopeful. My doctors advised me that studies have shown that it is the positive patients that tend to survive. I placed Scripture around our home to read, meditate, memorize, confess and pray. It kept my faith strong! There are healing Scriptures listed in the back of the book for a convenient reference.

The Powerful Weapon of Worship

Worship is Powerful and stills the enemy! It opens the door for God's presence and allows Him to do His work (see Psalm 50:23). In 2 Chronicles 20:18–22, Jehoshaphat was alarmed after being warned that an army of Moabites, Ammonites with some Meunites from Mount Seir was coming to make war against him. He called for prayer and fasting in all the land. Jehoshaphat stood up in the assembly of Judah and Jerusalem, at the temple of the Lord, and praised and worshipped the Lord and then reminded God of the promises He had made to the people. When he was finished, the Lord spoke back and gave him clear direction: not to be afraid or discouraged because the battle was not his, but God's. They took their positions, stood firm, and watched as the Lord brought deliverance. While they worshipped the Lord, the enemy was self–slaughtered.

Grumbling and complaining grieves the Holy Spirit. It's a hindrance to receiving the immediate blessings God wants to bestow upon us.

When Moses delivered the Israelites out of Egypt, it took them 40 years to make an 11 day trip. It was their ungrateful attitude that kept them in the wilderness. I make it a daily practice to thank God for all the wonderful people and things He has blessed me with in life. By doing this, it helps me stay in a thankful frame of mind and keeps me out of the self-pity rut that so many people fall into.

Self-pity can be an easy pit to slide into, especially if you have had one unfortunate thing happen after another. There is always going to be someone better off than we are and also someone who is far worse off than we. Being thankful not only gives you peace, it helps you be content with where you are until your circumstances change.

Prayer Brings Peace and Change

"Do not be anxious about anything, but in everything, by prayer and petition, with thanksgiving, present your requests to God. And the peace of God, which transcends all understanding, will guard your hearts and your minds in Christ Jesus." (Philippians 4:6, 7)

When we bring our needs, desires and wishes before God with a thankful heart, we are blessed with a sense of peace that is unexplainable. God hears our prayers and we can have confidence knowing, that if our requests are in God's will, we will receive those things without question (1 John 5:14, 15).

"Peace I leave with you; my peace I give you. I do not give to you as the world gives. Do not let your hearts be troubled and do not be afraid." (John 14:27)

It's nice to know that we can count on something in this world other than death and taxes. Although peace doesn't come from this world, we can still experience it. God freely gives us the peace we need, even during the darkest circumstances, when we seek Him. The key is to abide in Him, by keeping our eyes on God and His great ability to save, rather than focusing on the storms of life raging around us. This will help you remain in peace. A perfect example of this is when Peter got out of the boat to walk on the water toward Jesus. As long as he kept his eyes on Jesus, he remained on top of the water but as soon as he took his eyes off Jesus and focused on the wind storm around him, he sank. The good news is that when Peter cried out to the Lord to save him, Jesus immediately reached out with His hand and lifted Peter out (Matthew 15:22).

Are you like Peter? Do you have your eyes on the eye of the storm instead of on the one who can bring you through? It's not too late! Jesus is waiting for you to reach out to Him so He can lift you out of the storm you're in and walk you through to the other side.

Trip to the Genetics Counsellor

I was also referred to see a genetic counsellor to see whether or not I should be tested for the known BCRA1 gene or the BCRA2 gene. After thorough questioning regarding family medical history and habit patterns with in my own life, the genetics counsellor was certain that performing these blood tests, for these particular genes, wasn't necessary. She felt the cancer wasn't hereditary and the cancer factors must have come from toxins within my food, water and the environment, with stress mixed in, as a large contributing factor. During my career as a dental assistant I handled mercury on a regular basis and was sometimes exposed to unnecessary radiation.

I wasn't a smoker, but I had loved ones who were. For this reason, I was subjected to second-hand smoke consistently over my entire life, until about nine years ago. People in my work environment and almost all of my friends' parents were heavy smokers! I'm not blaming anyone. I'm just sharing the facts! Back then, we weren't aware of the health hazards, like we are today! Since then, tables have turned in society and smoking has been deemed almost socially unacceptable rather than the 'in' thing to do. Thankfully, the government has put laws in place to protect others from second–hand smoke in public buildings and restaurants. You can't control others' actions, but you can make choices that are good for you. If there are people smoking around you, you can put the ball back in your own court by avoiding such places because politely keeping your distance isn't enough.

Change of Plans

On May 3, the news from my oncologist hit me hard. The tumour was Her2 positive, which changed the diagnosis from a 75% survival rate to grim. With the antibody drug, Herceptin, it would bring the survival rate statistic back up to a 45% chance for 5 years and lesson the chance of re-occurance to 50%. The tumour, being Her2 positive, meant that my body, at that time, was producing too much of the Her2 protein. It was attaching itself to my cells, which is where the term mutating comes from. *Everyone diagnosed with breast cancer should be tested for Her2. Please make sure your doctor tests you.* I had a friend whose doctor didn't bother, until it was too late!

My doctor told me everyone has approximately two Her2 proteins attached to each individual cell. The tumour tested positive to having over 14 proteins per cell. This makes it more difficult for chemo to attack and destroy the cancer cells. The trial period for the drug Herceptin was closed for me because I had started with another treatment. My doctor was bringing a proposal to the government, along with some others on the hospital board, to make Herceptin a standard treatment, so that all patients needing this treatment wouldn't have to forgo this treatment due to cost. At this time, one year of treatment costs $45,000.00. I didn't want to be a financial burden to my family, but Rob would have found a way. Friends and family were calling or writing letters to our local Member of Parliament and government, for added support.

This is where I really needed to raise the faith bar, get my mind off the circumstances, and fix my eyes on Jesus. God can do so much more than we could ever hope, think or imagine, if we put our trust in Him. In Mark 9:23, Jesus said, *"everything is possible for him who believes."* Mark 10:27 states nothing is impossible with God and Mark 11:24 says that whatever you ask for in prayer, if you believe you have received it, it will be yours.

Sometimes, circumstances may seem hopeless. You may feel like giving up but you need to persevere so that, when you have done the will of God, you will receive what He has promised (Hebrews 10:36). The condition is doing the will of God. The Word says, *"My people perish for lack of knowledge."* Find out what God's will and wisdom is for your situation and be obedient. James 1:5 states that He gives wisdom to those who ask without finding fault.

No matter how many promises God has made, they are yes, in Christ. (In Christ refers to Jesus being your Saviour). Ask God for wisdom in your situation from His Word (the Bible) and wisdom will call out to you (Proverbs 8:1–4). Then these are 'yes' promises to you, in your situation. We need to receive them by faith. *"Now faith is being sure of what we hope for and certain of what we do not see." (Hebrews 11:1) Without faith it is impossible to please God, because anyone who comes to Him must believe that He exists and that He rewards those who earnestly seek Him.* The way we increase our faith, is by hearing the Word of God (Romans 10:17). If you don't feel like you have enough faith, get into the Word and ask God to increase it and to help you in your unbelief (Mark 9:23, 24). The Bible is relevant to our everyday lives. Regardless of your need, there are answers to every problem within. Gloria Copeland was instrumental in teaching me about faith, while Beth Moore stretched my faith to believe for those things that seemed impossible!

My doctor felt it would be wise to switch the type and length of my treatments. I was now going to receive four treatments of F.E.C. and four treatments of Taxol, to give a total of eight chemotherapy treatments. I had heard horror stories about this drug, in which you would have to place your fingers in ice water so your nails wouldn't fall off. Turns out, whoever told me this had confused it with a generic drug, Paxitacil.

I did have my large toenails lift off, only a third way down at the corners, but that's minor compared to the other story. The reason for the switch between F.E.C. and Taxol was that Herceptin and F.E.C. mixed can cause greater heart damage than with Taxol. This was a concern, due to the fact that my grandfather had died, at age 52, with a massive heart attack. My mother had experienced one mild heart attack and my uncle had a triple by-pass, before the age of 50.

The Lord showed me that we have to be very careful about the confessions we speak out of our mouths. In Proverbs 18:20, 21 it says, *"From the fruit of his mouth a man's stomach is filled; with the harvest from his lips he is satisfied. The tongue has the power of life and death, and those who love it will eat its fruit."* What we speak into our lives and the lives of others around us will affect them and us directly. You get what you speak. It is a matter of sowing and reaping (Galations 6:7); this is one of the foundational laws God created the world on.

Our words are like gates that open our circumstances, to allow either God or Satan to work in our situations because they both have the power to do so.[8] Whatever we complain or praise about is what we will experience. Our words fall directly back on us.[9] This doesn't mean a million dollars will drop out of the sky just because you go around claiming that you're going to be a millionaire.[10] It doesn't work that way! Satan takes the negative things we say and uses them for evil, while God takes His Word (Bible) and creates life with it.[11] God always desires the best for us, but Satan uses the words people speak to cause destruction. To put it simply, our words give either God or Satan the authority to bless or harm us.

When God created the heavens and the earth, He spoke them into existence (Genesis 1). God told Abram that He would be the Father of many nations, even though Sara and Abram's bodies were considered as good as dead. In the natural, it seemed crazy to believe such a thing because Abram was about a hundred years old and Sara was past child bearing years.[12] In Romans 4:17 it says, *God gives life to the dead and calls things that are not as though they were.* God changed Abram's name to Abraham, which meant "Father of Many Nations." Each time someone called him by his new name, they were speaking prophecy over Him. God is a God of the impossible. We need to line our words up with the will of God and guard our mouths from speaking negatively, so we are not allowing an opportunity for Satan to work. Proverbs 21:23 says, "He who guards his mouth and his tongue keeps himself from calamity." This doesn't mean we aren't to speak, but we need to choose our words carefully.

When Jesus was in the desert for 40 days, fasting, Satan appeared to test Him and Jesus spoke the Word of God right back at Satan. When David faced Goliath, he let Goliath ramble on with vicious insults but then David spoke right back at him, in full confidence, about what would become of him. You may wonder why Goliath didn't get what he said. David served Almighty God and it is our heritage, as servants of the Lord that no weapon forged against us will prevail and every tongue rising against us, God will refute. It is God's vindication to us when our hearts are pure (Isaiah 54:17). We must ask God to act on our behalf. Greater is He who is in me (God), than he that is in the world (Satan). When I accepted Christ as my Lord and Saviour, His spirit came into my heart to take up residency. It is through Christ that we are more than conquerors. We especially need to speak out after negative words (curses) have been spoken over us, or others. Whether it's a bad diagnosis from the doctor or someone saying your kids will never amount to anything (Isaiah 54:17), we need to reject the negative and speak life.

We need to think about what we are thinking because out of the overflow of the heart the mouth speaks (Matthew 12:34). We need to purposely refuse to think negative thoughts and think positively at all times, regardless of the situation. Philippians 4:8 says, *"Finally, brothers, whatever is true, whatever is noble, whatever is right, whatever is pure, whatever is lovely, whatever is admirable—if anything is excellent or praiseworthy—think about such things."* I realize this can be very difficult. We need to cast down all arguments and pretensions (imaginations) and bring them into obedience with the Word of the Lord. This means that if something goes against what the Bible says, whether it be thoughts or words spoken about us, our family, our lives, we need to choose to think, speak, and believe what the Word of God says in our situation, regardless of what the circumstances look like in the natural; we need to speak and believe the positive (2 Corinthians 10:3–5).

We are saved by the blood of the Lamb and the word of our testimony (Revelation 12:11). Romans 10:9–12 reaffirms this truth, for it says that it is by the confessions of our mouths that we are saved. The word "*saved*" taken from this text in Greek is "*sozo*".[13] The word "*sozo*" translated means: wholeness for our body, mind and soul.[14] The confessions of our mouth can bring healing, deliverance and salvation to our lives when our hearts are full of faith and aligned with the Word of God.

Just before Jesus drew his last breath on the cross, he said, "It is finished" (John 19:30). When something is finished, it means it's completed, with nothing else left to be done. There's no striving to add any extra last minute touches because it's finished! There is nothing to do. This is an amazing gift, wrapped up in one complete parcel, waiting to be received. It is yours for the taking; you just need to accept it. How do I do that, you might ask? You take it by faith.

The Power of Our Confessions

People can open a door for sickness by the confessions of their mouths and by what they believe. What you believe in your heart so shall be (Proverbs 23:7; KJV). Many people say, "In my family they eventually end up with cancer, diabetes, heart disease or arthritis," etc. They believe and say, "It's inevitable. They are genetically predisposed to these things and they are going to get it. It's just a matter of time." BE VERY CAREFUL! What we speak opens the door for the circumstance to follow. Yes, there is something to say about genetics, but you don't have to accept that. You could change the family trend of bad habits by choosing to eat properly. Maybe you come from a long line of smokers? You can choose to quit! God asks us to do the best with what He has given us and then He'll do the rest.

The Lord brought back to my memory a situation that happened when I was 13 years old. On this particular day, the youth group from my church was heading out to an event, in the city of Ottawa. My friends and I were jammed tightly together in the back seat of my friend's brother's car. Because of the lack of elbow-room, a fight broke out. One of the boys started throwing his arms around, in anger, and cracked me right in the boob with his elbow. I felt my face grow hot as I blurted out with anger, "Great, now I'm going to end up getting breast cancer you idiot!" Ok, maybe I was a little more dramatic than most girls. Some people may think this is just a coincidence but need I remind you of Proverbs 18:20, 21, the words we speak hold the power to either open up doors for good or bad. The King James Version of the Bible says, in Proverbs 13:3: *"He that keepeth his mouth keepeth his life: but he that openeth wide his lips shall have destruction."*

You may be thinking, 'great now what do I do?' If you have been someone that has spoken negative words over you, your spouse, children or even friends, don't worry, we can break that off. There is power in the Word of God, power in prayer, power in Jesus' Name and power in His blood. First I want to give you proof!

The Power of Prayer!

The Bible says it is the fervent prayer of a righteous man that is powerful and effective in James 5:16b of the New King James Version. God also promises that whatever you ask for in prayer, if you believe and don't doubt you will receive it and it will be yours (Matthew 21:21, 22).

There are significant keys to unlocking God's power, shown in the above passages, which reveal what makes prayer powerful. The first key has to do with the "fervent prayer." The word fervent means to be passionate and zealous about something. Therefore fervent prayer is being passionate and full of zeal about what you're praying for.

This second key "the righteous man," I believe is the most important. This is someone who is in right standing with God. We cannot hold iniquity in our hearts and expect God to listen to our prayers (see Proverbs 28:9). If I had cherished sin in my heart, the Lord would not have listened; (Psalm 66:18). We need to pray, as David did, *"Search me, O*

God, and know my heart; test me and know my anxious thoughts. See if there is any offensive way in me, and lead me in the way everlasting." Psalm 139:23, 24. If we want God to hear our prayers, we need to confess our sins to Him and ask for forgiveness, this includes forgiving those who have sinned against us (see Mark 11:25).

The next key is "to believe you will receive what you are asking for." God asks us to do our part by operating in faith (Mark 9:23; James 1:5, 6, 7). For our prayers to be powerful, they must also be in the will of God. How can we know if something is God's will or not? His will is revealed throughout the Bible. *Jesus said, "'If you remain in me and my words remain in you, ask whatever you wish, and it will be given you.'"* John 15:7. When we reside in a constant place with the Lord, spending daily time in His Word and talking to Him, He opens our eyes to the Father's will. It is then, that we can ask with confidence and receive.

Some people have misunderstood this concept and given this act the pet name, "name it, and claim it"! We must remember that God is Sovereign and has overall rule–ship over our lives. He asks us to watch what we say, so that He has the right words to work with. It's His choice to work with us. This is not a method to get everything we want. The things we ask for must be in His perfect will for His plans in our lives.

Praying God's Word

"For the word of God is living and active. Sharper than any double–edged sword, it penetrates even to dividing soul and spirit, joints and marrow; it judges the thoughts and attitudes of the heart." (Hebrews 4:12)

"So is my word that goes out from my mouth: It will not return to me empty, but will accomplish what I desire and achieve the purpose for which I sent it." (Isaiah 55:11)

When we pray God's Word, our prayers become even more powerful! I encourage you to ask God for Scriptures, regarding your situation, to use in prayer. Watch and marvel at the awesome things the Lord does on your behalf!

The Power of Jesus' Name

"The name of the Lord is a strong tower; the righteous run to it and are safe." (Proverbs 18:10)

"One day Peter and John were going up to the temple at the time of prayer—at three in the afternoon. Now a man crippled from birth was being carried to the temple gate called Beautiful, where he was put every day to beg from those going into the temple courts. When he saw Peter and John about to enter, he asked them for money. Peter looked straight at him, as did John. Then Peter said, "Look at us!" So the man gave them his attention, expecting to get something from them. Then Peter said, "Silver or gold I do not have, but what I have I give you. In the name of Jesus Christ of Nazareth, walk." Taking him by the right hand, he helped him up, and instantly the man's feet and ankles became strong. He jumped to his feet and began to walk. Then he went with them into the temple courts, walking and jumping, and praising God." (Acts 3:1–8)

When we pray, using Jesus' name, people are healed and circumstances change! But, I believe people can't misuse Jesus' name and expect to get their prayers answered![15] One of the Ten Commandments states, in Exodus 20:7, *"You shall not misuse the name of the Lord your God, for the Lord will not hold anyone guiltless who misuses His name."*

Do you allow the names Jesus, Christ or God to roll off your tongue, like they're any other word? You may think it's harmless, but it's not. By doing so, a person is taking a precious name and using it in a blasphemous manner. Would you appreciate someone using your name as a swear word all the time? We need to give honour to the Lord and Saviour of the world, by using His name respectfully! Do you need to ask the

Lord's forgiveness for not honouring His name? If so, now is a good time as any! He will forgive you, if you ask?

Dear God,

I confess my sin of using Your name in vain; I repent of it now and ask for Your forgiveness. In Jesus' name I ask this. Amen.

The Power of Jesus' Blood

What is it about Jesus' blood that makes it so special? Did you know that our sins actually separate us from God? God is holy, we are sinful. Sin and holiness are polar opposites that mix as well as oil and water. Even our good works are like filthy rags before Him (Isaiah 64:6). *"For all have sinned and fall short of the glory of God."* (Romans 3:23)

In the Old Testament, a priest would make sacrifices for his sins and the sins of the people. By doing this, their sins were covered and God was able to look upon them. This act wasn't enough to remove their sins once and for all. They had to sacrifice animals each time they sinned. What a dreadful, necessary job! We are so fortunate to now have a New Covenant with God. Because of God's great love for us, He sent Jesus, His son, to die on the cross for our sins. He became the perfect and final sacrifice for our sins and those who accept Him as Saviour are no longer bound by the law of sin and death. Ephesians 2:13 declares that we have been brought near to God through the blood of Christ (see 2 Corinthians 5:21; Ephesians 1:7).

In the Canadian Dictionary the definition of redemption states:

> 1. The act of redeeming or the condition of having been redeemed. 2. Recovery of something pawned or mortgaged. 3. The payment of an obligation, as a government's payment of the value of its bonds. 4. Deliverance

upon payment of ransom; rescue. 5. Theol. Salvation from sin through Jesus' sacrifice.[16]

The blood of Jesus protects us. How can that be, you might ask? Have you heard of the Jewish custom celebrated called "The Passover?" In the time when Pharaoh was king of Israel, Moses was sent by God to deliver the Israelite's who had been in captivity for 100 years out of the hand of Pharaoh. Pharaoh remained steadfast in his decision and refused to let the people go, even after God sent various plagues, revealing His great power. The Lord then spoke to Moses and Aaron saying that the Angel of Death was going to pass by and strike all the land. The entire first born of man and beast, of Egypt, would die. God gave Moses specific instructions on how to protect his people. The people were to kill a lamb, take its blood and apply it to the sides and tops of the doorframes of their homes. God promised them that when the Angel of Death passed through Egypt, the blood would be a sign to him to pass by the homes where the blood of the lamb was applied and not bring harm their way (Exodus 12).

Jesus is the reason we have a new Covenant with God. He is the literal and symbolic Lamb of God, our Lamb of sacrifice. His blood is a sign of protection for our lives that we need to apply to our lives, by faith (*Hebrews 11:28*). The devil is the destroyer and we need to apply the blood of the Lamb, in faith, for our protection.[17]We have the authority to do this, as believers in Christ (see *John 10:10*).

"They overcame him by the blood of the Lamb and by the word of their testimony." (Revelation 12:11a)

Prayer to Break Curses off! (Say Out Loud!)

"I renounce the curse of _____. (Say the negative word that has been spoken over you or your loved one. Be as specific as you can). This curse falls dead to the floor and

has no power over_____, (insert name). I speak life and blessing into this situa-
tion_____, (speak the positive of what you want manifested in your life or others),
this blessing, replaces the curse. In Jesus' name, I cover_____, (name) in the
blood of Jesus and ask You Lord to wash the circumstance clean with Your blood
and close and seal the door with Your blood so Satan no longer has rights in this
area. In Jesus' name, I ask. Amen."

This doesn't mean we should talk carelessly and then use this prayer as an eraser. We need to actively endeavour to do and say the right things. God's grace is not to be abused or taken for granted. God knows we are going to make mistakes and His grace and mercy will catch us when we slip up, if we ask Him.

It is important to replace the negative things we have said with positive ones. You don't need to be fearful wondering what things you might have said in the past. Ask God to reveal them to you. With His help, you can break free from these bondages. He loves you and wants you to live in freedom.

When I had cancer, I never called it "my cancer" because it wasn't something I wanted, nor wanted to be defined by. I didn't want to own it or keep it. I wanted to get past it to the point that, even when I was in treatment, I would say, "When I had cancer." I didn't want to be thought of as the victim, but rather a conqueror. With Jesus in my life, I have become just that.

"We are more than conquerors though Jesus Christ, our Lord!" (Romans 8:37)

When Jesus graciously died for our sins, He conquered death, sickness, disease, and poverty on the cross. Then He rose from the dead, on the third day, and sat down on the right hand of the Father to pray (intercede) on your behalf. With Jesus on your side, you don't need to fear!

Direction from a Dream

The Lord gave me a dream, the Spring before getting sick, about a particular stone home on the water, situated three houses down from the property, where I had grown up, in Iroquois, Ont. My mother was sitting at the kitchen table. This had great significance. My mother was a very busy lady with church, friends and with her work as Coordinator for the Food Bank. We often only saw her briefly about once a month, over dinner at our house. I felt we were missing out on valuable time together. As my mother and father were divorcing, Rob and I considered moving to that area so my mother could come live with us. My mom didn't want to move to Winchester and Rob and I had always hoped that someday we would move back to the water.

Curiously, I drove past this house several days later, to behold a glorious "For Sale" sign staked in the lawn. I was puzzled when it sold several weeks later because I really thought this house would be ours! Up until that point, I hadn't asked for discernment regarding the dream. Clarity came, as the new owners spent the next few months removing all the stonework from the outside of the house, rebuilding the frame, from the inside out, due to a serious mold problem.

I went to see a highly recommended Christian Natural Path Doctor. Dr. Ken, as we like to call him, performed an Electro–Dermal Screening test, to determine the reason I got cancer. This is a process in which information is gathered from the patient through what's called the bodies "information windows." Electrical current is applied to different pressure points on the body where the nerves run to and from different organs and collects data for evaluation, through a computer. The information is shown on a graph and indicates whether certain organs are out of balance. If there is an imbalance, the trained practitioner is able to treat with natural herbal remedies to bring balance back to the body.

The testing determined there was a fungus called Blastomycosis (a type of black mold) within my body, which stayed dormant for approximately 24 years. This meant I was thirteen at the time. The Lord brought back to my memory the time we had moved from our house in Iroquois to Morrisburg. I had gotten my fingers jammed in–between the panes of glass, in my bedroom window. There was a lot of black mold in my window from condensation. The fungus must have gotten into my system where the skin had scrapped off. My dad had to pull the windows apart to release my hand. This happened shortly after the incident in the car, when I was elbowed in the chest!

Do you see the connection? The dream of the house was not a literal manifestation, but actually symbolic! It represented the problem in my body (fungus caused sickness). The house (my body) was rebuilt from the inside out, due to cancer caused by mold, restructured by chemo. My mother, at the kitchen table, represented her partaking an active role in our lives. We began to see her more frequently. Mom helped out with early morning appointments by sending our boys off to school. She spent time with Spencer, when I was unable to get Respicare aid, and drove me to several chemo appointments.

All through Bible times, God used dreams to inform people of what was going to take place, to give guidance and direction, to warn people to change from their ways or to pray for circumstances to change. God still works the same way today. We need to be aware and be obedient to what God is asking of us! He speaks to us so we'll change our ways and not perish.

In the Old Testament, God declared that He would speak through dreams and visions, he said, "Listen to my words: *When a prophet of the Lord is among you, I reveal myself to him in visions, I speak to him in dreams.*" (Numbers 12:6)

"For God does speak—now one way, now another—though man may not per-ceive it. In a dream, in a vision of the night, when deep sleep falls on men as they slum-ber in their beds, he may speak in their ears and terrify them with warnings, to turn man from wrongdoing and keep him from pride, to preserve his soul from the pit, his life from perishing by the sword." (Job 33:14–18)

God said He would continue to speak to us through dreams right up into the end times. *"In the last days, God says, I will pour out my Spirit on all people. Your sons and daughters will prophesy, your young men will see visions, your old men will dream dreams. Even on my servants, both men and women, I will pour out my Spirit in those days, and they will prophesy."* (Act 2:17, 18)

God's Word declares that He instructs or counsels our hearts at night as we dream (Psalm 16:7). After reading these few Scriptures, I hope you understand and take your dreams more seriously. According to Mark Virkler, one-third of the total Bible recalls the stories and actions from the dreams God gave.[18]Hopefully, this will help those of you who are skeptical to see the importance and value of your dreams. Perhaps, its time you place more value and emphasis upon your dreams rather than blaming them on undigested pizza, from the night before![19]

The Gift of Baldness!

I didn't consider myself vain but, I did enjoy being complimented. As a tee-nager, to build myself up, I would often compliment others so they would, in return, say something nice to me. Or I would put myself down in hopes that they would say, "Oh no, that's not true." I started wearing foundation, blush, eye shadow, eyeliner, and mascara, "the whole nine yards" by grade five. I felt I was too ugly to go out anywhere without applying every prod-uct.

You'll be pleased to know, that as an adult, I've changed. I love making people feel good about themselves by giving compliments where they are due and I don't like it when others return the gesture, by saying nice things back, only because I've said something nice to them. My desire is for people to be truly sincere and only comment when it comes from their heart.

The chemo treatment that the health professionals administer for breast cancer always makes the patients lose their entire body hair, including eyelashes and eyebrows. Because I still carried my insecurity, I didn't want to subject myself to the humiliation of losing my hair. My sister-in-law, Laura, flew down for a week to give me a hand. While she was here, we went shopping to purchase a nice wig, some cute hats and a few head-scarves. I also attended a session of 'Look Good Feel Great' at our local hospital, to learn the tricks for applying make-up to help create the illusion that one still has eyelashes and brows.

I lost most of my hair just days before my second chemo treatment. The nurse had recommended that I cut my hair really short before this happened, thinking I would adjust better to the loss. I saw that as a complete waste of money. I wanted to keep the length of my hair as long as possible, knowing God would give me the strength I needed at that time. I lost the majority of it within three days. When the bald patches got too bad, my two friends, Mitch and Abby, came to my home to help me shave my head.

Carter, our second son, who had such a hard time initially with the thought of me losing my hair, became very angry with the girls when he realized what they were doing.

"I hate you. Stop! Stop!" he screamed, as he angrily pounded his fist against the locked bathroom door.

"Calm down, Carter, and Mommy will let you in." I replied from the stool.

"No Carter, you're not coming in until your mom's all done. Go away," Mitch hollered. The screaming stopped. Abby encouraged me to sit and relax so she could finish shaving my head. Everything within me wanted to go to Carter. Mitch stood guarding the door. Emotionless, I stared back at the stranger in the mirror. I felt completely naked. I brushed my hand over my head and decided I wasn't going out of the room looking like that and reached for my wig. As I stood adjusting it on my head in the mirror Mitch began to weep.

"I hate that wig, take that thing off!" She cried.

"Mitch, this is not about you and what you like. I'm the one with the bald head and if I want to wear the wig, I will!" I said as I headed toward the door.

As I gently opened the door, Carter pushed his way in." With feet set apart and both hands on his hips, his icy–blue eyes glared into Mitch's face.

"I hate you Mitch," he said.

"The girls are doing me a favour." I reassured him. "Everything is okay. Shaving my head was my choice." With tears trickling down his cheeks, he asked if he could see my bald head. He grasped my hand and watched as I pulled the wig off with the other. Carter giggled with delight. He thought I looked cute with my new "Demi Moore" look. Mitch was crying in the corner and I overheard Abby telling Mitch not to take our reaction personally. Carter reacted the same way most children would in the same situation. I apologized and hoped that she would eventually see the circumstance from our perspective.

I wore the wig for the first three months. When it got too hot and sticky outside, the kids spoke up and persuaded me to just wear my cap or go without the wig altogether. They were comfortable with the way I looked and thought nothing of it when their friends came over. The wig gave me the comfort and strength I needed to get through the transition, until I became more confident as a person.

Losing my hair was the last thing I ever wanted to happen but it turned out to be a real blessing in disguise. God has an amazing way of turning things around and using even the most unfortunate circumstances to bring good from them. It helped cement the reality that my value as a person doesn't come from my looks but from who I am on the inside.

Most people were very kind but I would always get the odd person who would avoid me like the plague. I realize that's how some people deal with uncomfortable situations, and that's okay. The last thing I was looking for was people's sympathy or attention because of it. I only wanted to be treated for the person I was.

I clearly remember the day I took Spencer to his new school, in Russell, for orientation. We gathered in the gym and even though the principal encouraged people to get to know one another, no one would talk to me. Picture me at this point; I'm dressed in a cute pair of baby yellow cotton shorts that's coordinated with a pink and yellow striped t-shirt, pink flip flops, bald and wearing a white ball cap. I tried to engage in friendly chat with several people; they were either cold or turned their backs. Finally, I went over and stood alone by the wall.

As treatment progressed, I grew tired. I was unable to perform my daily tasks with the same excellence I once did. Being positioned in a place of helplessness and having no other choice but to accept and learn to receive from others broke off my pride. I again learned that my value as a person came from who I am, not from what I do. In Isaiah 38, we read about King Hezekiah, who had become ill. He had an issue with pride because he had trouble receiving acts of kindness (pride can be a hindrance to receiving healing). When he repented, God added 15 years to his life.

I used to be performance-oriented and gained my value in what I could accomplish in a day. I ran on very little sleep and had expectations for myself and when I didn't meet those standards, I felt worthless and punished myself. It was very important not to make mistakes or I became depressed. I strived for affection and value from others for what I accomplished, always trying to get noticed. When I didn't receive attention, I felt devalued. I wanted to stand out and excel beyond others, so I purposely chose different hobbies than my sisters. When they took interest in my hobbies, I stopped. If I couldn't do something perfectly, I had no desire to do it at all.

I decided I didn't want to be a perfectionist and people–pleaser any longer. I still think it's important to do things with excellence, yet keeping a balance. When we become a people–pleaser, we lose our self as a person. We truly can't be the people God created us to be if we're always doing what others want so they won't reject us. We need to be obedient to God and do the things He wants us to do. If our motive isn't doing things for the Lord, then our good works will be of no worth.

When Friends Drop Out of Your Life

A stranger avoiding you is one thing but when someone you've known for years, one whom you've shared the intimate details of your life with, becomes cold and distant, now that hurts! Companions you've enjoyed spending time with, whether walking, shopping or having lunch, are now gone and you're left with an empty void that aches in its place. Even having the acquaintances that you've often shared very friendly chit chat with turn the other way or pretend they didn't see you can become a source of pain, if you let it. These are the times when you have to remember that there is nothing personally wrong with you and that is just how some individuals cope with uncomfortable situations.

My advice to the other people would be... don't avoid them, and say 'hello' rather than pretend they don't exist. Saying nothing can be just as damaging as saying the wrong thing! It only takes a minute of your time to give a smile or gesture a friendly hello! Besides, it makes you feel good and burns less energy than frowning.

I had two of my friends completely drop out of my life because they couldn't bear the thought of losing me. One friend ignored me completely. She either turned the other way or looked straight through me, as I'd say hello upon meeting her on the street. After numerous times of experiencing this type of encounter, she finally passed a message along, through a mutual friend via email, that she was sorry about my situation and that she cared. She wrestled with guilt, unable to give any support as she found it difficult enough to deal with the recent death of her father. She couldn't handle the thought of me being sick and was unable to even look my way without crying.

I wasn't looking for any support and released her from that expectation. We should never look to others to fulfill our needs, but to our Heavenly Father who is the giver of all good gifts. When we look to Him as our provider, He opens up the floodgates of Heaven to bless and meet every one of our needs. It's not necessarily in ways we would have imagined either, but better!

I'm sure it also hit home emotionally for her because she is also the mother of three young boys. I responded by writing a note, sincerely letting her know I appreciated the message, as it eliminated any feelings I had about offending her in some way. I communicated the fact that I understood and sympathized with her situation regarding her dad and that regardless of her inability to speak to me, I would continue to send a friendly smile or hello her way. By not doing so, it would go against the grain of my natural personality and it wouldn't have felt right! With this understanding, it allowed me to keep the proper perspective and made the uncomfortable situations that arose tolerable, by removing the sting from them.

If you're having a hard time coping with a situation of this nature, my recommendation to you would be to give the other person a hug or smile. Remember, there's two sides to the pain or discomfort being felt; let yourself cry if you need to because it's your body's way of dealing with pain. It's a good release and heals your body by discharging certain hormones that your body needs. If you don't allow your body the opportunity to properly grieve over loss or disappointment for a time, the pain will creep up later as a cry for help through the path of depression or addiction later on.

What makes people true friends is being able to feel comfortable enough to be real with one another. Being open and vulnerable, letting your guard down and showing your true emotions, whatever the situation, by laughing, crying or getting angry, if need be. Several people, who came to visit or call me, expressed afterwards that they were nervous initially; however, after spending time with me they felt very blessed. They thought they were coming to comfort and help me, but in fact, felt as though I was the one that encouraged them and brought them joy and hope. My thoughts are often caught up in those precious moments spent with those gracious people who sacrificed valuable time from their lives to share with me. I feel so much richer because of it.

I met some precious new friends along the journey and rekindled several old friendships. We had let our relationships slip away because of the busyness of our lives. Through it all, we were able to laugh and find humour in the midst of adversity and even had the occasional little cry, but rarely, because there was and is so much to be thankful for, even in the midst of darkness.

After a year had passed, my friend eventually became comfortable enough to talk with me on the soccer field but something had changed within my heart. An unexpected struggle arose within my emotions. I wanted to keep her at bay the way she did to me. She wanted me back in her life, now that I was better. I felt like I had to pretend that nothing had ever happened, that I was never sick, even though I was still walking daily with the reality of it! There is never a day that goes by that I don't think about my experience with cancer. Every time I think about putting something in my mouth I am faced with a decision that could alter my destiny. I try to make a conscious effort to choose only those things that will bring life and nourishment to my body!

Initially, it was easy to accept and understand the basis of my friend's reactions, but later when my friend had dealt with her issues, I needed to deal with the rejection I had endured. Regardless how understandable her reasons were, I needed to work through the offence I had taken on. Somehow along the way, the hurt must have grown into a bitter root because I had stuffed something down on the inside. I already had rejection issues from my past so I believe that this made me more sensitive in this area.

When someone decides they need to make another person pay for the wrong done to them, it's a clear sign of a deep-rooted problem called unforgiveness. There is nothing sweet about revenge. It just turns someone into a bitter, resentful, angry, grumpy person who can only see from one view, theirs! Sometimes, we're not even consciously aware we are trying to get even with the other person.

With that in mind, what do you think cold shoulders and the silent treatment are all about? Simple, isn't it? It all means the same thing. Unforgiveness! Unforgiveness is torment and you're the one being tortured. Do yourself a favour and let it go before it destroys you!

It's imperative to guard our hearts, by keeping a positive attitude at all times, and choosing forgiveness because by not doing so, we open the door to the sins of unforgiveness to develop in our hearts. Keeping this frame of mind and sticking with this decision is a conscious effort we must make in order to keep our hearts soft and open to love. For it is the pure in heart, that will see God. (Matthew 5:8)

We need to forgive to keep our hearts pure and clean. By forgiving we are doing ourselves a favour; getting mercy by giving it. When issues arise, we need to deal with them instead of stuffing them down because scientific studies show that issues that are not dealt with properly can cause illness later on in our bodies.[20]

A significant amount of time has passed since my particular struggle. You'll be pleased to know that I've been able to completely let it go and move on. Just last night, I had a very pleasant visit with my former friend at a school function; I can honestly say I'm at complete peace about everything that has happened. I wish her all the best. She is a lovely person and I know she never meant to hurt me!

The Lord has blessed me with understanding recently as to why a particular person kept their distance, during my walk with cancer. Although we were acquaintances that shared light conversation or a friendly hello, we were not close. She kept her distance because she didn't want to pry into my situation and appear nosey. Being the open book that I am, I never had that thought cross my mind. Things like that don't usually bother me. Then again, we're not all made from the same mold are we? Thank God for that! I don't know if the world could handle two of me!

However, in the past, she has had several delicate situations transpire in her life. With the first situation a particular person, appearing sincere, questioned her about very personal information and then in turn spread twisted facts across town causing great pain. Now, knowing her experience, I can clearly understand where she was coming from and why she treated me the way she did. What I perceived as being ignored was her way of giving me my space. It was out of respect! This proves that we should always give others the benefit of the doubt and choose to believe the best.

When people do certain things we think are unreasonable, there is usually a good explanation for the way they behave or react. We need to have compassion on others, even those by whom we feel mistreated, because only God knows each intricate detail in every situation. God sees and hears all and is the only One who knows the whole story. He and He alone is perfect and therefore has the only right to judge.

I wonder how many times people get their knickers in a knot, daily, over silly little things that would be more than alright, if they only knew the whole story! Are there situations that you are struggling with that would look different if viewed from another perspective? Perhaps we should try to keep an open mind!

Yes, sometimes the situation is more serious than someone just ignoring you. Maybe there is someone in your life who is not treating you or a loved one the best. Perhaps your child is being bullied at school by others who tear down his self-esteem, by yelling degrading remarks, teasing him over a poor grade, or by calling him stupid when he does something silly. This can be heart-wrenching as you watch your child suffer, especially if they begin to believe the insults being hurled at them. As a parent you want your child to be loved and accepted by all, and for others to see their qualities and strengths the way you see them, often wanting to spare them from the past hurts you've experienced and watch them enjoy life to its fullest.

You may have endured similar experiences as a child and know the damaging effects this can have on them. If so, you fear they'll close their heart off to the world of wisdom around them because they lack the confidence they need to try or succeed for fear of failure.

As a parent, you may be struggling with unforgiveness towards the other kids, or even the parents, involved. These people are likely hurting on the inside themselves and are lashing out at the closest available people because of the bottled–up anger or lack of self–esteem within themselves. Perhaps they feel the need to dominate others to gain power and control because they're lonely and afraid and haven't received the love and tenderness they needed. I find it helps, in situations like this, to ask God to help me see others through Jesus' eyes and love them the way He does, when others hurt or disappointed me. As I pray, my heart softens towards them and I can enjoy life in peace, while I sit back and marvel how God works in the situation and in these people's lives to bring about change.

God asks us to overcome evil with good by blessing those who curse us. By doing this, we open the door for God to work in their lives, rather than tying His hands to work on our behalf in the situation. He will bless you for your obedience.

Dear God,

Please reveal truth to me in my situations. Reveal the lies I believe and bring healing to those areas. Bind and remove all bitterness, anger and resentment from my heart and lose Your love, joy and peace and healing power into it. I pray in Jesus' name. Amen.

True Happiness!

Where does your happiness come from? True happiness can only come from within. Many people try to fill their lives with things to get a feeling of joy. Again, like comfort, this is only a temporary fix; one you'll continually have to feed to keep that happy high. Sooner or later when this need isn't being met by regular stuff, people turn to high ticket items or other addictions to attain their emotional high. This emotion can come at a greater cost that could eventually dig a deep hole of misery for yourself and your loved ones.

What's keeping you happy? Is it stuff, food, people, exercise, promotions or perhaps living your unmet dreams through the lives of your children? It's not my intention to make you angry but to provoke you to think! What makes you tick? What's going on deep down inside you? Getting in touch with your inner self could do you a world of good.

Are you wearing a mask to cover hidden sadness? In my small town, it is a common gesture to greet others with a "How are you?", when you're walking down the street. There are so many wonderful people where I live. Some genuinely want to know how you are but many will ask and continue on their way because they're asking out of a form of politeness. I am convinced that countless people say they are fine, regardless of how they are feeling. You can see it in their eyes and it's marked all over their faces. Do you say one thing but actually mean another?

Often people say they would be happy if their circumstances were different. There aren't too many people on the face of this earth that wouldn't change something, about themselves or their lives, given the chance but we only get one life to live, so we might as well learn to appreciate and enjoy it.

How about deciding to enjoy your life right here and now where you're at? I'm not telling you to settle for less but to enjoy each step on your journey. Remember the roses amongst the thorns. Sometimes our circumstances aren't necessarily the problem; it's our attitude toward the circumstances. Everything in life seems better when you look at it from a positive angle.

Everyone knows life isn't perfect! It doesn't take long to figure that one out. But our happiness doesn't have to depend on our circumstances. Seeing life from this angle can take tremendous strength. Being happy is a choice we make. You can enjoy your life and choose to be happy regardless of what is going on around you. It is actually a way you can gain control in a situation that you may feel you have little or no control in.

How is this possible? By not allowing your circumstances to rob you of your joy and by choosing to be happy no matter what comes your way! The answer is to draw your strength from the joy of the Lord (*Nehemiah 8:10*).

As a child, I had heard this Scripture used many times. We even sang songs about the joy of the Lord. It wasn't until this latest crisis in life that I finally realized what "the joy of the Lord" was all about. I should have recognized this unexplainable joy in action by watching my mother go through troubled times with a true smile on her face. People still comment about that even now. Yet, I was unaware. I was busy viewing life through a child's eyes. That is the key.

We could all learn from children. They take joy from every moment and it comes with such little effort. Give a child a menial task and they can turn it into a game. Not long ago, Carter was washing the back deck. He was having a whale of a time sliding and dancing with the mop, as if it were his date.

I love it when our boys break out with spontaneous fits of laughter. It brings a smile to my face even thinking about it. Spencer has this high pitched giggle that sends delight straight to my soul. Now I know why my dad said he always enjoyed lying in bed and listening to us laugh. It's nice. God created laughter, so why not loosen up and enjoy a good laugh.

We get far too stressed out about even the little things and take everything far more seriously that we should. God really is in control!

We are to look at the world with a child's perspective putting our total trust in our Heavenly Father, knowing that everything will work out because He is all we really need. The Lord wants to give you the oil of gladness instead of mourning, and a garment of praise instead of a spirit of despair. (Isaiah 61:3)

Look to Jesus and He will become your true source of joy. When you spend time in God's presence the weight that comes from this world will slide off your shoulders and you will be free to draw joy from the world He created for your pleasure.

Dear God,

Thank You for showing me I need to reframe each circumstance in my life with a godly perspective. With this new outlook, I pray that You would fill me with the joy of the Lord to give me the needed strength to endure whatever comes, with a thankful heart. In Jesus' name I pray. Amen.

---

[1] Canadian Medical Association. *Questions and answers on breast cancer: A guide for women and their physicians.* 2nd edition. (Ottawa, Canada: Health Canada, 2001). Strong, Amanda. Clemons, Dr. Mark. "The bone/breast Connection. What you need to know about managing bone health." in stride, Fall issue 2005, pp. 4.

[2] Joyce Meyer, "*Healing Scriptures*", Joyce Meyer Ministries, 1999, pp. 1-2.

[3] Leaf, Dr. Carolyn. *Who Switched of My Brain? Controlling toxic thoughts and emotions.* (South Africa: Switch On Your Brain, 2007).

[4] Ibid.

[5] Colbert, Don, MD. *The Seven Pillars of Health* (Lake Mary, Florida: Siloam, 2007).

[6] Ibid.

[7] Moore, Beth. Wednesdays with Beth; God of All Comforts Volume #6 (Fort Worth, Texas: Life Today Outreach International, 2008).

[8] Morris, Robert. *The Power of Your Words* (Ventura, California, USA: Regal Books, Gospel Light, 2006).

[9] Ibid.

[10] Ibid.

[11] Ibid.

[12] Copeland, Gloria. *The Unbeatable Spirit of Faith* (Tulsa, Oklahoma: Harrison House, Inc., 1995, Reprint 2001).

[13] Meyers, Joyce. "Healing And Wholeness" *Enjoying Everyday Life, Joyce Meyer Ministries Magazine*, March 2007, pp. 4.

[14] Ibid.

[15] Meyer, Joyce. *The Word, The Name, The Blood* (Fenton, Missouri: Warner Books, 1995).

[16] Nelson. *Canadian Dictionary* (Scarborough, ON: ITP Nelson. A Division of Thomson Canada, Ltd.), p. 1149.

[17] Meyer, Joyce. *The Word, The Name, The Blood* (Fenton, Missouri: Warner Books, 1995).

[18] Virkler, Mark & Patti. *Hear God Through Your Dreams* (Elma, N.Y: Communion With God Ministries, www.cwgministries.org, 1985, Revised 2000, 2003).

[19] Ibid.

[20] Leaf, Dr. Carolyn. *Who Switched of My Brain? Controlling toxic thoughts and emotions.* (South Africa: Switch On Your Brain, 2007).

Chapter Four
Herceptin

In his heart a man plans his course,
but the Lord determines his steps.

Proverbs 16:9

C hemo ended early September 2006. I started my initial Herceptin treatment three weeks later, in keeping with the regular schedule of chemo. I was able to receive these monoclonal antibody treatments at our local hospital. This saved quite a lot of money on gas, parking and meals, as it doesn't take long to add up! We incurred over $6,000.00 in added costs on these items alone.

Initially, I didn't want to burden my family financially if the treatment wasn't covered by insurance. Now I am able to see the whole picture from an entirely different view because of the spiritual growth that I experienced. Truthfully, I can now see that my death would have caused them far more pain than what a bit of debt would cause. Emotional pain and the dysfunction from the lack of a parent far outweigh the cost.

I still needed to be careful about being around people that were sick, which was hard for some to understand. Herceptin also shares a few common characteristics with chemotherapy, one side effect being that it knocks out the white blood cells that help the body fight infection and disease, putting the patient at a greater risk of infection.[1]

While waiting for the pharmacist to mix the dose of medication, the nurse always weighed me, asked a series of questions and took my blood pressure. The treatments were also given by IV (in my port-a-cath), which required one and a half hours to administer. I was then kept for an additional half hour for observation, to ensure that I didn't have an anaphylactic reaction. I was completely familiar with this condition because our oldest son Ben was diagnosed with an anaphylactic allergy to peanuts, milk and eggs. At a young age, he experienced numerous anaphylactic reactions, a few mild ones along with several frightening episodes, so I was a little nervous!

Anaphylaxis is a condition in which the body reacts to something harmless, as if it were harmful. The immune system sees the food or drug, etc., as a threat and goes into defence mode by shutting the body down into anaphylactic shock. It can be very dangerous if not treated immediately because the person can go into a coma or die. The first signs could be as simple as hives, swollen or itchy lips, mouth, face, eyes or tongue, tightness in mouth, chest or throat with difficulty breathing or swallowing. They may experience drooling, wheezing, choking, coughing, runny nose, voice change, vomiting, nausea, diarrhea, dizziness, rapid heartbeat, chills or loss of consciousness.

With Herceptin, many patients experience flu-like symptoms for several days after treatment. I was very fortunate and only suffered with arthritic cramping for several days, which transpired in my hips and down my thighs. It usually seemed to lessen and would occasionally dissipate with a short walk. Herceptin can also cause heart damage, so they kept a close eye on me with periodic gated cardiac scans.

After three doses of Herceptin, my oncologist cancelled the treatment because it had damaged my heart. It now pumped 10 percent less blood than before. The baseline, called the ejection fraction, began at 65 and had fallen to a mere 45, leaving me breathless and weary. She was concerned about the longevity of my life and health. She wanted to see me survive cancer and yet didn't want to damage my heart to the point that I couldn't do anything or worse, have me die due to heart disease or damage.

My oncologist booked a referral appointment with a heart specialist immediately. She was hoping my heart, over time, would repair itself and perhaps I would be able to resume treatments before my window of time was up. Studies indicate that Herceptin is effective while allotted in combination with chemo, or within 12 months after the chemo treatment has been completed.

I was distraught and sobbed periodically for several days following my appointment. The enemy tried to rip every ounce of faith from me. I began reasoning, trying to figure out why God would allow this. Then I realized, God wants what's best for me, this is not from God! The devil was scheming to plant a lie in my mind. Many times, people will try to reason and figure out what God is doing. Here's a great piece of advice: relax and trust God, it's not our job to figure everything out. You'll save yourself a lot of stress if you just rest in Him and be obedient to what He tells you.

I finally was able to get my head on straight and put my faith back in the right place. In God! I knew that God could use even this for His purpose. I surrounded myself with strong Christian friends to increase my faith, and decided to trust God by taking Him at His Word. I now believed God was going to heal me, regardless of how the situation looked!

I no longer had this miracle cure to rely on and had to put my complete faith in God for healing alone! He would now get the glory He rightfully deserved. I immediately received prayer at church for my heart and noticed a notable change in my energy level.

How many times has life taken an unexpected curve? You don't have to end up in the ditch, choose to trust God instead!

"Every valley shall be raised up, every mountain and hill made low; the rough ground shall become level, the rugged places a plain." (Isaiah 40:4)

Dear Heavenly Father,

As this life brings unexpected turns, help my new friend to trust You with each challenge they face. Bless them with the overwhelming peace and joy that only You can give. In Jesus' name I pray, Amen.

Resource: Herceptin information provided by the Ottawa Cancer Clinic: File #: 3–1–1–8–English MIS, for current medical information: www.cancercare.on.ca

Chapter Five
Radiation

Christ redeemed us from the curse of the law
by becoming a curse for us.

Galatians 3:13a

In the meantime, I started radiation. I attended an information session on radiation at the General Hospital. Basically, the nurse explained what to expect and things I should and shouldn't do. Doctors' opinions vary but mine only allowed a certain amount of vitamins E and C, concerned that high doses may interfere with the treatment.

The following week, I returned for a planning session. While lying down on the radiation bed, the radiation team worked together to line my body up with the machine using the precise degrees and angles calculated by the radiation oncologist. He mapped out a specific plan for my particular radiation needs. The radiation technicians tattooed four tiny black spots on different areas of my skin: middle of my sternum, stomach, bottom of rib cage on the right side and on my rib cage under my right arm, to use as an aid to quickly line the machine up to the areas needing radiation each day. The tattooing saves an incredible amount of time, enabling the team to provide more patients with the needed treatment. With all of this in place, I received 25 rounds of radiation, within a five–week duration.

Numerous radiation teams work together Monday through Friday during the day (unless an emergency), to administer treatment to all types of cancer patients. I drove myself into Ottawa (50 kilometres), for the majority of my appointments but as the end grew closer, I grew tired and concerned that I would get into an accident, so I accepted help when offered.

After approximately three weeks, the skin on my chest became red and itchy as a small rash began to develop. It later disappeared as the skin tone became dark and blotchy. The skin under my arm became almost charcoal black as the end of treatment approached. On the fourth week, my radial oncologist prescribed a special cream to administer to the area. The skin quickly peeled off in sheets, similar to what happens when you dip a tomato in boiling water and then run it under the cold water to skin it. The newly exposed flesh was red and jelly–like, resembling raw meat. With my skin in this condition, it became extremely uncomfortable to drive. The effects of the radiation continued to worsen even after the treatment had ceased, burning my skin and tissue as the radiation continued to cook! My energy level continued to decline. Two years later, it still hadn't returned to its original state. It wasn't until I started taking vitamin supplements that I noticed a huge improvement.

Two nights before I finished my last radiation treatment, I dreamt I was in the house where I grew up. As I walked into the kitchen, I noticed the current homeowner sitting at the table and a blood red porcelain bowl, streaked with black, sitting on the counter. The bowl was filled with beautiful, red delicious apples. In my spirit, I sensed it had something to do with Adam and Eve! A strong, yet gentle, masculine voice proclaimed, "The curse of sin and death has been broken."

The bowl cracked directly in half, symbolically signifying the curtain that was torn in The Holy Place when Jesus died on the cross, breaking the curse of sin and death for all who accept Him as Lord and Saviour. The apples rolled out of the bowl and I awoke immediately, knowing that healing was mine and I was going to survive! Several weeks later, the Lord confirmed this through Scripture during my prayer time.

Christ redeemed us from the curse of the law by becoming a curse for us, for it is written: *"Cursed is everyone who is hung on a tree."* He redeemed us in order that the blessing given to Abraham might come to the Gentiles through Christ Jesus, so that by faith we might receive the promise of the Spirit. (Galatians 3:13, 14)

As humans, we are sinful. There is no getting around that fact. It is impossible to obey the law perfectly. Therefore, because we cannot fulfill the law's demands 100 percent of the time, we fall under the curse when we rely on the law for salvation. Chapter 28, in the book of Deuteronomy, explains the different consequences for disobedience. Sickness, disease and poverty are a huge part of the curse but worst of all is eternal damnation! That is why Jesus died on the cross to redeem us from the curse by becoming cursed for us. When we accept Him into our lives, we can walk in freedom and blessing!

The Merriam–Webster Dictionary defines redeemed as a ransom by paying a price, to free from the consequences of sin.[1] The wages of sin is death but Jesus paid the price by dying for our sins, once and for all. (Romans 6:23) We are children of Abraham through faith, in Christ Jesus, according to Galatians 3:29, and heirs according to the promise. God made a covenant blessing with Abraham. We have right to claim that covenant for ourselves as believers. The promise of blessing is to prosper us in all areas of our lives including good health, financial prosperity, well-being for our family and salvation for our souls (Deuteronomy 7:12–15).[2] In Chapter 12, we will take a more in depth look at what we need to do to receive the blessings of the covenant. It's up to us! Many people are sick because they don't know what the Word promises them! They're not certain of God's will for their lives.

I recall the day I scanned my appointment card into the computer and decided to sit down on the north side of the waiting room, totally opposite from where I normally sat. While waiting for my radiation treatment, I noticed an elderly gentleman in a wheelchair being pushed down the hall, towards the department, his frail face concealed with an oxygen mask.

I felt the Lord speak to me saying: "He is going to come and sit beside you and I want you to pray for his healing."

This particular waiting room was a fair size with 35 to 40 chairs in total and only half were taken. Sure enough, he landed right beside me. *Oh boy*, I thought! I didn't want people thinking I was out of my tree! Placing the magazine over my mouth, I began praying quietly to myself that God would heal and strengthen him and improve his breathing. After the gentleman left to receive his treatment God spoke clearly to my heart saying, "I didn't mean pray for him, I meant pray with him!" I knew that! I purposely rationalized my way out of being obedient. I am an outgoing person but laying hands on a complete stranger out of a church setting was out of my comfort zone! Conviction rose up within me and I asked God for forgiveness and prayed that He would give me another chance.

Two weeks later, I saw the same elderly man from across the waiting room. He sat with a beautiful woman in her eighties, his breathing still laboured. I asked God to give me the strength needed to approach the couple. My body catapulted out of my chair, my legs carrying me halfway across the room to where they were sitting, before my mind could make sense of what I was doing. As I began to explain to the elderly gentleman what was on my heart, he was called in for treatment. Even though he had to leave right away, I was able to visit and pray with his wife. She was a woman of faith, her husband was not. She very much appreciated and needed the encouragement and prayer.

He was suffering from lung cancer and needed constant oxygen to breath. Radiation acts by burning the cancer cells out of the lungs; healthy cells are able to repair themselves but radiated cancer cells are not!

Several weeks later, I saw the same elderly man from a distance, shuffling his feet along using a walker rather than riding in a wheel chair. In reality, he should have been even weaker than before. A few weeks later, I again saw this man without any oxygen at all. Praise God! I never had the chance to speak with him again. That didn't matter! I could see that God was faithful in answering my prayers. He has entrusted me with a gift that I need to use and as long as I am alive, I will share it!

---

[1] Editors of Merriam. *Webster, Merriam-Webster Dictionary* (Springfield, Massachusetts, USA: Merriam-Webster Incorporated, 1997), p. 616.

[2] Snell, Jay. *How To Claim The Abrahamic Covenant* (Livingston, TX: Jay Snell Evangelistic Association), p. 5.

Chapter Six
Why Me?

When I pray, you answer me,
and encourage me by giving me the strength I need.

Psalm 138:3 (NLT)

I underwent an additional scan in December to check the ejection fraction of my heart. The results were forwarded directly to my oncologist and heart specialist. Although the tests confirmed the healing of my heart, I was still sent to the heart specialist for a referral appointment. Kelly, one of my best friends from high school, accompanied me. I had a pinched nerve in my back and could barely walk. We giggled like schoolgirls as we slowly walked up the sidewalk, arm in arm, resembling two little old ladies, stopping periodically to get the kinks out of my hunched back as it went into spasm. We must have looked so silly!

The specialist had his nurse perform an echocardiogram upon my arrival, which validated the earlier results—my heart was healthy!

"Why are you here?" the doctor questioned.

After explaining my medical and family heart history, he reviewed the test information sent to his office and advised me to be extremely careful about taking any more treatments that damage the heart. Otherwise, he felt everything looked good!

I returned to my oncologist in March. She strongly advised me to go back on Herceptin because of the aggressive nature and type of breast cancer, with which I had been diagnosed, as well as the survival and reoccurrence statistics without this treatment. Oh, what a decision to make! I felt I was healed and didn't need this medication, nor did I want to subject my heart to any damage. I was under a considerable amount of pressure from certain family members to resume treatment. The more I thought about it, the more confused I became.

As they conversed with me, my faith weakened. I knew my healing weighed heavily upon my faith, as stated in Matthew 12:24. A feeling of doom flooded my soul, dwindling any faith I possessed. I had confidence that I would experience complete healing in the end because of what God showed me. I was reminded that sometimes visions and dreams manifest themselves right away and other times it can be years before they transpire.

I had one week to make this life or death decision. Feeling the pressure, I began to panic, doubting my own ability to hear from God. I sought out those in different healing ministries to provide the answer I needed from God. Using great wisdom, they prayed in agreement with me and asked God to provide me with the wisdom needed for the decision at hand (see James 1:5). Clarity resumed as I prayed to God about what direction to take. I now realized the importance of hearing from God myself. Many people have good intentions and advice, but the point of view I needed was from the One who knows all, from beginning to end!

How to Hear from God

"Ask and it will be given to you; seek and you will find; knock and the door will be opened to you. For everyone who asks receives; he who seeks finds; and to him who knocks, the door will be opened." (Matthew 7:7, 8)

The first thing we need to do is ask. The Bible tells us we have not because we ask not. (James 4:2) God wants to bless us but first we must humble ourselves and ask. To hear from God we need to be listening and looking for His direction. Many times, He's trying to get our attention yet we are not recognizing the signs and wisdom He is sending our way. We've become so caught up in the business of life that we're not focused on what's going on around us. If we would still our hearts, turn off the distractions and tune into the peace and quiet, we would be able to feel His presence and recognize the answers when they come. If you would eliminate a fraction of the constant noise around you, for a few moments each day, it would help tremendously. You may even decide you enjoy the quiet.

"Be still and know that I am God." (Psalm 46:10a)

Sit in a quiet place with no distractions and clear your mind of everything. Some people find this difficult at first. It helps to keep a paper and pen handy to jot down any pressing matters that may come to mind to do later. This keeps you focused and acts as a reminder. This will enable you to relax. Don't get frustrated or overwhelmed; this is a discipline and skill that comes with practice.

Focus your mind on God. Thank Him for the blessings in your life. You may be going through a very difficult time right now. Try to think of something positive, even if the only thing you can think of is the beauty of creation. Thank Him for the birds, grass and the magnificent sky, that in itself is an awesome gift. As you Praise God for the good, as well as the bad, God will turn it around. Praise will open the door to God's presence.

Ask God for the solutions in life you want to know. "If any of you lacks wisdom, he should ask God, who gives generously to all without finding fault, and it will be given to him." (James 1:5) Seek God for the answers you need within your situations and circumstances. It doesn't matter what kind of trouble you are experiencing, God cares and wants you to come to Him.

"Be still before the Lord and wait patiently for him." (Psalm 37:7a)

When you've finished praying what's on your heart, sit quietly in God's presence and wait for His reply. This is where patience comes into practice. Solutions will come to you that you may not have even considered. You may be wondering, "How do I know if it is God speaking to me?" After the resurrection of Christ, God promised to send His Holy Spirit here on earth to counsel us (John 14:26). In John 10:26 it says, "My sheep listen to my voice, I know them, and they follow me." God will not tell you anything that does not line up with the Bible. As you learn His Word you'll learn to recognize His voice. As God speaks to you, you will be filled with an amazing peace. It's like a calm stillness that accompanies an assurance within your heart.

If you have questions or doubts popping up in your mind like "I wonder....?" those thoughts are not from God! God leads you in the way of peace (1 Corinthians 14:33). God is not the author of confusion, Satan is!

One of the ways God speaks to us is through His Word. The Bible is living and active, it may be an ancient book but it is still relevant to our everyday lives. When you read the Bible, God will speak to your spirit giving you a deep desire to do certain things. You may even have a Scripture almost jump off the page at you; it speaks to your heart and gives you a strong sense that it's meant for you. A gut feeling you can't explain! When this happens, you may find underlining it or writing it down helpful. This is also a good time to meditate on that particular Scripture and memorize it. Later if you attend church or watch a service on television, the pastor, preacher or evangelist may use that exact same Scripture reference or the message you felt the Lord trying to speak to you.

You may pick up a magazine or a book and stumble upon the same topic with the wisdom you have been seeking. God has perfect timing, the answer doesn't always come immediately, so be patient! I've been told that when I don't feel like I'm getting an answer, it often indicates that I'm to continue to do as I have been doing.

God speaks to us through our circumstances. One example from my own life was when I believed my oldest sister was more favoured by my father than I was. For years it seemed to be all he talked about whenever I visited or called. I felt hurt and frustrated. It seemed I could have stood on my head and spit nickels and he wouldn't have noticed. Then after going through some difficulties with our oldest son being bullied at school, I myself became totally consumed with his welfare. This is where I felt God speaking to me. My sister had been through several years of great suffering. My Dad, concerned for her welfare, stayed focused on her. The lie that I was not valued came through a wound and I allowed it to become truth in the situation. Many times when we become offended it is through misunderstandings. By not seeing the complete picture, we carry biased opinions and lay blame on others, formed by inaccurate judgments. When we can consider the situation from additional angles, it can be seen clearly. I realized that I was wrong concerning my father, and was reacting out of my own insecurities. I love each one of my children equally, even when they make mistakes. I have one child that has been more of a challenge at times; nevertheless, he has blessed me in amazing ways. God has used him in a very necessary way to sand off my rough edges. Each one fills my heart with overwhelming love and joy.

Other times, the Lord sends people your way that have experienced similar challenges to help guide and direct you onto the right path. I believe there is no such thing as a coincidence.

When I stopped looking to others for the answer to my question and asked God, He placed Nancy Thrasher into my path, a woman healed of an incurable condition! Nancy had suffered from daily Grand-mal epileptic seizures for 17 years. Without me revealing any information concerning my situation, she began to tell me of her healing experience that took place 10 years ago.

Nancy went forward for prayer one Sunday night at church to receive prayer for healing. As the pastor lightly laid hands on her to pray, she felt a surge of power (the power of God) hit her entire body with great force throwing her back three to four feet from where she was standing. In midair, she panicked, wondering who was going to catch her. Her body hit the floor and slid directly underneath the front pew without incurring any rug burn or injury in any way. As she lay on the soft carpet, a brilliant bright light, whiter than any white she had ever seen, surrounded her. She saw something in the spirit (vision) that looked like God's hand holding a sterling silver surgical instrument with two fingers. As He cut a portion out of her brain, she felt a dark force leave her body and flee from the church, with a psss... sound.

She had only been a believer for approximately six or seven weeks and became concerned that she had made a spectacle of herself. Afraid the people would throw her out of the church, she quietly sat up pulling her legs tightly into the fetal position. A woman from the church quietly walked over and gently rubbed her back, without saying a word.

The minister spoke, "Remember it wasn't me that healed you, but God."

She sat quietly thinking to herself, *I must really be special that God would do this for me.* Upon returning home, her daughter immediately asked what had happened to her. She looked different! Her face held an aura of glory and appeared almost in a trance! Even though she knew something significant had happened, she continued her medication for six months, until she felt the Lord specifically tell her "Your faith has made you well, go to the doctor and tell him you think God has healed you."

Under the doctor's supervision, some neurological tests were performed and confirmed her healing. Her doctor then weaned her off the medication and she has retained her healing, showing no trace of epilepsy. Nancy advised me that it is very wise to take the doctor's advice and to always be sensitive to what the Lord is saying to us.

In the summer of 2006, I made a new friend who was huge into the faith movement and like myself, loves Jesus. God used her tremendously in my life to help strengthen my faith and pull me up when darkness tried to grip me. She also believed and insisted that after someone receives prayer once they should step out in faith and stop all treatment and not bother going to the doctor. *Word of caution, we need to use wisdom and only stop when tests prove we are healed!* Going to regular check-ups doesn't mean you lack faith, it shows responsibility! I am not knocking faith! We need it! It's important to have faith because faith pleases God, and anything that is not based on faith is sin (Hebrews 11:6; Romans 14:23). Remember, God has a unique plan and path for each one of us. We need to hear directly from God ourselves about our situation and act in faith on what He shows us rather than on what others think our direction should be.

Be careful not to take Scripture out of its context. Many people will take bits and pieces from Scripture and mold it trying to make it fit their circumstance, rather than asking God what His will is for their situation. The Bible says we should seek godly counsel when we need guidance. Just because the person is godly doesn't mean it's the counsel God has FOR YOU! Pray about it, He will show you and peace will guide you. I do believe that God gives us medical technology to help heal us. There is nothing wrong with using doctors in conjunction with faith. Faith is very important! We need to put our faith in God and trust that He will heal us, whether it's through medical treatment or divine healing, depending on the path along which He is leading you. God is all-powerful and is well able to perform miracles without treatment.

The miracle Dodie Osteen experienced comes to mind. Dodie was diagnosed with liver cancer and was given only two weeks to live. She confessed the healing Scriptures from the Word of God over herself day and night. She never complained about being sick or feeling tired and guarded her mouth from speaking negatively over her situation. She carried on with life, helping those in need around her and refused to behave like someone who was sick. Dodie gradually began to feel stronger day by day. Years later, doctors performed tests for other reasons, which confirmed her healing. There are other countless documented stories to prove that miracles do happen.[1]

At times, God chooses other avenues for us and it is important to understand what the Lord is calling us to do in our situation. Some are blessed with instant miracles, while others are called to walk through circumstances, receiving their miracle in the end. In some cases someone's miracle may be to receive the grace to walk through the adversity at hand, moment by moment. This can be a place of learning and growth if embraced. Sometimes these circumstances can be used to help and encourage others through their difficult experiences by being able to offer compassion and a listening ear with someone who can relate.

This painful journey has seemed endless at times, but in reality it's a small sacrifice in the long run. Our lives are but a whisper in the wind. When I've been tempted to complain, I remind myself that I have no right to. It's nothing like the suffering Jesus endured for us so that we could receive the free gift of salvation. He was mocked, ridiculed, rejected, beaten beyond recognition and nailed to a cross to suffer and die because for our sins. He loved us so much that He gave His very own life.

I often asked God why I had to go through this! This revelation came to me as I attended appointments in crowded waiting rooms with long waiting times. The people were always so pleasant and eager to visit. On many occasions, I've had the opportunity to share my testimony of the wonderful things God has done for me, which has filled others with hope and faith.

As I waited in the hallway for a post surgery appointment, a very pleasant, middle age woman asked me why I was there visiting the clinic. Apparently, we were both in the same predicament. I however, had great peace in my heart because of the initial dream and Scriptures God gave me. God blessed our family with a previous miracle that first revealed itself through a dream. I explained my initial encounter with dreams through the following story about Ben's healing of food allergies. Ben's doctor actually laughed at me when I asked him if he thought Ben would grow out of his peanut allergy. He informed me on three different occasions that all peanut and nut allergies are lifelong with an extremely rare chance of growing out of them. A peanut weighs a gram and it only takes one millionth of a gram to cause an anaphylactic reaction. To make matters worse, a peanut trace can stay on a surface for up to six months.

At age three, Ben had grown out of his milk allergy. We were told not to return for testing until age five because of the severity of the egg allergy. The doctor said he would probably be 11 years of age before he grew out of this, if at all. I wrestled with the thought of sending Ben to school but I felt in my heart that he needed the social stimulation.

One night, while Ben was in senior kindergarten, (age four, he's a November baby!) I dreamt he was eating pumpkin pie, which has cooked egg in it. When I awoke I told Rob about my dream, his immediate reaction was a certainty that Ben wasn't allergic to egg anymore.

I took Ben back to the specialist to be tested even though it was earlier than they had suggested we return and sure enough he had grown out of the *cooked* egg allergy. The raw egg still registered a minute amount, which meant we still needed to be careful about dips, salad dressings, mayo, meringue, and to be sure the egg yolk and white were thoroughly cooked, not runny, when served.

On March 5, 1999, I had another dream. This time a man with a crippled hand was preparing food for Ben out in the desert in a grass hut. I was panicking and asked him to please wash his hands before preparing the food and to be careful of the ingredients because of his peanut allergy.

"Do not fear for the Lord your God will heal your son of his allergy," the man replied.

That morning, my Bible reading came from Luke 6. It was the story of Jesus healing on the Sabbath day. The man Jesus healed had a shrivelled hand. That next day, I received a call from a friend saying, "This might sound strange to you but I had a dream about a man with a crippled hand and I feel like I'm suppose to tell you to read Luke 6." The hair still rises up on my body when I think about it. This confirmed what God had shown me in the dream and that it was His promise to me.

Ben had several different reactions over the years due to his allergy to peanuts, resulting in hives, swollen face and boils, projectile vomiting and diarrhea. On April 10, 2000, I received a call at work, from Ben's school to inform me that his throat had begun to close from eating an Easter egg off a friends decorated hat.

With tears streaming down my cheeks, I cried out to God, "I thought you said you would heal Ben of his allergy, why is this happening? Please protect him Lord!" Regardless of the situation, I chose right then and there to believe in my heart that Ben would be fine because of the dream God had given me and continued to hold onto God's promise.

He was rushed to the hospital, given three doses of medication, placed on oxygen and kept for observation by the doctor for several hours. At home we administered Benadryl to reduce other symptoms like watery red eyes and hives over the next few days. The Lord gave me the understanding that this reaction had to occur to remove all skepticism and to prove beyond a shadow of a doubt to others that Ben really was allergic. I wasn't just an over-reactive mother as some may have cared to believe.

In November 2000, (grade 1), the same calendar year, we headed back to the specialist for our yearly routine testing for Ben. We were feeling hopeful that there would be a change with his raw egg allergy. Ben tested negative to eggs and also showed no sign to his peanut allergy either. The specialist retested the peanut with a stronger solution of the protein and still no reaction occurred. The doctor was very pleased, but still needed to be extremely cautious. He sent Ben to a special lab in Ottawa for a special IgE. blood test for peanut allergy. The test returned negative. Our hearts flooded with joy. We were again asked to return in a month's time for retesting and if the result was still negative the doctor would do a food challenge!

On December 17, 2000, Ben had yet another skin test that produced a negative result. The specialist conducted a food challenge in which Ben was fed 10 peanuts over the course of two hours. The specialist had Ben blow in a special machine to register his breathing to ensure no reaction was occurring. At the end of this procedure, the specialist stated that he believed Ben was no longer allergic to peanuts. We were instructed to return home and feed him at least 10 peanuts each day, for a week. At the end of the week if no reaction occurred, than Ben wouldn't have to carry his Epi-pen, showing he was clearly free of any allergy. (An Epi-pen is a needle which is given during an anaphylactic reaction to re-open the air way and provides approximately 15 minutes to get to the hospital where additional medication can be given.)

Ben was and is totally healed. Carter who also had a mild walnut allergy was retested and is free as well. We are so thankful to God for His goodness. Miracles are real, and still happen today!

Just as I began sharing this experience, a beautiful young blonde lady came and joined us in the hall. Upon finishing, she began to apologize saying, "Sorry, I couldn't help but eavesdrop. I don't think my being here today is a coincidence! I have an 18 month old baby boy who is anaphylactic to sesame seeds and nuts. I have been just beside myself wondering what I should do." She was a school-teacher and was scared half-to-death about leaving him in daycare and was finding food preparation a challenge. We talked for quite awhile. I was able to provide her with the name of a good food allergy support group, as well as my phone number in case she had any questions!

These are only a few incidences that God used to show me the reason I needed to walk through this journey. It is a blessing to help others and it is a privilege to lead them to Jesus. He is the way, the truth, and the life. God should receive the glory He rightly deserves!

Sometimes in life we go through difficulties that prepare us for other stages in life. If I hadn't gone through the struggle with Ben's allergies, I wouldn't have known the healing Scriptures and the truth in God's Word to get me through my own health issues. This trial in life became a stepping-stone to victory for a greater purpose in life and in the process I am able to help others.

Let these challenges mold your character for the better. There are two ways to look at every situation in life. The right way, which is the positive, or the wrong way, which is the negative. The positive way points you in the direction to a joy filled, abundant life that leads to promotion, while the negative leads you to a path of misery and destruction. You get to choose. No one can do that for you.

God often uses these situations to refine us. Frequently, when people face life and death situations it causes them to take a good hard look at life and evaluate their priorities. They tend to sift out the unnecessary, meaningless things and take more time for others and themselves. It's amazing what hitting rock bottom will do. Many search for spiritual answers they once ignored and turn away from such things as independence, rebellion, pride and selfishness. Suffering causes us to turn away from sin (1 Peter 4:1).

Suddenly, material things don't matter like they once did. The only thing that goes with you to eternity is your soul. You can't drag your stuff along with you. I certainly would rather leave behind cherished memories with my family and friends than collect things that don't last. I would rather touch the hearts of the lonely and needy than to fill a fleshly desire that is forever hungry and never satisfied. I know that I am not perfect and I make mistakes, but my heart is moving in the right direction. I plan to continue to travel on this road, it's much more satisfying!

A little tired and wanting a change in scenery, I took Spencer to the Early Years Center to play. It's a lot like an organized play-group that is funded by the government. It provides parents with resources and acts as a preschool setting where children can interact and moms can visit if they so choose. As I sat quietly enjoying a cup of herbal tea, I listen to two of my friends complain about their weight, and how they were having a hard time staying out of their children's snacks. Oh, I wanted to scream! Wake up and smell the coffee! Both of these girls look great! Neither of them was overweight. There I was, just diagnosed with cancer, recuperating from numerous surgeries and waiting to start chemo and I had to sit there listening to a conversation about how they wished they had a magic pill to fix their cravings. We all have a magic pill, it's called self–control. We need to stop making excuses and act on it. We have a choice!

We need to think about what is really important! The part that upset me so much is that there are some people who do really struggle with their weight. It's a matter of life and death because their weight is a health hazard. I don't take this lightly. I'm concerned because many times this problem stems from painful emotional issues that need to be addressed. Let's think about what is really important and let go of the meaningless things. Let's stop worrying about broken fingernails and big noses and start repairing relationships, mending broken hearts, helping the hurting and the needy. That's what's important! That's the heart of God!

When bad things happen we often think that God is punishing us for something we've done wrong. God does correct His children because He loves us, but not by making us sick (1 Corinthians 11:32; Proverbs 3:12; Hebrews 12:6, 10). God's plans are to always prosper us, not to harm us; to give us hope and a future (Jeremiah 29:11). It is Satan who plans for your destruction.

This does not mean that every time something negative happens it's because we're being corrected. God is a God of love and He does not treat us according to what our sins deserve (Psalm 103:10). We live in a fallen world with the enemy on the loose.

In John 16:33 Jesus said, *"I have told you these things, so that in me you may have peace. In this world you will have trouble. But take heart! I have overcome the world."* God doesn't promise us that when we follow Him we will not have difficulties in this life. Yet, He does promise that He will bring us through victoriously (see 2 Corinthians 2:14a). He always has the answer to our problems.

You may be thinking, well if God loves me so much, then why have all these bad things happened in my life? In the beginning, God made the heavens and the earth. Along with the heavens, He made heavenly beings called angels. He set apart the most beautiful angel, named Lucifer, and put him in a special position of authority. If you recall, Lucifer became proud and jealous in his heart and had to be removed from heaven by God with a tenth of the angels who were his followers. He no longer had authority or strength. God then gave man authority and dominion over all the earth. Lucifer, now called Satan, devised a plan to get his authority back. Imagine for a moment, back to the beautiful Garden of Eden, that we previously talked about in Chapter 2. The Garden was filled with amazing fruit trees that bore every kind of fruit imaginable. Adam and Eve were allowed to eat of every tree, except from the forbidden tree in the centre of the Garden. Satan devised a plan to use doubt and temptation to deceive Adam and Eve to gain back authority by causing man to sin.

"Now the serpent was more crafty than any of the wild animals the Lord God had made. He said to the women, "Did God really say, 'You must not eat fruit from the tree that is in the middle of the garden'?" The woman said to the serpent, "We may eat fruit from the trees in the garden, but God did say, 'You must not eat fruit from the tree that is in the middle of the garden, and you must not touch it, or you will die." (Gen. 3:1, 2)

Satan convinced Eve that they would gain knowledge if they ate of the forbidden tree (Genesis 3:4–6). When they saw the fruit looked good to eat and believed they would become wise like God, Adam and Eve gave in to temptation and ate the forbidden fruit. By doing so, they handed the authority back to Satan through their sin. God created us for His pleasure, so we would have a relationship with Him. He wanted each of us to have our own free will; He did not want to own a bunch of puppets. Although God gives us this choice, it's His desire for us to submit and follow Him. When Adam and Eve sinned, they were removed from the Garden of Eden. As a result of sin, the land became cursed with thorns making it more difficult for men to work the earth, and women's pain increased during childbirth. God told them not to eat of the fruit for their protection and benefit. It is the bad choices of man that affect our lives and the lives of others. God is very aware of the choices we'll make and is able to override them because of His sovereignty, yet He chooses to work with us according to our choices!

God in His goodness put His next plan in action. This time He sent Jesus, His only Son, to earth to destroy the work of the devil and return the blessing back to us through the blood covenant of Jesus. When we make Jesus the Lord of our lives by submitting our body, mind and spirit to Him, we take our God given authority back from the devil. Temptation no longer has the same hold when we submit to God (see James 4:7, 8a). He is available to help us through these times when we reach out to Him.

Jesus said there would be tribulation in the world, but to cheer up because He has already overcome the world. Jesus said, in John 10:10, *"The thief comes only to steal and kill and destroy; I have come that they may have life, and have it to the full."* God wants us to live and enjoy our lives. What Satan (the thief) means for harm, God will use for good! He is our Redeemer!

In Genesis, we read an account of the story of Joseph where many unfortunate events happened to him. Joseph was the youngest of 11 brothers and was especially loved by his father, Jacob. His father showed him this love and favour by making him a beautiful coat of many colors. His brothers were extremely jealous and became very angry with Joseph after he told them about the dreams God gave him. In one, his sheath of wheat stood tall while his brothers' sheaths bowed down to his. In the second dream, the sun, moon and 11 stars bowed down to him (this represented his family). In their anger, they threw him into a pit and then sold him to some Midianite traders who were passing by.

The traders took him to Egypt where he was sold as a slave to Potiphar, an officer of Pharaoh the king. Potiphar recognized the Lord's favour on Joseph. He placed Joseph in authority over all his possessions, everything within his household and fields, except his wife. Potiphar's wife was attracted to Joseph, as he was very handsome. She tried to seduce him daily but he always refused.

One day, when no one else was in the house she snatched his robe and cried rape because yet again he refused to sleep with her. He was wrongfully thrown in jail for a crime he didn't commit. The Lord showed Joseph mercy by granting him favour with the prison guard. The guard put Joseph in a position of authority in the prison and again, whatever Joseph did, he prospered.

During this time, the butler and baker offended the king and were thrown into prison. While there, each had a dream and became distraught because they were unable to interpret them. God enabled Joseph to interpret these dreams and Joseph asked the butler to remember him to Pharaoh after he regained his position in the kingdom. Joseph was forgotten until two years later when Pharaoh had his own dreams that no one in his kingdom could interpret. God gave Joseph direction through his own dreams and told Pharaoh about the years of plenty and the years of lack and famine the country would have. Because of his wisdom, the king placed Joseph second-in-command over the entire kingdom. Through this, Joseph saved the lives of many people including his own family, the very ones who sold him and said he was dead!

Everything the enemy sent Joseph's way to bring harm, God used to prosper him. The trials of opposition trained and equipped him for promotion.[2] Joseph kept a good attitude and continually stayed in relationship with God.[3] God always promises to bring about good in every situation for those who love Him (Romans 8:28). Like Joseph, God's plans are always to bring about blessing in our lives. If you are still struggling with this issue, please read ahead to God's will to heal. It will provide you with a solid foundation on this truth.

"In this you greatly rejoice, though now for a little while you may have had to suffer grief in all kinds of trials. These have come so that your faith—of greater worth than gold, which perishes even though refined by fire—may be proved genuine and may result in praise, glory and honour when Jesus Christ is revealed." (1 Peter 1: 6, 7)

It shouldn't be a great surprise when trials come; they are inevitable. God only allows what we can handle in our lives to purify our hearts, attitudes and motives, test our faith and to draw us into a closer walk with Him.

Are you prospering spiritually? That is what really matters! Jesus asked this question in Mark 8:36, *"What good is it for a man to gain the whole world, yet forfeit his soul?"* Many people are filled with frustration and loneliness as they spend years searching for happiness in all the wrong places. People spend time climbing corporate ladders only to discover, when reaching the top, that they are unfulfilled; the empty void within them remains as they still find themselves unhappy and full of regret.

If you follow God, you will be filled with unexplainable love, joy and peace. There is no need to strive in your own ability or chase riches because as you pursue God and His righteousness, success and all God's blessings will fall into place (see Matthew 6:33).

Back to My Story

I felt God directing me to resume the Herceptin treatments. My medical oncologist hoped to tack on the three missed treatments, due to heart damage, to the end of the allotted time, on condition that my heart stayed strong. Herceptin was administered every three weeks as before, while my doctor continued to keep a close eye on my heart. After six doses of Herceptin therapy, my doctor decided to discontinue the treatment, this time for good! The ejection fraction of my heart had greatly decreased (down to 45) and my doctor wasn't willing to risk the health of my heart any longer. Feeling exhausted had become normal, so I hardly noticed the symptoms of heart damage except when I became out of breath from climbing stairs or was gasping for air while having a conversation. Blacking out became a regular occurrence and the boys were aware that when I stared lethargically into space or started blindly grabbing hold of things within my reach, they need not panic. I was trying to brace myself to refrain from passing out because I had gotten up too quickly. I learned to press past these symptoms and continue with everyday tasks.

I had a confidence within me that this time, I was healed from cancer! The Lord gave me a dream in which I boarded a long, yellow school bus (symbolizing a long journey). I stood at the front talking with one of my former school teachers, who had suffered with breast cancer as well. I gave her my prettiest pink hat with the sweet rose bud on the front that I wore during chemo, and told her that I wasn't going to have to wear it again!

More Dreams

On December 5, I had a vision in the night that I sat up in bed to look into a mirror and saw the Glory of God on my face. God is so... Holy! Terrified, I bolted straight up into a sitting position and clutched the blankets, stirring Rob from his deep sleep. He quickly dozed off again after I assured him that everything was okay. I then fell asleep and dreamt of a baby girl wrapped in white linen lying in a wooden cradle on the left side of my bed. I sat up, touched her and then lay back down to rest! I sensed God telling me that He was giving me a new beginning and to rest in Him, knowing He was taking care of me. It was important to continue to walk in obedience to the wisdom He had given me. God confirmed this numerous times over the next month through Scripture! (See Isaiah 43:19a; 1 Peter 1:3–5; 2 Corinthians 3:18.)

When we allow the negative elements in our lives to work for us rather than against us and cooperate with God by giving Him the authority to operate in our circumstances, He removes the junk that corrupts our souls, and He refines and purifies our hearts. Our character begins to take the moulded resemblance of God's beauty as it emanates from our very being.

---

[1] Osteen, Dodie. *Healed of Cancer* (Houston, TX: Lakewood Church Publication, 2003).

[2] Bevere, John. *The Bait of Satan* (Lake Mary, Florida: Charisma House, A Strange Company, 2004).

[3] Ibid.

Chapter Seven
Fear

For God has not given us a spirit of fear,
but of power and of love and of a sound mind.

2 Timothy 1:7 (NKJV)

There is nothing more gripping than fear. It has the power to stop you in your tracks, freeze and overtake your body, mind and soul leaving you breathless, if you succumb to it. What is it that makes people do the strangest things? Have you ever thought of fear as a spirit? (Job 4:12–16) The spirit world is very real; one that many choose to ignore. The thought of demons is rather scary to them, but that does not change the fact that they exist. When Jesus walked the earth, He delivered people from evil spirits many times during His ministry. In the passage below, you will see that sickness and fear are a direct result of oppression from the devil.

"When evening came, they brought to Him many who were under the power of demons, and He drove out the spirits with a word and restored to health all who were sick." (Matthew 8:16; Amplified)

Again, we see this truth revealed in Mark 5, when Jesus traveled across the lake by boat, to the region of the Gerasenes. He was met at the shore by a man who was possessed by evil spirits. This man lived in the tombs and would scream and cut himself with stones. The people were unable to restrain him because of his great strength; even chains couldn't hold him. When this man saw Jesus, he ran to Him, threw himself at His feet, cried out to Him and asked Jesus what He was going to do with him. Jesus then commanded the evil spirit to come out of the man. The spirits recognized Jesus as the Son of the Most High God and pleaded with Him not to torture or send them away from that place. Jesus addressed the evil spirits, who referred to themselves as "Legion" because there were many of them, and not the man. They pleaded for Jesus to cast them out into a large herd of pigs that were grazing nearby. After Jesus gave them permission, the demons went into the pigs. They rushed down a steep bank and drowned in the lake. Those who witnessed this event ran to tell others within the town and countryside. Curious and wanting proof, the people flocked to see the man themselves. When they arrived, the people saw him sitting with Jesus, completely dressed and with a sound mind. The man later returned home to live with his family and share about the amazing things the Lord had done.

Another example of sickness relating to oppression from the enemy is shown in Matthew 15:21–28. A Canaanite woman came to Jesus crying out in desperation for her daughter that had an evil spirit tormenting her. Because of the mother's act of faith, Jesus told her that her request was granted and that her daughter was healed.

One Saturday evening, an elderly gentleman came to preach at a local church for a healing service. After sharing from the Bible, he invited those needing prayer to come to the altar. He walked directly in front of me, looked straight into my eyes and said, "The cancer is gone, but you have a spirit of fear that is tormenting you." He placed his hand on my head and with authority he said, "I bind the spirit of fear and command you to come out of her, in the name of Jesus." Cold chills ran up my spine and out the top of my head. I know it sounds odd, but it's true. The fear that tormented me was now gone. Moments later, joy burst within me like an explosion of bubbles. I left the service with the assurance I was healed and with a giggly disposition for the night.

My radial oncologist has such a heart of compassion for his patients! On the last day of my radiation treatment, he thoroughly examined me and commented on how pleased he was to see that I was adjusting well emotionally. He warned me that when cancer patients have finished with all their treatments, a great number are often filled with a sense of hopelessness. This is because they are no longer taking an active role in battling the nasty disease. Many experience depression and fear. The strong support that once surrounded them like an iron wall has diminished to a mere trace, leaving a crumbled foundation where the fortress once stood. They're left to quietly cope on their own. They feel burdened and believe they are expected to carry on with life, like nothing ever happened. They're left to process the remainder of the mass confusion that the whirlwind of cancer left behind. They are often tired, bewildered and overwhelmed with what has happened. Initially, they are often much stronger during treatment than their loved ones around them, who have been blind-sided with the news. The minds of the loved ones are filled with fearful thoughts of losing their loved one, while the patient's mind is fixed in "survival mode." I remember saying to Rob one day, that in spite of the circumstances, what we were going through wasn't that hard! He looked at me in astonishment and replied, "What do you mean? This sucks big time!" In my mind everything was kosher; God had given me amazing strength, He was meeting all of our needs, the kids, for the most part, seemed to be coping very well and in my mind I thought everything was great!

Making a Choice

Approximately one month after treatment had ended, the numbing blow from shock started to dissipate. The reality of what had happened finally set in. My mind began to process the information and I was forced to deal with my suppressed emotions as I sorted through each event. The time–clock ticked loudly, the waiting game had begun. The outcome was soon to be revealed as to who had won the battle, the cancer or me? Nagging questions began to loom in the back of my mind. What if it comes back? Each ache or pain I felt was triggered with wonder. Could this pain be related to cancer? How much longer do I have to live? Will I get to see my children or grandchildren grow up, graduate, get married and have their own babies? These tormenting thoughts began to overwhelm me the majority of the time. I kept quiet, putting on a brave face for all to see, not wanting to trouble my family by putting fear into them. I began to hibernate when feeling this way to avoid being asked how I was feeling because I couldn't be untruthful and didn't want to speak negative into my situation. I had allowed fear to creep its way back into my head by giving precedence to negative thoughts. They were crippling my life. Something had to change. It was time for a life altering choice that would begin each morning and continue each moment throughout the day!

I could allow these thoughts to rob me of my joy and steal the precious moments I do have left or I could choose to think positively and enjoy each moment for the treasure it is. Life is such a prized gift! People often take their health for granted, not realizing how important it is until it's threatened or worse, gone! There is great wisdom in the advice of taking life one day at a time. Each day has enough trouble of its own in itself, so don't worry about tomorrow (Matthew 6:34). Make the most of each moment.

We have a choice as to where we allow our minds to go. To take control of our thoughts we first must identify and be aware of what thoughts are coming into our head. I'm not telling anyone to ignore pain; it's very important to get those things checked out. What I am saying is that we shouldn't allow fearful thoughts to consume and overtake our minds. Worrying amplifies life's problems, steals our peace and joy. It doesn't change anything! However, using our concerns to motivate ourselves in a positive way (without being obsessive) can be a blessing when we stay in balance.

I've often heard the word FEAR described as False Evidence Appearing Real. Think about it! Do you want to spend your days worrying about something that might not even happen? This type of mental agony will weaken your soul; it's self-destructive and defeating. My Nanny always said it was a proven fact that nine times out of ten what people worry about never happens. So why waste precious time! If the things you worry about transpire, deal with your issue then. You can't control life but you can control your reaction to it. Why not put your concerns in the Lord's hands and allow Him to work out the details. God wants us to hope and believe for the best. Worry can cause physical tension, anxiety, depression, premature aging and sickness due to stress.[1] It is also the open door that allows Satan to torment you. Fear and worry are the opposite of faith and trust. We can't trust and walk in fear at the same time.

I think if you worry about something long enough, it may actually happen by drawing the negative to your situation through worry, doubt and unbelief. Unbelief may be the opposite of faith, but it is still faith believing the negative or opposite of what you desire to happen. It's sort of like faith working backwards or against you. Faith allows God to work in your life, while doubt and unbelief slam this door shut. This enables the negative possibilities to happen because it cripples the positive. When you doubt, you believe that the undesired result will happen, allowing the enemy to work in your life. That's why the Word of God says we will not receive what we ask for when we doubt (James 1:6, 7).

It's Satan's intention to implant lies into your mind. He wants to control your life through negative thoughts. It's his desire to destroy our lives, if he can. Job was a righteous man in the eyes of God but he allowed fear to overtake his life. He continually made purification sacrifices on behalf of his children for fear that they had sinned in their hearts toward God. Eventually, the very thing Job feared most came upon him (Job 3:25), he lost all that he had, including his wife and children. Fear can paralyze someone until it becomes a reality. Fear can seem real and has the power to deceive. We must remember it only has the power we give it! Thankfully, God in His goodness restored Job with double for his loss!

"Come to me, all you who are weary and burdened, and I will give you rest. Take my yoke upon you and learn from me, for I am gentle and humble in heart, and you will find rest for your souls. For my yoke is easy and my burden is light." (Matthew 11:28–30)

Rather than wearing yourself out with worry and frustration, try putting that energy into asking God for help. He will give you peace and guidance. While God is working on your behalf, think of some way you can help someone else. I have found this to be extremely beneficial. By doing this, you are sowing seeds to reap a harvest in your own situation (Isaiah 58; Galatians 6:7). I don't know about you, but it always makes me feel so good to help others. It's a win–win situation. You can't lose. When you help others, you are filled with amazing joy and a sense of purpose and meanwhile, God works on your behalf. That old saying, "What goes around comes around", is true! A man does reap what he sows! What can you do today that will make a difference in someone else's life? Keep your eyes open for clues. It can be as simple as a smile, opening a door, carrying someone's bag, praying for someone, buying a coffee or lending a compassionate ear. It may seem like such a little thing to you, but to someone else it may be huge!

Types of Fear

Most fear is the absence of faith. People who suffer from fear consider and expect unwanted circumstances as a probable outcome. There are several different types of fear. Terror is often the first kind that comes to mind. I had a frightening experience just the other day while out for my daily exercise. A young girl was playing with her Burmese Mountain dog in her front yard while a guardian stood close by raking leaves. I have to give them credit for keeping it on a leash but when the dog saw me approaching with my Golden Retriever, it came barrelling across their lawn, dragging the young girl over the grass, towards me. It looked like something you'd see on "America's Funniest Home Videos", except I wasn't laughing. Finally, losing her grip, the dog circled around mine barking and giving Rosie the old sniff over while she stood frozen like a statue. The large dog ran away for a moment and then came charging back again. Thank God there was a seven–foot wire fence for me to climb. Yes, I climbed it, screeching like a chimpanzee, maybe not as skillfully but I did manage to climb it! Talk about a humbling performance. You may be asking yourself, "What was so scary about that?" Well, I'm not finished yet, just stay with me here.

As a child, I was bitten several times by my best friend's dog, leaving me skittish of small, fluffy, white beasts. Unfortunately, over the past few years I have experienced numerous dog attacks, leaving me less than brave. My real fear evolved eight years ago as I set out for a nature walk up the road from my father–in–law's house, near Charleston Lake. A black lab from a nearby house came tearing across the road with great speed, baring teeth and snarling as I was walking down the opposite side with Chelsea, my trusted Chesapeake Bay Retriever. The attack lasted several minutes but felt like an eternity, the other dog getting the upper hand or paw, you might say, biting chunks out of Chelsea's fur.

My dog, regardless of her large stature, rolled over on her back showing submission. The black lab was relentless. She pounced on top of Chelsea and went straight for her neck, puncturing her throat. I believe it was my screaming that brought the neighbours out to our rescue. The dog's owner bolted out of his house, yelling obscenities at his dog. She submissively crouched low to the ground with her tail between her legs, as he kicked her with great force back onto his property and chained her up. That was probably a good indication of why she was so vicious!

My vet seemed to think Chelsea's wounds would heal but the exuberant spirit Chelsea once possessed never returned. She became quite nervous and trembled when I even mentioned the word "walk". Several months later she rapidly regressed and stopped eating and drinking. Hip-dysplasia, which was only a mild problem before, set in full-force and we had no choice but to have her put to sleep. It was one of the most difficult things I've ever had to carry out. From that moment on, I became terrified of being attacked by dogs, especially when walking.

Eventually, we ended up getting a new puppy through the Humane Society. In the summer of 2006, I had another unfortunate incident happened, while walking my dog. Two dogs attacked my Golden Retriever, Rosie, after escaping from their owner's house. The lady called her large female Golden Retriever and male Dalmatian over to Rosie thinking it would help her and her daughter capture their loose dogs. Her plan worked in one aspect but backfired in another. She was able to get hold of her dogs, but I was injured in the process. As the dogs attacked, I kicked at her Golden Retriever to push her away from Rosie, to give her a chance, as she was only a year old at the time. Rosie bolted away, dragging me down by her leash to the hard pavement, badly bruising my hand, spraining two fingers and injuring my hip and back in such a way that it pinched the sciatic nerve down my right side. The lady felt so bad about what happened. I trusted her sincerity and reassured her that I forgave her. Stuff happens!

It wasn't until about an hour later that my back seized up. Unfortunately, I was unable to walk for about six weeks. Thankfully, I was able to get a little exercise by riding my bike for about fifteen or twenty minutes before my right leg went numb. After a month of numerous trips to the chiropractor, I finally decided to try physiotherapy. My condition greatly improved within two weeks and I was able to resume my regular walking habits. I was so fortunate that my husband's benefit package from work covered the majority of my treatments.

A dog attack is only one fear out of hundreds that people suffer from in today's society, preventing them from enjoying their everyday lives. The anxiety experienced causes them to avoid certain places, people or circumstances. These fears and phobias are developed from negative past experiences, natural environmental conditions or illusions created through imagining unpleasant happenings. Some may appear silly to you, but to the person affected, they are very realistic and relevant. There are people afraid of endless things. The depth of fear experienced can range from being mildly afraid to being absolutely terrified. You can even suffer from fear and not even be aware. I was plagued with the fear of rejection for years and hadn't realized it!

Hollywood movie producers and publishers make millions of dollars from people who enjoy being scared! It amazes me how many people love to be literally frightened out of their wits and pay good money to do it! It's like an addiction. If you are someone who struggles with fear, it's important to guard your heart. This is accomplished by being careful about what you feed your spirit. Horror movies, thrillers, novels and scary programs open your heart to fear and put you in a vulnerable place. Even the news can cause anxiety. Be your own judge. If certain programs make you anxious or fearful, you may consider not watching them, because your eyes are the very window to your soul. This is why David vowed not to allow any vile thing to come before his eyes. (Psalm 101:3) He knew the importance of feeding your heart and mind with good things.

As humans, we should all have a healthy fear of God because He is all powerful! The Bible instructs us to fear God by having a holy reverence for Him. This was meant to keep our lives on track. Many people have allowed the wrong type of fear towards God to separate them from Him. They believe He is angry with them. You need to realize that God is not angry with you; He's angry with sin! He hates it because it goes against His very nature. Yet, He desires to have a relationship with us sinners. For this reason, He paid the penalty for our sins Himself.

God has also given us a healthy fear known as your "gut feeling" or "sixth sense" to warn or protect us during times of danger. This is God speaking to our conscience to reveal the safe path to proceed. Listening to this inner voice connects us to His perfect will. Sometimes we ignore our inner voice and do what our flesh craves anyway. At times, it's out of sheer laziness or rebellion that we pay no attention. If I had seriously listened to my gut feeling about avoiding sugar in my diet, I may not have had to travel along this twisted road, embellished with pink ribbons.

God created our brains to store memories so that when something bad happens, our bodies will warn us by becoming stressed and anxious.

God has placed this essential safety mechanism within us as a means of self-protection. Regrettably, the enemy has taken advantage of this. If people haven't received healing from past traumas this can cause them to be anxious and stressed to the point that they are fearful all the time. This was never God's intention. Later in this book we will look at ways to reduce stress and anxiety.

In conclusion, God has given us His Spirit to warn, guide, comfort and protect us. We must be open to receiving His direction to enjoy these benefits of relationship. Ask Him to lead you by His Holy Spirit.

Overcoming Fear

"Finally, be strong in the Lord and in his mighty power. Put on the full armor of God so that you can take your stand against the devil's schemes. For our struggle is not against flesh and blood, but against the rulers, against the authorities, against the powers of this dark world and against the spiritual forces of evil in the heavenly realms. Therefore put on the full armor of God, so that when the day of evil comes, you may be able to stand your ground, and after you have done everything, to stand." (Ephesians 6:10–13)

What are you afraid of? Getting in touch with your inner-self, by reflecting on your actual thoughts and behaviour, will reveal the root source of your fears. Once you have established and identified the basis of your anxieties, you will then be able to deal with them. You will gain victory as you face each fear prayerfully. Confessing and meditating on the Word will also provide added strength. Be determined to press forward, even if you are afraid.

Part of overcoming fear is facing those things that frighten you. By making a choice to do these things, even though you're afraid, you will eventually conquer that which brings torment. It's a matter of taking little steps and trusting.[2] God has provided us with the armour to aid us in overcoming fear. Spiritual battles require spiritual weapons and fear is a weapon the enemy uses. God gave us this armour so we can remain strong in the Lord's mighty power and so that we can stand against the enemy's schemes. When we put on the armour of God we are then equipped to stand our ground firmly. Just as Roman soldiers needed armour in the ancient times to protect themselves during war, Christians need armour to protect and guard themselves against an attack of fear!

Put on the Armour

God has also given us this spiritual armour to cover and protect us. Soldiers are called to be brave and face their opposition head on. Instinctively, many people would like to run and hide from life's problems but that doesn't solve anything. You might as well face your problems head on by dealing with them, because ignoring them won't make them go away either! Everytime I've been tempted to run from my problems or from what God is calling me to, He always reminds me of the story of Jonah. God asked Jonah to go to Nineveh to deliver a message to the people, to stop their wicked ways. Jonah didn't want to go because he feared them; they were ruthless and bloodthirsty. Instead, he ran and boarded a ship destined for Tarshish. Meanwhile, a storm evolved, almost capsizing the ship. Jonah was thrown overboard and was swallowed by a whale. After spending three days in the belly of the big fish, the whale spit him up onto shore. Once again, God asked him to go to Nineveh. Only this time, he listened and went. If you don't face your fears, they'll just keep rearing their ugly head until you do!

"Stand firm then, with the belt of truth buckled around your waist, with the breastplate of righteousness in place, and with your feet fitted with the readiness that comes from the gospel of peace. In addition to all this, take up the shield of faith, with

which you can extinguish all the flaming arrows of the evil one. Take the helmet of salvation and the sword of the Spirit, which is the word of God. And pray in the Spirit on all occasions with all kinds of prayers and requests. With this in mind, be alert and always keep on praying for all the saints." (Ephesians 6:14–18)

The Belt of Truth

The belt of truth is the most essential piece of armour because all the other pieces depend on it for their operational success. It is the written Word of God, the actual words given to man inspired by and breathed of God (2 Timothy 3:16). We can trust His Word and stand on it, for it is truth! God is unable to lie for He is pure and holy. There are Scriptures in His Word for every situation we face. We need to have a solid knowledge of the Word to be powerful. It has the ability to stand above all else, counteracting and defeating the enemy's plans.[3] If God gives us a particular promise for our lives, we need to act on it by obeying His commands and walking in faith and in love until we receive the promise.[4]

When negative reports were given by the doctor, symptoms appeared or discouragement tried to set in, I would then take the healing Scriptures to meditate on them and pray. This gave me the strength to reject any information that opposed God's promises. Focusing on God's ability, His love and His Word will help overcome any fear, doubt and worry you may experience.

Breastplate of Righteousness

"Do not let this Book of the Law depart from your mouth; meditate on it day and night, so that you may be careful to do everything written in it. Then you will be prosperous and successful." (Joshua 1:8)

By wearing the breastplate of righteousness, we are able to overcome evil with good. This will overturn all of the enemy's schemes. God reveals righteousness to us when we read His Word. He speaks to our hearts. Righteousness is choosing God's way above all else. This is the way to true prosperity and blessing beyond compare. When we renew our minds and meditate on His Word, it becomes part of us, the new natural way to think. Because our actions always follow what we believe, it is important to read His Word daily!

There are those who honour God with their lips because they know it's the right thing to do, but yet their hearts have not connected (Matthew 15:8). Some people have confused obeying the Law with having a relationship with God. The Law was given for our protection from the enemy and it is important to follow it for our blessing (John 13:17). Yet some believe Christianity is based on following rules! I personally had a hard time differentiating between the two because I was missing a solid foundation concerning God's grace (see Titus 3:4–7). Jesus died so that we could have a divine connection with the Father. He wants to speak to each one of us individually and for us to live and breathe each moment through Him. It's all about having a relationship! That is why He created us.

We show God our love for Him by being obedient to His Word. Although He gave us free will, He desires for us to follow Him. One way we can triumph in this area is to be kind and loving toward those who are not. We all have people in our lives that can be difficult. Following this path may seem hard, with the pressures of people's opinions ringing in our ears and our screaming flesh, but the end result will bring about a positive reward. In Romans, the Lord promises to work on behalf of those who choose righteousness. When we are kind by blessing and meeting the needs of those who mistreat us, it is as though we are throwing hot coals upon their heads. This love melts even the coldest of hearts. How can they withstand such love? God's way is the right way, even though it seems opposite or upside down from the ways of the world.

We must walk in love to walk in faith. Our faith carries us through to victory as we learn to trust God and walk in righteousness. It's simple, if we do not love others we are short of loving God, because God is love. If we are unable to love those that we walk, talk and spend time with each day or on occasion, how can we say we love God! We haven't even seen Him! As our love for our fellowman increases, it is then we aspire to love God.

"God made him who had no sin to be sin for us, so that in him we might become the righteousness of God." (2 Corinthians 5:21)

One of the enemy's schemes is to make people believe they're so bad that God wouldn't ever accept them. They live in constant condemnation and guilt, thinking they have to strive and struggle for God's acceptance. Believe it or not, God is not legalistic. Yes, He created rules, but He also gave us free will. Legalism is abiding by rules to earn God's favour. God's love for us is not determined by our righteousness. He loves you because you are His child, that's it! He sent Jesus to die for your sins because He wants you to be free, not bound by the curse of the Law (Galatians 3:13). God gave Moses the Law for mankind's protection, to show us right from wrong. God made the way to have a relationship with you. If you have asked Jesus into your heart, you are in right standing with God. Believe it! There is a prayer at the back of the book for those who would like to take that step.

If people could only see themselves through what Jesus has done for them rather than looking through the magnifying glass that amplifies their sin. They would enjoy the abundant life Christ died to give them. Did you know God has His own magnifying glass? After we accept Jesus Christ as our Lord and Saviour it becomes filtered. From that point on, we are considered righteous in God's eyes. He now sees Jesus in us. How cool is that? Our sin is washed away by the precious blood of Jesus, while His Holy Spirit dwells within us to change us from the inside out. I realize this still doesn't make us perfect, but God's love doesn't change. When this truth settles in our hearts and minds, we are able to rise up to make the right choices with the boldness and determination we need to win the battle. The Breastplate of Righteousness is meant to guard your heart. Remembering these truths and acting upon them will do just that.

Shoes of Peace

"Peace I leave with you; my peace I give you. I do not give to you as the world gives. Do not let your hearts be troubled and do not be afraid." (John 14:27)

God has blessed us with peace to walk through life's stormy weather. These shoes work in conjunction with the helmet of salvation. Are you agitated, disturbed or unsettled about things you have little or absolutely no control over? Making a decision not to allow your situation to steal your joy is powerful. Often it is our emotions that the enemy will try to attack because he knows if he can disturb our peace, he can uproot our faith as well.[5] It's our faith that keeps us stable. When mixed emotions and uncertainties cloud your mind, this is a clear indicator that these thoughts are not from God. Peace is our spiritual coverage that comes to protect us against anxiety, fear and worry when we leave our problems at the feet of Jesus.[6] He cares about us and wants to carry our burdens. When our thoughts are fixed on God's ability and love, our emotions stabilize and we are able to experience the calm serenity that comes from God's presence. This peace gives us the confidence we need to not be moved by our circumstances.

Roman soldiers wore leather boots with three inch spikes on their soles. This gave them a firm footing and stance. When times of doubt and discouragement attack your mind, wear the shoes of peace as the Roman soldier wore his spiked boots and dig your shoes of peace into the firm foundation of God's Word as Rick Renner encourages us to do in his book "Dressed to Kill."[7]

One of the most important keys to walking in peace is to cast your care on God through prayer and trusting Him. As Christians, we are to live at peace with all men and aggressively pursue it (Psalm 34:14; Romans 12:16–18, 20). God doesn't want us arguing with one another. It is important to know when to say something and when to stay quiet. We would be farther ahead to pray for the individual rather than prove our point. It is important to share your feelings and not to "stuff them down", but when the other person is not open to hearing what you have to say, you need to let it go. Remember, God always has an open ear for you. Let peace be your guide! If you become agitated, confused or anxious, this is a sign that you're not in the will of God.

Shield of Faith

The shield of faith is our protection to extinguish all the fiery darts the enemy shoots at us. To be successful, we must walk in faith and not doubt. God has given each one of us a measure of faith which increases as we read and hear the Word of God (Romans 10:17). It gives us the encouragement and strength to press past our situation and believe the desired outcome, rather than what is happening in the natural. However, when we become neglectful, we can easily be led by our emotions.[8] Emotions feed off our thoughts and it is our thoughts that our behaviour follows. Therefore, it is crucial to pay attention to what thoughts we are allowing into our minds.[9]

If you permit negative, irrational, unrealistic fears, doubts or worries into your mind, you should get a handle on them! If you don't control your thoughts, your thoughts will control you. These are the darts the enemy uses to disarm your faith. Talk to yourself if you have to! Get together with positive people and other Christian friends to lift your faith. Moreover, choose to listen to what the Word of God says about you and your situation. Our flesh is weak and needs the strength that comes from reading the Scripture. Our minds also need daily renewal to keep our emotions from ruling over us. When we submerse ourselves in the truth of God's Word we are able to hold the shield of faith up high because faith connects us to God's power. It is here that we become immoveable.[10]

Ben, my oldest son, made quite a reputation for himself playing Pee Wee Hockey. Although he wasn't overly tall, he was exceptionally fast and very solid on his feet, which earned him the nick-name "the human tank." Since no one got hurt, it seemed quite humorous when large players would skate at Ben thinking they were going to take him out with a body check, only to find themselves flying through the air and landing flat out on the ice. Once a player even did a summersault in the air! When we stand with our shield of faith in hand and our shoes of peace securely fastened into the Word of God, we become as immovable as a human tank. This is when the enemy is unable to succeed!

The Helmet of Salvation and the Sword of the Spirit

"You will keep in perfect peace him whose mind is steadfast, because he trusts in you." (Isaiah 26:3)

The helmet of salvation is based on knowing what the Word of God says and applying it to our lives; the helmet and the Sword of the Spirit, which is the Word of God, work together hand-in-hand. The enemy's weapon is deception, therefore it is imperative to know the truth and walk in it. As you become aware about what you're actually thinking, it's your job to choose to think positive thoughts and reject the negative ones that go against what God's Word says regarding you and your situation. Again, it's important to know what the Bible says; your entire life depends on it! Meditating on Scripture will transform your mind (Romans 12:1). Thinking positive thoughts and having the right attitude during difficult situations are mighty defensive weapons. It puts the puck in your possession and the stick in your hand!

One of the benefits of living in Canada is that we get to enjoy a long season of hockey. Not wearing your hockey helmet would be extremely dangerous; you just wouldn't do it. Without your stick in hand, you wouldn't be able to score any goals. Wearing the helmet of salvation will protect your mind and give you peace as you take the Sword of the Spirit and utilize it. The Sword is a mighty weapon in the spiritual realm that will score the goals for God's team! Having strong players that know how to skate a fancy dance, handle the puck and score goals is crucial, but it doesn't matter how good the team is if they lack confidence! If they don't believe they can win, they probably won't and if they go out with a passive attitude, they can easily be beaten. With these mindsets, they are defeated even before they step out onto the ice! On the contrary, if the players are determined, and go out believing they can win, anything can happen. Our mind also needs to have this type of offensive/defensive mindset!

The armour God has provided is comparable to hockey equipment. It's important to wear each piece for your protection. Each one has a specific purpose and all are meant to be used in conjunction with one another. In hockey, if you're missing any one piece of equipment, you aren't even allowed out on the ice to play. However, life is not a game and you are faced with a real battle whether you wear all your armour or not. Meditating on the Word has the power to break habitual chains of behaviour, wrong thinking patterns and bondages (see Hebrews 4:12).[11] Bondages can be anything that has a strong hold on you; things that seem difficult to let go. It not only refers to addictions like over–eating, drugs, alcohol, smoking, compulsive lying, cheating or gambling, but also strong emotions such as fear, or even negative thinking, worry, hate, laziness lack of confidence, etc., the list is endless!

"The weapons we fight with are not the weapons of the world. On the contrary, they have divine power to demolish strongholds. We demolish arguments and every pretension that sets itself up against the knowledge of God, and we take captive every thought to make it obedient to Christ." (2 Corinthians 10:4, 5)

God's Word is active and full of life! It has the ability and power to discern our innermost thoughts, attitudes, desires and motives.[12] When we choose to allow God's Word to judge and work in our hearts here on earth, our conscience is filled with peace because it's the issues that we have not dealt with that we will have to give an account for later! Furthermore, getting connected with God will provide us with the discernment we require in all circumstances.

Confessing the Word

Confessing God's Word brings the desired results. In *Chapter 3*, we discussed how our words affect our lives! Grumbling, murmuring and complaining are also negative confessions that will hinder the positive results we wish to attain, just as unbelief and doubting do. Confessing the Word of God equips the angels to act on God's behalf. See the following Scriptures below to gain a clear view on how confessing Scripture is a mighty weapon.

(See: Psalm 103:20; Proverbs 18:20, 21; Isaiah 46:9–10; Isaiah 55:10, 11; Romans 4:17; Romans 10:9–10; Hebrews 1:14; Hebrews 4:14; Hebrews 10:23; 2 Corinthians 4–5; 2 Corinthians 1:2.)

In Matthew 4, Jesus went to the wilderness to fast for forty days and nights. Here Satan twisted Scripture to manipulate Him. Knowing Jesus was hungry, Satan insisted Jesus prove that He was the Son of God by turning the stones into bread. Jesus spoke back to Satan using the Word of God. Jesus was in constant fellowship with God the Father and therefore was imparted with the wisdom and strength He needed to withstand Satan.

This is where positive confession comes in! This builds up your faith in the situation. When you speak something, it goes out into the air and right back in through your ears. From your ears, it goes down into your heart and becomes part of your actual being. As discussed, faith is built by hearing! What are you listening too? Are you listening to everyone else's opinion or what God has to say?

Your mouth needs to speak positive suggestions to your heart. Your heart is the life source of your whole being. Have you ever considered why someone who has had a heart transplant begins to have cravings, dreams and memories of the donor's life, revealing details they wouldn't have known? It is because the heart is the well–spring of life! (Proverbs 4:23)

In conclusion, we need to continually feast on the Word until it manifests within our hearts so it naturally navigates out of our mouths, in our time of need! You don't have to be a victim. Just because someone makes a comment to you doesn't mean you have to accept it as truth. Instead, reject it and replace it with a positive confession based on the Word.

Prayer is a Weapon

"And pray in the Spirit on all occasions with all kinds of prayers and requests. With this in mind, be alert and always keep on praying for all the saints." (Ephesians 6:18)

Prayer is a wonderful weapon that connects us with the One who is our Saviour in battle. We pray to overcome obstacles and to ask for the basic needs in our lives. It releases the power of God to stop the enemy in his tracks. It's quite simple; you talk to God the same way you would talk to a friend. It's not complicated. All we need to do is come to our Heavenly Father with child–like faith and ask Him for help. He wants us to come to Him with our needs.

"Do not be anxious about anything, but in everything, by prayer and petition, with thanksgiving, present your requests to God. And the peace of God, which transcends all understanding, will guard your hearts and your minds in Christ Jesus." (Philippians 4:6–7)

There are Several Types of Prayer

- Prayer of Adoration or Worship (honouring God for His attributes)

- Confession (acknowledging our sin and asking for forgiveness)

- Thanksgiving (thanking God for all things)

- The prayer of supplication (prayer for spiritual, emotional and physical needs of others, then for yourself)[13]

When Jesus died for our sins on the cross, He took back the authority Satan stole. Therefore, we can come boldly before the throne of grace with our petitions to God. I always start with a prayer of thanksgiving. This brings you face to face with God in an intimate way. I believe showing gratitude is important and it welcomes His presence. It brings us pleasure to be recognized when we give to others. God deserves our thanks! Thanking Him in advance for hearing our prayers and answering them is a token of appreciation and humility. Asking God for help in areas of weakness gives us greatly needed strength. He provides a way out when faced with temptation and aid in times of crisis, or during emotional, or spiritual need. God is not limited!

"If you remain in me and my words remain in you, ask whatever you wish, and it will be given you." (John 15:7)

God promises that if we abide in Him and His Word abides in us, we will receive whatever we ask. When we meditate on the Word of God it transforms our minds, hearts and our prayers. People are often skeptical or even afraid to ask God for certain things because they're unsure whether their request is in His will or not. Reading the Bible gives us a clear knowledge of God's desires and provides us with the confidence to pray boldly!

We are called to intercede on behalf of others and ourselves to gain or maintain victory. Often the Holy Spirit will give us wisdom as we pray, bringing Scriptures to our minds about issues we wouldn't have thought of on our own, giving the reassurance that builds our faith within our circumstances. The Holy Spirit even prays on our behalf when we don't know what to pray for (Romans 8:26).

We are told in Ephesians 6:18, to pray continually, small prayers throughout the day when a situation or person comes to our mind. These prayers do not need to be long or drawn out to be effective! Quite often, I will wake up in the night with a strong urge to pray for an individual. God even reveals circumstances or people I need to pray for in my dreams. God is so good! You would be amazed to know how many people are praying for you because God has placed you on their hearts. Perhaps you'll find out in heaven!

We all make mistakes and do things we wish we hadn't. All the wishing in the world won't make our sin go away. But Jesus' blood can wash it away! When you realize you have sinned, pray and ask God for forgiveness; this will make your heart clean. That's it, you don't have to punish yourself with guilt or do penance, just be sincere and ask God for the strength to not repeat these sins again.

Pray with authority (knowing your place in the kingdom) and believe you'll receive what you ask for. As you focus on God's greatness and use Scripture in your prayers, they become more powerful. Staying alert and being watchful to pray will put you in the proper position for battle!

"But when he asks, he must believe and not doubt, because he who doubts is like a wave of the sea, blown and tossed by the wind. That man should not think he will receive anything from the Lord; He is a double-minded man, unstable in all he does." (James 1:6–8)

God works in our lives through faith. It is the open door He uses to deliver what we're asking for. He gives us wisdom when we ask and believe, not when we've done everything correctly. All we need is a positive, hopeful, expecting attitude. Are you someone that is tossed to and fro or are your feet planted firmly on the ground, confident that you'll receive what you ask for? Sweetheart, it's time to dig your heals in and fix your mind on what you want to happen! You need to become sure and steadfast by resting in God, knowing He's in control.

Jesus didn't perform many miracles in His hometown because the people lacked faith (Matthew 13:58).

"For we also have had the gospel preached to us, just as they did; but the message they heard was of no value to them, because those who heard did not combine it with

faith. Now we who have believed enter that rest, just as God has said." (Hebrews 4:2, 3)

Do you realize that unbelief is a sin? What is not of faith, is sin! We can't enter the rest of God unless it comes together with faith. (Hebrews 3:19) Faith is the active ingredient God uses to answer our prayers. Let's compare faith with baking a cake. What would happen if you left out the baking powder? It's simple! All your hard work would go to waste because it would turn out flat as a pancake, right? Now, when you pray, ask God with the ingredients of His Word, and active faith stirred into the mix. Give this mixture to God and wait patiently for Him to bake it. You'll be pleased with the results.

Facing the Battle

As we take the focus off of ourselves and our situation and place our thoughts on God's ability, we then position ourselves for victory. When we triumph over the spirit of fear in an area, we need to stand firm in our faith to continue maintaining that territory. Sometimes, we can overcome one problem but still have bondage in another. Questioning our thoughts and the reasons for our behaviour can expose unacknowledged reservations. As these areas of struggle are revealed, ask God for the strength and courage to rise above. With God's help, you will be able to regain ground in those places you once struggled. Enjoy life the way God intended. Keep pressing on, it's worth it!

I've learned that dogs feed off the negative energy of others, by watching "Dog Whisperer". All this time, the dogs were reacting to my own internal fear. They were merely invited by my own anxiety and insecurity. I've learned to pray for protection and ask God to fill me with His perfect love that casts out all fear. It's also my responsibility to wear the armour and trust God to protect me, as I stand guard watching my emotions, to ensure that I don't allow fear to creep back in. It took me almost two weeks before I could get up the nerve to walk past the house where I had my fence–climbing incident, but I decided it would be the best thing for me!

Almost a year has passed and that house has continued to be part of my daily route. While walking last week, I noticed the back gate was wide open. Guess who came to see Rosie and me? Our old friend the Bernese Mountain dog came trotting out of the back yard, along with a yellow lab, to greet us. This time, I remained calm, remembering the dog only wanted to engage in harmless play during the last encounter. I reassured myself it would be okay and let go of the leash, as the mountain dog quickly ran towards Rosie. I quickly learned that this was nothing like the last attempt at puppy play. The mountain dog bounded around, snarling and snapping its teeth, while the lab barked and lunged at Rosie's side, mouthing her fur. My heart felt as though it was going to pound right out of my chest. Feeling jarred, I slowly walked sideways to move away from the dogs. It didn't matter where I turned, they circled back towards me. I quickly prayed, asking God for help. I knew with every ounce of my pounding heart I was being called to stand my ground. I leaned in towards the dogs and yelled repeatedly at them to go home. They eventually backed off and ran into their backyard.

This is a prime example how we can experience deliverance with the Lord's help! Please don't take this example out of context. Caution must be used at all times. It would be foolish to start petting strange dogs to challenge this principle. Always follow the leading of the Lord and you too can experience freedom from fear.

"This is what the Lord says to you: Do not be afraid or discouraged because of this vast army. For the battle is not yours, but God's." (2 Chronicles 20:15b)

"You will not have to fight this battle. Take up your positions; stand firm and see the deliverance the Lord will give you...Do not be afraid; do not be discouraged. Go out to face them tomorrow, and the Lord will be with you." (2 Chronicles 20:17)

In this passage, Jehoshaphat was seeking God's direction because he had just heard that a huge army was about to come against him and his people. The Lord tells us not to be afraid, to take up our position and to put our confidence in God, by fighting the good fight of faith. Are you holding up your shield of faith?

God gave Jehoshaphat very specific instructions for the battle he was to face. He desires the same for us. He wants us to seek His direction and walk in obedience to overcome our fears. Often, when we experience fear, our initial reaction is to run and hide. We hope the problem will fix itself or go away altogether. Life is not like that. We can't be like the ostrich from the cartoons that sticks its head in the sand. You cannot gain victory by avoiding the circumstances! You'll never enjoy life to its fullest. Fear will always manage to rear its ugly head when you least expect it. Facing your fears is the only way to overcome them. Hold your head up high with confidence; the Lord wants you to win. Is it time for a little confrontation? Hesitation is common to man but it doesn't have to be your norm. Be strong and courageous. You're not alone; God is with you and He wants to lead you into victory. Will you let Him take your hand?

"Jehoshaphat bowed with his face to the ground, and all the people of Judah and Jerusalem fell down in worship before the Lord. Then some Levites from the Kohathites and Korahites stood up and praised the Lord, the God of Israel, with very loud voice." (2 Chronicles 20:18, 19)

As discussed in Chapter 3, worship is a very powerful weapon that the Lord has provided to defeat our adversary. When we humble ourselves in worship to God, He fights our battles on our behalf. There isn't any problem on earth the Lord can't defeat because He is greater than the one

(Satan) that is in the world. We are blessed beyond measure to have this power available to us anytime. When we ask Jesus into our hearts, His Holy Spirit comes and takes up residence in us. It is the power of the Holy Spirit that strengthens us as we worship and walk in love, obedience and prayer helping us face and conquer each fear. It seems particularly difficult to worship during times when situations look bleak. How can we ask our feelings to agree when it feels so amiss? That is why it is called the sacrifice of praise. There is a wonderful blessing that comes with praising the Lord. It removes the dark clouds that hover over our hearts and minds.

God's Love Drives out Fear

"There is no fear in love. But perfect love drives out fear, because fear has to do with punishment. The man who fears is not made perfect in love." (1 John 4:18)

Love shuts the door on fear because fear is unable to reside with love. Fear is dark; love is pure and good. Love is God's character; the very essence of His being. His love is perfect and it is this genuine love residing in us that casts out fear. The enemy uses fear to torment people, but when we come to a full knowledge of the love that God has for us, there is no longer any room for his torment. It doesn't matter what happens in life, God promises that He will be with us and work everything out for our good. (Romans 8:28)

Reading the Bible and praying will increase your knowledge of God's love for you. The better you get to know Him, the more you will realize you can trust Him. He gave us His very best! God gave us Jesus, His one and only perfect Son as the Sacrificial Lamb for our sins. Now that's what I call love!

"For God so loved the world that he gave his one and only Son, that whoever believes in him shall not perish but have eternal life." (John 3:16)

Knowing God's goodness invited peace and joy into my soul. I now have the confident assurance that my time is in God's hands. Whatever happens in our circumstances, He will bring us through to victory. In Philippians 1:21, Paul said, *"For me, to live is Christ and to die is gain."* While I live, I can enjoy the awesome life the Lord has given me, and when I die, I'll spend eternity in paradise with Him, where there is no sorrow, sickness or pain. Either way, I win!

When we draw close to God, Satan has no other choice but to flee from our presence, taking his nerve-racking fear with him (James 4:7). As I began choosing to take God at His Word and trust Him, believing that His intentions toward me are always for my good (Jeremiah 29:11; 3 John 2), I found myself at peace, knowing my time is in God's huge, capable hands. Did you know that He measured the waters of the earth in them? (Isaiah 40:12)

It is my prayer that you too will come to this same knowledge of understanding of the Father's love for you. May it give you the assurance you need to trust Him. May you be filled with amazing peace and walk with Him in victory.

"And so we know and rely on the love God has for us. God is love. Whoever lives in love lives in God, and God in him." (1 John 4:16)

To be perfected in God's love, we must be filled with it. What does that mean? We need to live in love, to live in God. This is because God is Love! When we choose to love others, in spite of their shortcomings, we are filled with the love of God. We show God our love by being obedient to His Word and putting Him first, above all else. Then we must love others and ourselves equally. We all have people in our lives that are easier to love than others. Try loving those who treat you badly. It's more difficult loving selfish, arrogant, the impatient or gossipers who slander you or yell in your face. That's difficult! However, it is possible with the power of the Holy Spirit. This is done through prayer. Praying for these individuals is an essential key to the solution, as it keeps your heart from being bitter. A soft heart can't help but love them! As we follow these steps, we are filled with love, joy and peace. It is in this place that fear is unable to reside.

We are all in a spiritual battle, whether we're aware of it or not. Our battle is not with people, but with principalities and powers and wickedness in high places: Satan and his dark angels. Satan is the master of deception, a liar and a cheat! It's his plan to thwart all the good things God has for us. He hates God and he knows the best way to get back at Him is by getting to His children. When people mess with me, it's one thing but when they mess with my kids, the mother bear comes out in me! We need to take this same aggressive stance to defeat the enemy's plan. Let's put on the armour of God and take back possession of the things we have allowed the enemy to steal from us. Remembering that people are not the enemy and walking in God's love defeats Satan's plans, causing them to backfire. Lastly, walking in love covers a multitude of sin. This protects us. God promises that He will always make a way for you, He loves you! Don't be afraid. You can trust Him because He's faithful.

Resting in God

"And God raised us up with Christ and seated us with him in the heavenly realms in Christ Jesus." (Ephesians 2:6)

After Jesus died on the cross and rose again, He sat down at the right hand of God (Hebrews 1:3). This is where He intercedes for us. The fact that Jesus sat down is very significant, as it represents that everything that needed to be done was done. In Ephesians 2, we're told that we also are seated with Jesus in the heavenly places. This means we're to take our place of rest in Him!

"Find rest, O my soul, in God alone; my hope comes from him." (Psalm 62:5)

Focusing on God and His goodness will put our minds at rest. We don't need to worry, reason, strive or fret in our minds about those things that cause us stress and anxiety. God wants to take care of the details. It's our job to have faith. Trust and rest in God by putting Him in control of our lives. This process may take time. Rome wasn't built in a day, and neither is anything else that has any lasting value. Thoughts that have become a life–time pattern will take time to dissipate. God will help you overcome your enemy of fear, doubt and worry little by little, if you are determined to be set free.

Refuse to allow your mind to be filled with overwhelming or confusing thoughts that steal your joy. Promise yourself to keep peaceful thoughts and enjoy a little heaven on earth. At times, I would get frustrated and upset to see other people abuse their bodies and not get sick. I wondered why I had to go through health issues. It didn't seem fair. Perhaps you may have felt the same exasperation. We begin to play judge, when it's not our place! This is one area we shouldn't allow our minds to go! Also, it isn't our responsibility to figure everything out. There are always going to be questions you'd like answers to. We need to act on what God tells us in our own situations and pray for those who frustrate us. Give these issues to God and let Him deal with the things that aren't our business.

"You will keep in perfect peace him whose mind is steadfast, because he trusts in you." (Isaiah 26:3)

Decide to concentrate on God's goodness and heavenly things, rather than on depressing situations (see *Colossians 3:1, 2*). If we would become more heavenly–minded, life's issues would have less of an effect on us and many of our choices would be different! Have you ever wondered what heaven was like? The Bible speaks of its extravagant beauty with golden paved streets and gates of pearl. We don't have to wait until we get to heaven to see God's beauty; it's all around us. Take a look at all the amazing things God created in nature. Nature is the very expression of God's beauty. (Isaiah 6:3)

Take a moment to imagine the most beautiful scenery you've ever gazed upon, either in real life or from a picture or magazine. Perhaps you envisioned the massive snow-tipped Rockies, a vast evergreen forest with eagles flying high above the trees, or the rushing of crystal clear spring water as it flows down an amazing waterfall into a stream below. Now picture yourself present amongst God's creation. Feel the breeze caress your face, hear the rustling leaves as they eloquently express their joy, feel the warmth of the sun soak deep into your skin. Breathe in through your nose and slowly let it out of your mouth. How do you feel now? Are you relaxed, refreshed and full of peace?

God wants us to keep our minds on Him and on eternity in heaven because it brings our minds to a place of peace. I'm sure the beauty on earth is of no comparison to the beauty of heaven. There is no sickness, pain or suffering there, only eternal peace and joy in God's presence.

Overcoming Anxious Thoughts

Chances are if you are reading this book, you are in need of healing! Are you prone to migraine headaches or do you need healing from something as serious as cancer? Doubt, worry and fear are common to every man; we all struggle with these things from time to time. I want to show you the steps to overcoming these things so you can experience peace and victory.

To start, it's important to discard the negative thoughts, one at a time, and meditate on positive ones. The next step is to envision your desired goal in your mind. You need to be filled with determination. God wants us to find the positive perspective in our situation. Don't be afraid to speak it. If you tell yourself you'll never be able to do it, you won't. When you tell yourself something often enough, you'll begin to believe it. (Proverbs 23:7a; NKJV)

"For out of the overflow of the heart the mouth speaks." (Matthew 12:34b)

What you believe in your heart always comes out of your mouth, and when it does, it returns right back into your ears and reaffirms your beliefs. It's a cycle that sets your actions in motion. Your words are powerful (Proverbs 18:21). Therefore, be careful what you speak over yourself. Your thoughts have a direct impact on how you feel about yourself. This impacts what you say, which directly affects the way you act or behave. Over time, this determines the habits you develop, whether good or bad. Do you need to reprogram your thinking so that what comes out of your mouth will benefit your future? If so, this can be done by renewing your mind daily from the Word of God (Romans 1&2).

Do You Consistently Worry About Whether You Will Have a Long Life?

I've gained great peace from meditating on the Scriptures that promise a long life. God created the world on a foundation of laws. Most of the promises operate on a condition. There's an "if" involved. If we want to reap the benefit, we need to follow through with the guidelines for that condition. When we do our part, He can do His. God wants us to be blessed but it's our sinfulness that gets in the way! Promises of long life are no exception to the rule (Exodus 23:25).

We all make mistakes in life! If we ask for forgiveness, God's grace will cover our errors but we do need to be actively trying to do what's right. I encourage you to get into God's Word so you can learn what behaviour reaps a good outcome. We cannot plead ignorance as an excuse. Remember, people perish when there is lack of knowledge. (Hosea 4:6)—(See Hebrews 10:36; Galatians 6:9 and Hebrews 10:23.)

"Let us hold unswervingly to the hope we profess, for he who promised is faithful." (Hebrews 10:23)

To hold onto something unswervingly means to not let go, no matter what! To do this, we need a firm grip. Do you see a connection here? We need to follow the will of God and not give up. God's will is mapped out very clearly for us in His Word. We need to read and follow it. It's important that we do not become like the man who looks into the mirror and then forgets what he looks like; this man is deceived. By looking into the mirror of God's perfect law that gives freedom, and following its instructions, the man becomes blessed in whatever he does (James 1:22–25).

"Honour your father and mother, as the Lord your God has commanded you, so that you may live long and that it may go well with you in the land the Lord your God is giving you." (Deuteronomy 5:16)

The Bible tells us that when we honour our father and mother we will be blessed with a long life, and that life will go well for us. Although we're going to take more of an in depth look at this promise in Chapter 9, I wanted to mention this because of its great importance! When we don't honour our parents we open ourselves up to the curse of disobedience.

"Because he loves me," says the Lord, *"I will rescue him; I will protect him, for he acknowledges my name. He will call upon me, and I will answer him; I will be with him in trouble, I will deliver him and honour him. With long life will I satisfy him and show him my salvation."* (Psalm 91:14–16)

Do you love the Lord? Do you acknowledge His name? God will deliver you from harm and place you in a spot of honour, if you love Him with all your heart, soul and mind. Scripture says if we are embarrassed of Jesus He will not utter our name before the Father and we will be disowned. (Matthew 10:33, 34)

"Jesus replied: 'Love the Lord your God with all your heart and with all your soul and with all your mind.' This is the first and greatest commandment. And the second is like it: 'Love your neighbor as yourself.' All the Law and the Prophets hang on these two commandments." (Matthew 22:37–40)

Exodus 20:8 tells us to, *"Remember the Sabbath day by keeping it holy."* Studies have shown that people who attend church live longer, which also proves that there is life in the presence of God.[14] God gave us the Sabbath as a gift to rest. Even God took time to rest after creating the world. It took Him six days to work His wonders and then He took the seventh day off to relax and enjoy what He had made. We need to recharge our energy by giving ourselves a break once a week. You'll be healthier and more productive as a result.

If we want to take cover under God's umbrella of protection and blessings, then we need to walk on God's path, by following His commands. It is God's will for us to be healed. When we don't follow God's guidelines, the enemy takes legal right through sin, to put sickness on people. Instead of worrying about whether you're doing everything right, develop a relationship with the Lord and seek Him. When you seek Him first, everything else falls into place.

Dear Heavenly Father,

Perfect me and fill me completely with Your love so that there isn't any room for tormenting fear within me. Deliver me from all fear and doubt. Help me to live in peace, power and love (Psalm 34:4). Guard my mind with thoughts that are pure, good and holy. Your Word promises that through Christ I can do all things! Enable me to walk in faith and in Your power to face and overcome those things that frighten me, and to be obedient to Your Word. In Jesus' name I pray. Amen.

(Scriptures for Combating Fear: Psalm 23:4; Psalm 27:1; Psalm 91:4–6; Psalm 112:7, 8; Proverbs 29:25; Isaiah 41:1; Isaiah 54:14; Luke 12:32; Hebrews 13:5, 6; 1 John 4:18; Deuteronomy 20:4.)

———————————————————

[1] Colbert, Don, MD. *The Seven Pillars of Health* (Lake Mary, Florida: Siloam, 2007).

[2] Meyer, Joyce. *The Spirit of Fear.* 6 Disc Set (Fenton, MO: Joyce Meyers Ministries).

[3] Renner, Rick. *Dressed to Kill, A Biblical Approach to Spiritual Warfare and Armour.* (Tulsa, OK: Teach All Nations, Rick Renner Ministries, Inc., 1991, New Edition 2007).

[4] Ibid.

[5] Renner, Rick. *Dressed to Kill, A Biblical Approach to Spiritual Warfare and Armour* (Tulsa, OK: Teach All Nations, Rick Renner Ministries, Inc., 1991, New Edition 2007).

[6] Renner, Rick. *Dressed to Kill, A Biblical Approach to Spiritual Warfare and Armour.* (Tulsa, OK: Teach All Nations, Rick Renner Ministries, Inc., 1991, New Edition 2007).

[7] Renner, Rick. *Dressed to Kill, A Biblical Approach to Spiritual Warfare and Armour* (Tulsa, OK: Teach All Nations, Rick Renner Ministries, Inc., 1991, New Edition 2007).

[8] Meyer, Joyce. *Managing Your Emotions: Instead of Your Emotions Managing You* (Tulsa, Oklahoma: Harrison House Inc., 1997).

[9] Renner, Rick. *Dressed to Kill, A Biblical Approach to Spiritual Warfare and Armour* (Tulsa, OK: Teach All Nations, Rick Renner Ministries, Inc., 1991, New Edition 2007).

[10] Renner, Rick. *Dressed to Kill, A Biblical Approach to Spiritual Warfare and Armour.* (Tulsa, OK: Teach All Nations, Rick Renner Ministries, Inc., 1991, New Edition 2007).

[11] Ibid.

[12] Meyer, Joyce. *The Word, The Name, The Blood* (Fenton, Missouri: Warner Books, 1995).

[13] Renner, Rick. *Dressed to Kill, A Biblical Approach to Spiritual Warfare and Armour* (Tulsa, OK: Teach All Nations, Rick Renner Ministries, Inc., 1991, New Edition 2007).

[14] "Going to church may help you live longer." *post-gazette.com living.* 30 Sept. 2007 (http://www.post-gazette.com/pg/06094/679237-51.stm).

Chapter Eight
Reconstruction

*Instead of their shame my people will receive a double portion, and
instead of disgrace they will rejoice in their inheritance; and so they
will inherit a double portion in their land, and everlasting joy will
be theirs.*

Isaiah 61:7

My Oncologist referred me to a plastic surgeon after discussing the
ways I could protect myself from re–occurrence. She called the
surgery, "stacking my deck." Literally, it was! I attended a seminar in Ottawa with approximately a hundred other people. My friend Angela
drove me into my appointment and watched Spencer along with her little fellow, out in her van. Meanwhile, inside I listened to the plastic
surgeon give a presentation of the different types of reconstruction surgeries, giving the pros and cons of each type.

We viewed, on overhead, actual before and after pictures of women
who had undergone this type of surgery. After the presentation, he answered questions for approximately half an hour. I was extremely overwhelmed with the wealth of information and had a little cry on my way
home. There was so much to digest and the thought of it all, made me
feel sick to my stomach. The doctor purposely displayed actual pictures

of not only of his successful cases, but of the imperfect examples as well, to give each person a realistic view of what to expect. He is a fine doctor who performs with amazing skill and produces some pretty great results. Unfortunately, the results of patients that have had radiation, like me, aren't necessarily as perfect because of the skin he has to work with. When skin is radiated, it becomes thin, loses its elasticity and sometimes becomes hard with indents. All the cases were an improvement but they certainly weren't perfect! In my mind, I had pictured the dream God had given me in which I was perfectly restored. I had high standards and imperfection didn't sit well with me.

Rob was anxious for me to have this procedure done and had begun asking, on a daily basis, when I was going to contact the doctor to have reconstruction. I wasn't mentally ready at that point. Because he wasn't able to take time off work to come to the seminar, to observe the graphic images I saw, he had difficulty understanding this. I was becoming quite comfortable with my new body and wasn't ready to experience anymore pain.

I warned Rob one day, that I wasn't ready to go there. I wanted him to leave me alone, to stop questioning me about it, and to allow me to proceed when I was good and ready. I expressed to Rob that I needed to know that he truly accepted my body at the stage it was at. If he couldn't accept me at that point and then started chasing me around all frisky-like later expecting action, real resentment would have set in. Rob, being the kind, loving sweetheart that he is, loved me tenderly and waited patiently.

I think his biggest desire behind wanting me to have the surgery was to rid himself of the constant reminder (scars) the cancer had left behind. It hindered us intimately as I was extremely self-conscious in the bedroom, always needing to be covered up, with the lights out. In my mind, I had placed a wall of protection up with the excuse that Rob didn't want to see my missing breast. In reality, it was my insecurity and fear of being rejected that hindered my freedom. I assumed that he was the one uncomfortable with my imperfection, when all along it was me.

I started hosting a prayer group in our home every second week, at the request of some friends. Our leader lent me a book and some CD's by a man named Todd Bentley. Todd is an anointed, healing evangelist who travels the world. In these services, hundreds of thousands of people get healed of incurable diseases; the blind regain their sight, the ears of the deaf are opened and the crippled walk. Millions of people give their lives over to Christ after witnessing these miracles. My oldest brother, Peter, knew him personally and had attended several of his crusades. Peter went to one of his meetings in Toronto, on my behalf, and Todd prayed for me over his cell phone. When he did, I felt a heat permeate across my chest.

On one of the CD's I listened to, Todd spoke of a woman who suffered from breast cancer and had a mastectomy three years previous.[1] She screamed out during a healing crusade in Africa because her breast grew back. I know it seems hard to believe. I would have been skeptical myself but when I was a young girl, my mom took us to a healing crusade where we witnessed, up close, a women's leg, that was several inches shorter than the other, actually grow even in length with the other leg. She was able to walk out without her cane and special, thick-soled shoe.

A friend encouraged me to ask and believe God to perform a miracle and recreate my breast. I knew God was and is all powerful and He, being the Creator of the universe, could do this no problem. Through months of prayer and basking in God's presence, I actually had muscle tissue that was removed during my initial surgery, grow back. I had to purchase a smaller prosthesis cup to replace my larger one, so I wouldn't appear lopsided. I had quite an indent before but it had changed to a small mound, a definite difference. I have pictures to prove it. I went through the summer with no additional change in my chest, and decided to ask the Lord for wisdom in this situation. Each time I did, I received a call from the plastic surgeon. I now had an indent form on the left breast and it had become quite itchy, just like the problem I experienced on the right side. In the spring, at my doctor's request, I had an ultrasound preformed. The technician said that there was only a three percent chance of it being cancer. I would have preferred a zero percent chance! All the same, I put it behind me and tried to remain in faith. Meanwhile, at this time, I was still receiving Herceptin therapy.

One night, I dreamt that I was sitting in a waiting room, filling out a questionnaire with my mother and her friend that had survived major surgery. Then two male surgeons, dressed in scrubs and white lab coats, pushed me down a corridor, on a hospital gurney. One doctor was much older than the other. As they were wheeled me down the hall, the questionnaire I held took the shape of a light bulb. Everywhere around me became illuminated by a bright light and a masculine voice spoke, "Do not fear, you'll be surrounded by angels."

Upon awakening, I knew in my heart that this was the direction I had sought God for. I called the doctor's office right away and received an appointment that Friday. Rob and I had met with the plastic surgeon and discussed the "ins and outs" of the procedure I had chosen. The plastic surgeon agreed that direct implants with expanders were my best option because of having such a young family. Bi-lateral Free TRAM or latissimus dorsi surgery would be much more extensive, with both hospital stay and recovery time being longer. It also limits what you can do after surgery because of the incisions across the abdominal area, where they remove skin, flesh and muscle tissue to use in the reconstruction. If the implants were unsuccessful, I could always fall back on this option. The necessary measurements were then taken. I was shown God's favour when the plastic surgeon opened additional surgery dates and requested that I choose one at our family's convenience. My surgery was scheduled for the following month, placing me ahead of other women who had been waiting for over a year for their reconstruction.

The medical surgeon—the second doctor in my dream—would be performing the mastectomy on the left side, while the plastic surgeon observed. After the mastectomy was completed the plastic surgeon would step in and do the implants. I met with the surgeon at his office and went through all the necessary preliminary pre-op steps. He decided to squeeze me in during the lunch hour for an emergency mammogram to the left side because of the lumpy tissue, indent and skin irritation. The results would determine whether I would be able to receive reconstruction or have to endure more cancer treatment. I was beginning to become accustomed to the emotional ups and downs of the whole process, so I was trying not to let it bother me too much. I decided to wait and see what the results were before getting all upset.

The mammogram clinic was down in the basement of the building. Although I really wasn't hungry, I grabbed an egg-salad sandwich on whole-wheat from the cafeteria to eat on the way down. I only had half of it eaten before the technician called me into a cold, small room that was furnished with two hard chairs (in case you want to share the humiliation with someone else), a desk and the mammogram machine. She asked me a few questions and handed me a thin, white paper vest to change into. You know, I never thought I would lose that uncomfortable feeling you get when you have to bare your all to a doctor, but after a few hundred times, it doesn't bother me a bit! Just remind yourself of that old saying, "If they've seen one, they've seen them all!" Obviously, there are many shapes and sizes, however it's your face they'll remember, not your nakedness. I do, however, feel sorry for the student doctors who aren't as conditioned to this. This mammogram, much like my first, took minutes to perform. The technician grabbed my breast as if it were a stress squeeze–ball and strategically placed it on the shelf of the machine. She then lowered another paddle down to squeeze the breast, making it as flat as she could, and then locked the shelves in place to keep my breast from moving. As if it was going to go somewhere! I never knew I had the ability to be a contortionist. They should call this stunt "boob gymnastics". She had no trouble twisting my floppy, sock–boob out of its natural shape. I spent the next twenty–minutes praying while I waited for the images to be processed and read. Thank God, the results were clear, regardless of the funky symptoms my body was producing. I was able to proceed with surgery, two days later, as planned.

On November 10, 2007, I had my surgery and returned home the same day! I must say, Ottawa hospitals are completely different than the one in our small town, even the doors were high tech. I felt like I was in another century. I said goodbye to Rob in the waiting room, as family members weren't permitted in the pre–op rooms, and I was escorted to a change room. After putting on my hospital attire, I was assigned a bed close to the nurse's station. I filled out some forms and I quietly read sitting on my bed. While going over my forms, the head nurse noticed that I had checked off the box regarding an overnight stay and came to talk to me. She explained that they didn't have a bed for me. I said that was fine but that there must have been some sort of mix–up because the plastic surgeon had told both Rob and I, at my initial appointment, that I would be accommodated with an overnight stay. He suggested this because of our distance away in conjunction with the age of our children. Not wanting to make an issue about it, I asked to speak to Rob, so that he didn`t leave right away after my surgery and could make arrange-ments for my mom to stay longer with the boys. Sensing that I was telling the truth, she decided to take matters into her own hands and confront the doctor about his empty promise. They argued back and forth on the phone for about five minutes.

"You tell her then!" she retorted as she walked over and handed me the phone.

"Hello", I said hesitantly.

"Listen, we don`t have a bed for you. Do you want the surgery or not?" He questioned with an intimidating voice. My heart pounded frantically. My mouth was so dry I could hardly get the words out.

"Yes, off course I want the surgery. I didn`t want to make a big deal out of this. I just wanted to talk to my husband, so he could make changes to our arrangements. That's all!" I replied. The last thing I wanted to do was upset the man who was going to cut into me.

"She's just doing her job and looking out for her patients. If you need to stay past eight o'clock, we'll put you down in emergency for the night." he said, with a little more compassion.

I handed the phone back to the nurse and then asked to speak to Rob. She called the waiting room and got Rob on the line. My nerves were shaky but I managed to tell him what had happened. He made the necessary arrangements with my mom and assured me that every-thing would be okay.

The nurse wheeled and placed my stretcher along the wall just outside the operating room until the staff had finished prepping. My plastic surgeon came to ask me some last minute questions before going in. Nervous about what had just happened, I started to cry.

"Hey, there's no crying in sport!" he said and then asked me if I wanted to see what the implants looked like. Moments later, the O.R. staff rolled me into the room and had me sit on the side of my bed. I dropped my gown, to allow the plastic surgeon to draw on my chest and remaining breast where he wanted the surgeon to make precision cuts. After he finished, I laid on my back staring up into the familiar bright lights waiting for the anesthesiologist to place the mask on my face to inhale a garlic tasting vapour. I quietly prayed and reassured myself while I focused on my dream of angels surrounding me. As music played in the background I watched the doctor bounce up and down in my peripheral view like a boxer, getting ready for a fighting match; ten, nine, eight... dreamland.

This treatment was the most painful. It felt like I had an elephant sitting on my chest and my body ached as if I had been hit by a cargo truck. I returned four days later to the plastic surgeon's clinic for re-examination. The doctor entered into the room to see me sitting on the edge of the examination bed grinning from ear to ear. I was quite surprised and almost taken back when my doctor asked me if I was on something.

"What do you mean, "On something"?" I asked.

He clarified by asking me if I'd taken a happy pill! I knew exactly what he meant the first time but I couldn't believe that he actually thought that!

"I'm happy I finally have cleavage!" I said. Apparently, he's not accustomed to happy patients or ones that are able to look past the pain right away and focus on the end result before things are perfect! I was surprised that with the number of appointments I'd already had with him, that he didn't know my character better than that! Even people who don't know me call me "Sunshine"!

When he finally got around to examining me he was astonished!

"Who beat you up?" he questioned. There was a huge degree of bruising on my chest. I was covered with an array of beautiful shades of blood red, deep purple and a little green, amongst the swelling. With a little questioning, my doctor determined that I hadn't stopped taking my vitamin E soon enough. I took it daily because it helped keep my port–a–cath from clogging and had great antioxidant properties. This is a natural remedy used to thin the blood, rather than the over–the–counter rat poison version! Yes, I said rat poison! The commonly used drug "Warfarin" is a small dose of what they use to kill rats. It thins the blood but can also cause cancer. The last thing I wanted to do was put something in my body that caused the very thing I was trying to avoid!

I returned three weeks in a row without the plastic surgeon being able to add any fluid to the implants. The swelling hadn't gone down and the bruising was still very bad. I was sentenced with a few weeks of couch rest, with strict instructions not to use my arms at all; only being able to watch movies or read. I begged the kids to play cards and checkers with me or to let me read to them.

When I was going through chemotherapy treatment, the boys had learned to pitch–in around the house and were quite happy about earning a little extra allowance. Although, after my chemo treatments ended, they returned to their regular chores as the novelty of earning some extra cash had worn off and I was able to resume my duties. The trouble was that now I needed them more than ever. I couldn't use my arms at all and I couldn't risk the surgery having to be redone. Because the boys had heavier loads at school, their responsibilities remained almost the same. Rob declined any overtime offered to him, so that he could look after the family. Declining overtime was very difficult for Rob because it provided the means for me to stay home with our children and look after our family's needs! He also takes great pride in his work and doesn't want to let anyone down. I learned to ignore the mess, while Rob managed to do his best at getting most of the meals on the table. Like many women, I wrestled with the guilt that tried to attach itself to my spirit because I was unable to fulfill my usual responsibilities. Very few people knew about my reconstruction because I wanted to keep it quiet. The few friends that did know surprised Rob by dropping off a few meals to help Rob out. Once the swelling went down, the doctor was able to gradually fill the implants by adding small amounts of fluid, every few weeks. The skin needed time to stretch after each allotment. Breathing and sleeping became difficult for several days afterwards because of the sharp pains, due to the muscles and skin being stretched. Once the incisions were healed, I was able to resume my Tuesday morning ritual of swimming at a local indoor pool with Spencer and some other moms and tots. After almost six months of traveling in and out of Ottawa to even out the implants, an ending seemed to be in sight.

Unfortunately, I formed a scab, on the radiated side along the scar line, due to my swimsuit rubbing across the area where the port tube ran along under my skin. I accidentally scratched and ripped off part of the scab, while drying myself. After returning home, I realized I had a hole, the size of my small fingernail, in my skin and could see the implant underneath. I called the doctor's office and scheduled an appointment to have it checked. He didn't seem to be alarmed; he added more fluid, said it would heal and sent me home. His receptionist called me to set up an appointment to have the fluid evened out and have the ports removed. Although the scab healed quite quickly, my bra ripped it off again.

This time it didn't close up and it became very infected. My shoulder blade became extremely sore. The incision was red and oozed yellow fluid. The scab was green and I could still see the implant tubing underneath. I was coughing up green chunks from my lungs, at this point, and found it difficult to sleep because of the pain. My family doctor put me on a very strong antibiotic of 500mg Keflex tablets, four times a day for seven days. I returned to the doctor's office, the following Monday, to be measured because he said I needed to have the implant changed as my radiated skin wasn't allowing the implant to drop down like the other side. One side was up high and the other down low. Both were different in size, far too obvious when wearing anything, especially a t–shirt.

All I really wanted was to look normal and not be self–conscious all the time. When the doctor saw how infected the right side was, he had me return to the clinic the next day to have the ports removed and some infected scar tissue cut out as well. A male, student doctor came in, along with the plastic surgeon, to observe the procedure. As I lay on the table under the examination light, the plastic surgeon first extracted fluid from each implant to give them a softer more natural feel. He then removed more from the left to even it out with the right side and sat me up to determine his accuracy and then instructed me to lie back down. I let the doctor know that typically from past experiences, whether dental or minor operations, I've needed additional freezing. His response was a quick, "No you don't!" *Okay now what?* I thought. *Maybe he thinks I'm a chicken!* I didn't know and I wasn't about to ask! I had often found myself defending him to other patients who commented on his terrible bedside manner. Even my oncologist had warned me, yet I always tried to keep a positive attitude and overlook his comments. I wanted to be a godly example for him! This was becoming quite a challenge! Now, every ounce of my flesh was clearly agreeing with their point of view!

With the needle, he injected freezing all along the scar and port areas, on both sides, where he was going to be working. He probably inserted twenty needle injections per side and then left the room for a minute, to allow the freezing to take effect. *That was painful!* There's nothing to numb the stabbing pierce of needles. I'm not a wimp, unless it involves cold weather! I actually have a very high pain threshold.

When the doctor re-entered the room, he promptly began his work by cutting along the scar line to remove the scar tissue and some infected flesh. I clenched my teeth and closed my eyes. With each cut of the scalpel, I experienced an overwhelming burning, stinging sensation. Just as I opened my eyes, the doctor handed the student a shinny, silver instrument.

"Here, retract the tissue back with this," the doctor said. Then looked straight into my eyes and told me to forget that he had help!"

I shut my eyes again. This time, my mind raced as to why he would make such a statement! Your guess is as good as mine. Maybe it's because he wasn't licensed or perhaps his ego? It didn't matter to me, as long as he did a good job. The port was like a tight suction plug that took quite a few attempts to remove, by tugging. He then capped the implants so the fluid wouldn't leak. The long tube that filled the implant had over time, attached itself to my tissue. It became part of me, regardless of the fact that it was a foreign body. It basically had to be ripped out. I also felt this because there was no way to freeze for that. He repeated the same steps on the left side and then stapled each side up. I only felt a few of the staples pinch. The doctor said they were some of the easier ports he had removed. The student doctor bandaged my wounds and then sent me out the door, with instructions to return the following week. At that appointment we would determine whether we were happy with the results or whether we needed to go with a second stage implant.

My voice quivered as I tried to make my follow-up appointment.

"Are you all right?" The receptionist asked.

"I just need to get out of here," I said. My eyes flooded with tears. I couldn't get out of there fast enough. I can't remember a time in my life where I felt more shaken. I quivered from shock as I rode the elevator back down to the main floor. It was an extremely painful experience; one that I would definitely like to forget. Traumatic would better describe it! Thoughts of self-pity engulfed my mind but, as I pushed open the final door to the outside, God once again put everything back into perspective. To my left sat a woman in a wheelchair with two bare stumps. She had no legs, no artificial limbs, nothing! Forget the pain; at least I now had two artificial breasts! Thankful, I drew a breath of fresh air into my lungs and left with my mom by my side!

As I lay on the couch, I tried to make sense of this whole thing. I was in so much pain I could hardly pray. I doubled my dose of painkillers, two hours earlier than what the directions stated. For me to take something, it has to be bad! I asked the Lord if anything good was coming out of this because I just couldn't see it.

That night, I dreamt about watching an adult golden retriever walking through a green, hilly park with a golden retriever puppy by its side. The pup explored and sniffed, as it continually found places to defecate (get rid of its filth). All of a sudden, I was no longer watching the dream, I was in it. As I sat in the grassy meadow, my right breast opened up and out spilled fresh, red raspberries and chunks of fine white china.

Right away I prayed for discernment and this is what God impressed upon my heart: The large dog represented the Lord, our faithful companion. No matter where we go or what we do, He always sticks by us through everything! He doesn't leave our side, not even for a moment. Guess who the cute little puppy, pooping all over the place, represented? Me, of course! God was using each part of this journey to reveal and remove hidden sin in my life. Like the puppy, sometimes we make a mess out of things. This doesn't change the Lord's faithfulness; He still brings good out of the bad. He doesn't always necessarily clean up our mess but He will guide us through it. When bad things happen, God hopes that the memory from these situations will ingrain in our minds, so that we will turn from our sin and not fall back into our old ways.

We are also to learn from the mentors God places in our lives. They're there to teach and help us. The grassy park signified the place of rest we have when we trust Jesus as our Lord and Saviour. The 23rd Psalm tells us that the Good Shepherd (Jesus) makes us lay down in green pastures and leads us beside still waters, especially when things around us are dark and scary. The Lord wants to lead and guide us through the messes in our lives, even the ones we make. His intentions are always good. When we trust Him, we realize that the trials we face are meant to yield good fruit (fresh red raspberries). Even though He did not cause this sickness, He used the suffering to get rid of my sin and to refine me. Now let's talk about the china. There is quite a process to making china. *Clay is a mixture of bone ash, feldspar, clay powder and flint, mixed with water. When this product attains the right consistency, it's put through a filter press and then extruder to get rid of any excess water or bubbles and is placed into a mold. This is put into a kiln at 2200 degrees for nine hours. When finished, the form is sanded, glazed, fired again, inspected, filed down if necessary and then put through a vibrating vat of stones to smooth and polish.*[2]

This long and arduous process could be compared to trials. The clay, like us, starts out soft (weak) and has impurities in it until after it's been squeezed, moulded, sanded, polished and put through the fire. It takes many hours of refinement before the clay becomes a strong, beautiful piece of art. We too can be like the beautiful piece of china if we attain a positive attitude and learn from the trials we face.

In the past, when I got dressed, I wanted to be noticed and to show off my figure. There is nothing wrong with wanting to look beautiful or dressing nice. Our motive needs to be in-check and we must dress to please the Lord. God doesn't want us attracting attention from others, making ourselves an idol or stumbling block for other men. God wants us to be discrete, pure and holy.

It's hard work for men to keep their minds pure, especially when their minds are wired to store images that can pop up at anytime. Many men may not want to admit it; however, it often happens when a husband is being intimate with his wife. If the wife knows this, it can be very degrading, leaving her with a sense of low self-worth or wondering what's wrong with her and why she doesn't add up. A woman needs to feel set apart from others, special, beautiful and noticed by her man.

In today's society, it's considered acceptable to shop around with your eyes as long as you don't touch. This is how some men and women can become dissatisfied with their spouses and sometimes become addicted to pornography and lust. God said if a man even looks at a woman with lust in his eyes he is committing adultery. The same can be said for women! This was grounds for divorce in Bible times. It's okay when we notice that someone is attractive but it's wrong to lust about others or entertain wrong thoughts in our heads. Since I didn't get the attention and love I desired from my father, I searched and looked for love and affection in ways that were inappropriate to fill this void. My thinking pattern about my self-worth evolved from the abuse and rejection I suffered while growing up. I was told and believed that the only personal quality I had of any value was what I had to offer in service to a man.

The time I spent trying to discretely hide and cover up the fact that my chest was uneven became a training session. God used it to change my attitude and motives before I received my new figure. Now when I dress, I question myself about whom I'm dressing for and let my conscience be my guide. Are you dressing to entice or capture other men's attention or do you dress to please God?

After this procedure, I felt pretty shook up and had a lot of unanswered questions about this situation. I wondered if somehow I had caused this to happen. Then I had to remember that it's not my job to figure everything out. I need to trust the Lord and rest in Him. God gives good gifts to His children, not bad ones, and my thinking about this was a little mixed up. God says to give thanks in all situations! This is something I needed to do because I was starting to feel pretty sorry for myself. I actually had to go back and re-read part of this book about reframing my thoughts. I began to thank the Lord for the good He was about to do. I knew it was all going to work out because, right from the start, He had shown me in a dream that I would be restored. Why do we worry so much? All we need to do is trust the Lord. It sounds so easy and yet, sometimes, it's so hard because of our fear!

Near the end of reconstruction, my emotions went up and down like a roller coaster. One week I was told the implant wasn't going to work and it needed to be replaced. The following appointment, the doctor unexpectedly added more saline to the implant, telling me it looked like it might work. Two weeks later, I returned to the clinic and was told the implant wasn't going to work, due to the infection, and I was given an appointment to be measured for a new implant. When I returned for the measuring, the doctor examined me and booked me the following day as an "emergency" to have the ports removed, due to the severity of the infection. The next day when I returned to have the ports removed, the doctor told me the results looked favourable and to return the next week so we could make a decision then. For two months, I went through this emotional roller coaster ride. What a work-out for my faith. I'm glad that's over! They're not perfect, but after all I've been through, they're still better than they were before. I'm not about to put myself, or my family, through anymore grief just for the sake of beauty. Besides, my husband loves me just the way I am, imperfections and all. Now that's love! I think he's great!

The Final Touch

I always swore I'd never get a tattoo. I really don't like the look of them. I'm sorry; I don't mean to offend anyone, it's just my personal preference. The thought of sticking needles into skin to inject dye to create a picture on a body part that will someday shrivel up, sag and fade, just doesn't appeal to me. There's something so attractive about soft, smooth, bare skin that shows defined muscle.

The last procedure of reconstruction is where the good doctor actually tattoos your areola onto your skin and twists and stitches the center to create a nipple. I do feel this type of tattoo is entirely different because it is to create the illusion of a missing body part. It costs an additional $500.00 and is *not* covered by OHIP (our Ontario Hospital Insurance Plan). Why? It's purely cosmetic! If I'm going to do this, it needs to be for myself and not because of others. It doesn't matter to my husband whether I have it done or not and I don't feel like any less of a woman without it. I guess that's my answer. The only reason why I contemplated this procedure was to avoid being the center of a gawk show in public change rooms. Tattooing for some, may help bring closure to a painful chapter in their lives!

You need to decide what is best for you, in your situation. Many people will offer advice. Take all the time you need to weigh the facts and don't let anyone push you into doing something you're not comfortable with. It's your body and you have to live with the results! If people are being pushy and you don't want to hear what they have to say, just tell them you don't want to talk about it! It's really not their business!

---

[1] Bentley, Todd. *The Voice of Healing* CD's (Vancouver, BC: Sound of Fire Productions, 2003). For additional information or material call 250- 355- 9096.

[2] "How Fine China is Made." *How Stuff Works Videos*. Dec. 2007 (http://videos.howstuffworks.com/howstuffworks/51-how-fine-china-is-made-video.htm).

Chapter Nine
Inner Healing

The Spirit of the Sovereign Lord is on me, because the Lord has anointed me to preach good news to the poor. He has sent me to bind up the brokenhearted, to proclaim freedom for the captives and release from darkness for the prisoners, to proclaim the year of the Lord's favor and the day of vengeance of our God, to comfort all who mourn, and provide for those who grieve in Zion—to bestow on them a crown of beauty instead of ashes, the oil of gladness instead of mourning, and a garment of praise instead of a spirit of despair. They will be called oaks of righteousness, a planting of the Lord for the display of His splendor.

Isaiah 61:1–3

Before you read this chapter you need to know that it is told from my little girl perspective. I know my parents did the best they knew how at the time and what I'm sharing with you is not meant to bring dishonour to them in any way. The things I share are for the mere purpose of helping you get a clearer view of where my thoughts, fears, and struggles stemmed from so that you are able to get a clearer picture of God's redeeming power. It is my hope that you'll be able to see how God has healed my life and given me a new outlook. He has taken the pain of my past and turned it around to help others find acceptance, freedom, and healing in Jesus.

Growing up was hard! When I was two, my father abandoned our family and left my mother with five young children to raise on her own. Our ages ranged from six months to 12 years old. As I grew older, I learned that he went out West with another woman. I wondered what was wrong with us, that he would choose someone else over his family. My mom received funding as a mature student to return to school during the day and she worked at a convenience store at night. Every day when I got off the bus, my mom would be driving down our long gravel driveway to go to work. She always stopped for a quick hello and kiss. I was too young to understand why she had to go. My heart ached every time she left as I feared she might decide to leave too! It seemed like she was never home.

My oldest sister, Debbie, kept house and took care of all the motherly responsibilities while Mom was away. Although we lived in a big, beautiful house, there were times we didn't have much to eat. Deb would collect things from the garden and mix it with whatever we had in the cupboards to create the most interesting meals. She always managed to make it taste good! I'll never forget the look on my sister's face the day my mom brought home a five gallon pail of peanut butter to feed us economically. Not long after, a big tub of honey followed. I never realized there were so many ways to serve peanut butter!

My younger brother liked to fight with me, and mom had a hard time getting us to stop. I didn't much care for her methods of punishment. As if anyone likes it! I don't know which was worse: getting our heads knocked together, being pulled around by our ears or being sent to the den where we were spanked with the wooden spoon. As we got a bit older, she allowed her friend to spank us with a wooden paddle that had holes drilled into it. I often sat on mom's lap pestering her for kisses or to have her run her fingers through my hair. One night, my mom sent me to bed and said she'd come tuck me in shortly. I stood at the top of the stairs and cried as loud as I could, for what seemed like half an hour, hoping she would remember me. I finally gave up, crawled into bed and cried myself to sleep, feeling as though she didn't care. Regardless of how loving she was, I often carried that underlying feeling with me.

Around the age of six, someone began to physically and sexually abuse me, without my mother knowing. With our big house, it was difficult to hear everything that went on. One day, my sister, Susan, heard me screaming from the bedroom. I tried to escape but he had pushed the bed up tight against the door. She beat the door with her fists and yelled but was unable to help. I lived with constant shame and the longer the abuse continued, the deeper the self-hatred and lies I believed about myself embedded into my soul. I hated life and I hated myself! I often wished I'd never been born. One night, I awoke to see a hooded demon at the doorway of my room. I trembled with fear as its red eyes blazed like fire and then I pulled the covers over my head. Frozen stiff, I sputtered the name "Jesus" out past my trembling lips and peeked past the covers to see if it was gone. Relieved that it had disappeared, but still afraid, I pulled the covers back over my head and remained that way until morning.

Peter, my oldest brother by eight years, always seemed to be angry. He listened to raunchy music and didn't have anything nice to say. One day, when my sister was babysitting, Peter took our string of Christmas lights my younger brother James and I were using to decorate our homemade fort with and strung them up over his Kiss poster in his room. It was a close-up of Gene Simmons's eye, the guy who always stuck his pointy tongue out. I always ran past the door when it was open because it gave me the creeps! Not wanting to mess with Peter, I went back to my room to play. James, however, quickly ran to tell Debbie. She came up and demanded that he give the lights back. They argued back and forth until Peter punched her in the mouth. Deb fell back and slid down against the wall holding her mouth as the blood streamed through her fingers. Peter fled the room. Debbie withdrew her fingertips to see the damage and cried for a facecloth. She'd recently had her braces removed and all four wisdom teeth extracted. Shaken, I quickly scampered to the blue bathroom, one room over to fetch it. Thoughts of guilt scurried through my head. Moments later, I returned with my peace offering and was relieved to find her teeth still straight. However, he did manage to put them half way through her tongue which required stitches. She happened to be biting it when he hit her. From that day forward, I worried about being a bother and avoided asking others for anything or getting in their way. Peter ran away from home shortly after this incident.

At school, I spent most of my time in class daydreaming of an imaginary world I wished I lived in. In doing so, I missed most of the foundational teaching I needed for a solid base in learning. I struggled with math and reading, and because of the circumstances, I never received the extra help I needed. However, I do remember my sister Debbie reading "Scat, Scat Go Away Little Cat" to me. I often identified with that curious, fluffy white kitten. My mom saw it best to hold me back and repeat my grade one. I felt dumb when the other kids moved on and I had to stay back.

The other kids at school would question me about my dad and certain circumstances I knew little or nothing about. How could I answer their questions when I never even knew him? Mom didn't talk about him and I'd never received as much as a letter or a phone call from him. Sometimes, I would sneak into the den to look at the little picture of him that sat on the shelf, and secretly wondered what he was like. I longed to be loved by him and to be held in his arms and to be told everything would be alright.

When I was nine, my dad came back. In my excitement, I announced it in front of my class and then had to turn around and tell them a month later that he had left again! Mom and dad got in a huge fight and dad went back out West. My dreams of having a dad were crushed. I tried to run after him but somebody grabbed me and held me tight, so I couldn't. I cried for the longest time, curled up in a ball on the couch. I couldn't believe he'd left me again! My daddy didn't love me enough to stay. From that moment on, I believed I wasn't good enough and decided I wasn't worthy of love!

Six months later, my dad pulled up in our driveway in an old Volkswagen van. He'd sold everything out West and had come home to stay. I vowed in my heart to do whatever I could to ensure that he didn't leave again.

As a home-coming gift, my dad gave me a beautiful white jewellery box, lined with red satin. I neatly arranged the few earrings I had along the top row, and placed some trinkets in the bottom. I loved it! Curious, I snuck into my sister's room to see what hers contained. Although she'd had one for years I never took much interest. Just as I lifted the lid enough to catch a glimpse of the pretty things inside, Susan came in and caught me. After explaining myself, I left thinking everything was cool! Apparently, it wasn't! Minutes later, Dad came to my door demanding that I hand over my jewellery box. Grabbing it out of my hands, he shook it up and down and then threw it up against the wall.

"That will teach you to go into your sister's things!" he yelled. I quickly ran over, picked it up from where it had landed and sat on the edge of my bed sobbing in bewilderment. Were all fathers this angry and violent? Was I bad? I now feared doing the wrong thing. The last thing I wanted to do was upset him or others. Another part of my heart died that day.

One day at school, one particularly bright girl taunted me during recess, saying, "You may be good at sports, Nancy, but being smart is what's important! You're stupid!" This started after my teacher embarrassed me in front of the entire class because I hadn't done my speech assignment according to her expectations. I did it about birds in a creative storytelling method which, in her eyes, was unacceptable for grade five. The three years she taught my class felt like an eternity! I was convinced she hated me. Over time, I began to believe the insults hurled at me, which increased my shame and lack of self-worth.

Numerous times during my school years several different friends stole from me. I learned to trust no one! I was extremely skeptical and questioned everyone's motives, as well as my value as a friend.

It's customary each year for grade eight graduation, for the teachers to select students for specific awards. My teacher asked the class who they thought should win the athletic award. Most of the kids called out my name. The award was to be based on whoever made the most teams in combination with whoever had the best ability. I was the only girl on every team, which included gymnastics and cheerleading. If all went according to the rules, I would be the winner! As I sat anxiously waiting for the announcement, the boy behind me leaned over and suggested that I go ahead and get up because it was obvious that I had won. I anxiously waited in my seat. My name was not called. They'd chosen someone else! I felt robbed! In high school, my gym teacher continuously begged me to join the sports teams, but I refused! Instead, I joined the cheerleading team! I was finally popular and loved the attention I received!

My father's temper seemed to flare up from time to time. We just never knew what would set him off. His very presence intimidated me, yet at times, he resembled a big, lovable, teddy bear. Once when I had several friends over after church on a Sunday, my father grabbed my mother by the scruff of her sweater and dragged her across the dining room table and punched her in the face for making a comment about money that he didn't like. Dad stood yelling at her in front of the picture window, while mom held the side of her face.

"I think my jaw is broken," she cried. He grabbed her arm to coax her towards the basement stairs.

"Let go of me. I'm not going over there! You just want to throw me down the stairs," she sobbed as she struggled to break her arm free. My mind filled with fear as I recalled the story I'd heard about his attempt to choke her to death. Adrenaline surged through my veins. My body thrust out of the chair and over in front of them. I burned with rage. With clenched fists, I leaned forward and yelled in his face.

"You take your hands off my mother right now." I screamed. One of the neighbours across the street ran through the ditch with a frying pan in our defence. While I ran to the neighbour's house, my sister called our pastor and within minutes, he and his wife arrived to help work things out. Things seemed to settle down, but I remained unsettled in my heart. I feared his retaliation and worried about what he thought of me because I came to my mother's aid and I avoided him as much as possible.

My journey through life for years represented one who walks on broken glass with tender, bare, feet. My family never again discussed what happened that day, nor acknowledged or expressed their emotions.

As a teenager, my dad told me that he never wanted me, that I was a product of a night of too much alcohol and that my mother basically tricked him into getting her pregnant. He said the original plan for building such a large family home was so that his parents could eventually come to live with them and implied that my mother stopped this from happening by ensuring all the bedrooms were occupied. These words embedded themselves into my heart, leaving me feeling even more rejected and unworthy. I gravitated to anyone who would accept me, even when they were verbally abusive. I naturally put up with it, thinking I deserved that type of treatment! I always viewed myself through the abuse and mistakes I'd made. This caused me to constantly strive to earn God's forgiveness. I worried all the time and in the process developed a bleeding ulcer.

I always had a boyfriend because I needed someone to help me feel good about myself; although I never really believed I was likeable. After about five years into a certain relationship, I began to have flashbacks about the abuse. I told my boyfriend, hoping to receive some sympathy. Instead, he became angry with me and told me it must have been my fault. Around this same time, another girl came to live with us in Morrisburg. She had been molested and raped by her two brothers and then was kicked out of the house by her father, after telling someone. My own father remarked that she probably asked for it by teasing them with her breasts and most likely enjoyed it! How could I ever tell what happened to me, when my own father held this type of attitude? I learned to suppress my feelings and feared that all men believed women were only good for one thing: sex! I started to believe that my abuse must have somehow been my fault and that I deserved to be punished. In anger, I often punched myself in the head or pulled on my hair until I got a headache.

The Bible says that whatever we believe in our hearts will become as truth to us (Proverbs 23:7). That is why Satan will work overtime to implant lies into our minds, during the hurtful times, to cause deception. The lies hold power over us until they're broken, because we act on what we believe. If we believe these lies, they will always take precedence over the truth, until we recognize them and replace them with the truth. If the Bible tells us to guard our hearts, how can we do this without placing up walls? The answer is revealed in Proverbs 4:20–22, which tells us to meditate on God's Word. It contains directions for every situation we face. When we do this, it trains our hearts with truth and in return, retrains our thinking patterns and therefore guards our hearts! This is imperative because our heart determines the outcome of our lives.

"Above all else, guard your heart, for it is the wellspring of life." (Proverbs 4:23)

I built walls of self-protection and had difficulty establishing healthy boundaries in relationships. When others didn't honour the boundaries I'd set, I'd secretively get angry with them for not respecting me and furious with myself for not speaking up about it. Because I felt so guilty about my past, I tried to make up for it by becoming extremely good. I became a perfectionist and a people-pleaser to ensure everything around me stayed safe and secure; to not allow others the opportunity to reject me again. Addicted to people's approval, I put others' needs before my own and even my family's, thinking I was doing the right thing. Just because something is good, doesn't mean it is God's will for you. It took me a long time to realize that. We need to be true to God and ourselves and honest about our feelings with self and others before committing to things. If we'd take the needed time to pray about matters beforehand, we'd save ourselves from a great deal of hurt and confusion!

Part of my struggle with perfectionism led me to believe that I also had to be the perfect size, so in my late teens I started skipping meals whenever I could and sometimes purged. Even as an adult, I walked on eggshells with everyone for fear that my world would crash around me. I kept people at arm's length and controlled situations the best I could.

The fact is, people are human and we all make mistakes. We need to trust God to protect us and ask Him to heal our hurts when bad things happen. Sometimes we question whether others have ulterior or wrong motives. Only God knows people's hearts and the complete story behind all things. Only God has the right to judge. By judging others, we open hurtful doors for ourselves because when we judge, we are judged in the same manner (Matthew 7:1–3). Let me encourage you to take down the self–protective walls and trust the Lord to protect you and ask God to work within the hearts of others. When you feel as if their motives are wrong, ask God to be your vindicator. He will! God has a purpose for our lives and we each have a destiny to fulfill. If we get hurt along the way, which we will because that's just part of life, God will heal those hurts if we allow Him too. Sometimes it's a daily struggle to keep the walls down and to trust God to protect me, but it's much easier when I put it in His hands.

In the fall of 2004, a huge emotional bomb dropped on our family again! My mom and dad separated again, after forty–seven years of marriage. Although, they'd had their ups and downs, I couldn't believe it! I took responsibility for this on my own shoulders. Regardless of my age, I thought as many children do, that somehow it must have been my fault! My father had confided in me that he planned to go through the motions of marriage counselling and that no matter how long it took, he would wait until the therapist told them to get a divorce. This way, he would get what he wanted without looking like the bad guy. Naturally, I wanted to protect my mother from enduring any more pain, so I told her. My father belittled me for telling her and implied that their break–up was my fault. Of course I wanted to protect her because she had faithfully looked after me from day one! My father seemed cheerful about the entire break–up, while my mother wept endlessly and I wrestled with guilt. It was difficult for me as I watched her struggle. She had stood by my father through many difficult times and to me it seemed like all was for nothing! She now had to leave her home and give up her dog.

I helped my mother pack her possessions and move them into storage, as well as look for an apartment and house-hunt. I made her burdens my burdens and resented the lack of help from others. As I grew tired and stressed from the pressure, repressed anger and guilt began to percolate within me. Thoughts and fears that my father would shut the family out of his life again brought the feelings of abandon-ment flooding back into my soul. The scabs off past wounds started to ooze. The statement I had heard Joyce Meyer use many times, "Nothing buried alive ever dies," became a reality! The issues we repress will re-surface one way or another, whether in attitude, deed, addiction or sick-ness!

"See to it that no one misses the grace of God and that no bitter root grows up to cause trouble and defile many." (Hebrews 12:15)

How does this verse pertain to our lives? Our bitterness can cause trouble in our lives and cause other people to sin because of our bitter-ness. God's grace gives us the ability to react to situations with mercy. When we stuff issues down and ignore them, bitter roots form in our heart. We react out of those bitter roots and defile our relationships and situations with our sinful attitudes. Whereas when we are merciful, bit-ter roots are unable to form and are unable to destroy our relationships or lives.

"Honour your father and your mother, as the Lord your God has commanded you, so that you may live long and that it may go well with you in the land the Lord your God is giving you." (Deuteronomy 5:16)

The Bible clearly states that we are to honour our parents and when we don't, things will not go smoothly! The scales finally dropped off my eyes as God's Word penetrated my heart. I hadn't honoured my father. Honour means to esteem highly and to speak well of, and I had not done that. I finally recognized how bitter and angry I'd been towards my father. I needed to stop rehashing past hurts and injustices and stop picking the scabs off the wounds that God was trying to heal. God began revealing things to me. My father was harshly disciplined as a child and was sent off to boarding school, while his sister was highly valued, and a great amount of time, effort, and money were put into developing her skills. He developed schizophrenia as a young adult and just couldn't cope. He felt he had no choice other than to leave. I gave my dad what I felt was a heartfelt letter expressing my love about how I forgave him for everything that had happened. I opened up about my fears, hurts and how his abandonment and their break-up had affected me. Crushed by my letter, he sealed it up and vowed to never to look at it again. My letter had backfired. What I thought would bring healing in our relationship had brought about more pain. Several weeks later, he decided he owed it to himself and his children to reread it. His reaction gave me the understanding that he truly had no idea the impact his decisions had on our lives. All his choices were made through the eyes of his pain and its perception. I know he never meant to hurt us. We can all get a little self-absorbed when things are rough. Unfortunately some people reside in that place. Do you ever lose thought of how your actions affect others? Millions of people live with regret about the decisions they've made. We surely appreciate hindsight. It's time to give some people the benefit of the doubt! I needed to think positively, knowing my father truly didn't have the ability to love within himself to give at that time. If parents are wounded themselves, they aren't able to call their children to life as God intended.[1] They can't give away something that they haven't received themselves. He was hurting on the inside himself and didn't know how to be any other way. I needed to repent for all the ungodly responses and judgments I'd made towards my father. With the help of the Holy Spirit, prayer, repentance, and forgiveness I'm finally able to separate my father's sickness from the person he is. It's a good thing, because one day I'll stand before God's throne, the same as everyone else, and give account for my own actions, no one else's! We're responsible for our responses regardless of what others have done to us.

Do you honour your father and mother or are you critical, pointing out their faults or commenting on what you would do differently? Why is it that we are to place our parents in a status of honour? God appointed them to be our parents for a reason. It was His doing, and to question that would be like saying God doesn't know what He's doing. God detests grumbling and complaining, especially when we rebel against authority (Romans 13:1, 2). The Israelites spent 40 years wandering in the wilderness because of this very reason. A trip that should have taken only 11 days! If we want to receive blessing, we need to place our parents in a position of honour and keep them there. I am not saying to idolize them—only God is to be worshipped and nothing and no one else should ever take God's place! You might be thinking, "Oh no, that's too hard, you have no idea what I went through as a child." I understand and realize that not everyone had it rosy! Some parents are better than others, but no one is perfect. We need to extend grace and forgiveness to them for the mistakes they've made and choose to bless them with honour for their strengths and for the right choices they've made. Be thankful for the positive aspects they've brought to your life and choose to make changes in the areas you wished were different. This helps stop the cycle of repeating similar mistakes.

We often think it's our job to make people pay for what they've done. We feel justified, don't we? I agree that sometimes circumstances aren't fair. Jesus knows all about that! We're all sinners! It wasn't fair that Jesus had to be nailed to the cross for our sins either and yet He willingly laid down His life anyway. Who had the greater price to pay? James 2:13 warns us to be merciful because those who judge without showing mercy will not be shown mercy themselves. It also tells us that mercy always triumphs over judgment! Are you ready to give a little mercy?

My dad has some wonderful qualities and has done many honourable things. Coming back to set things straight after leaving and having to face people after the mistakes he made took amazing strength. It wasn't easy for him either! My dad has expressed that he is now thankful for each child and loves each one of us. I truly love my dad with all my heart. I like to visit him whenever I can. He's getting older now, so I like to help him with errands and chores. That's how you honour a father! We all have good traits; search for them in others, take note, and honour them for those things.

I'm sure there are many who have experienced similar stories of parental abuse, neglect or abandonment and haven't had the luxury of their relationship being restored. Perhaps you're adopted, or your parents just aren't interested. My heart truly goes out to you. Don't be discouraged, you do have a parent that truly loves you. Your Heavenly Father is interested and always will be. He promises that even when our earthly parents reject us, He is there to receive us. For it says in Psalm 27:10, "*Though my father and mother forsake me, the Lord will receive me.*"

Our lives were far from picture-perfect growing up, but mom did the best she could at the time. I admire her for that; she really is an amazing woman. Now that I have my own children, I realize how challenging and frustrating it can be sometimes with all of life's demands, especially when I'm tired. Even though she was gone a lot when we were little, she always had our best interest in mind. Single parents deserve a huge pat on the back! It's not an easy lifestyle; one many wish they didn't have. After dad returned, mom made up for lost time and spent as much time as she could with us, volunteering at our kids' clubs and youth group meetings. She even got me a tutor for chemistry when I was in high school. Unfortunately, it was a lost cause because I still was unwilling to try!

Recently, some teachers and students from my old high school organized and put on a cancer fundraiser. I was asked, along with other local survivors, to walk a victory lap around the school track to kick-start their event. We waited at the reception area until the event started and then crowded in front of a platform to hear a guest speaker. My chin dropped when they announced and welcomed to the platform the teacher who humiliated me in school. Right away I thought, *"oh great"*! I felt resentment rise within, but as I listened to her story about her own pain and suffering, the bitter feeling I had melted away like ice on a hot summer day. God gave me empathy and a new respect for her. It was as though He whispered to my heart, "she too is human." Her initial mistake tainted my every view. Could it be possible that she intended to be encouraging the times I perceived her as criticizing? When she corrected me, was it out of compassion rather than dislike? Perhaps she wanted me to fulfill my potential, something I couldn't see for myself! I, as well, would have been frustrated with someone who didn't listen or try! Most teachers want their students to excel and do well in their classes. Perhaps some have lost sight of the reasons why they started and their passion to make a difference. They need our prayers more than ever. The children in today's society are faced with more than we ever were. This teacher was the same one I had dreamt about giving my favourite pink hat to on the bus. I could now see that giving her the pink hat was a symbol of peace! A healing had taken place in my soul. When we judge situations from one view, we allow unnecessary hurt into our lives.

My abuser came to me and asked for forgiveness when I was a teenager. God had gotten a hold of his life, convicted his heart, and drew him into repentance. I said yes then but, honestly, it took years for my feelings to completely fall into place. However, even if he hadn't changed, I needed to forgive him for my own sake! Unforgiveness will eat away at your soul like a cancer. I went to counselling before I had children because I wanted to make sure I had dealt with this issue properly. I didn't give it much time because I didn't think I had a problem. My abuser himself was a victim of abuse and was wacked out on drugs when he was hurting me. He, too, had a great amount of hurt in his life. It's no excuse, but it helped bring understanding. Even though I forgave, it wasn't until after I had cancer that I realized I'd never dealt with my emotions. You see, I was numb and didn't even know they existed!

After having my own children, I realized that kids say a lot of things they don't necessarily mean, even though their words are hurtful. Many times, the insults they hurl reflect how they feel about themselves and are not about you at all! For example, in grade five during winter carnival, we had an arm wrestling contest: girls against girls and boys against boys. After winning first place in the girls division, somebody decided that I should compete against the winning boy. Feeling very confident, I agreed, competed, and won! For the longest time, the boy razed me and called me "brute". As an adult, I have the ability to reason and see how it must have made him feel to lose to a girl and how it probably tarnished his reputation as a tough guy. At the time, I never once gave that any thought. I only took his words to heart. Let's face it, when we're kids, it's all about us. Some adults still haven't gotten past that. The girl who insulted my intelligence did have two left feet and was likely trying to make herself feel better about not being athletic. It's good to be able to understand situations from another person's perspective and may even remove a layer of its painful sting. However, I want to caution you in this. Ignoring your true feeling will not fix things. Reasoning and justifying others' actions may be part of the forgiveness process, but you must also allow the "hurt child" within you to be healed by God, to experience true healing. Otherwise you'll continue to walk around in life with actions based on the old lies from these painful memories, still compelled by the remaining suppressed emotions. The brokenness we experience as a child still remains as truth until dealt with. We must come to God as that broken child and express our fears, anger, disappointment, and whatever other emotion we've bottled up inside to be healed completely. Until you acknowledge and express your feelings and then forgive and release, you will be unable to move forward as the whole person God intended you to be. Instead, you are left wandering through life aimlessly trying to cope and wade through past garbage that weighs you down. Like luggage, this baggage can be seen by others because it comes out in our attitudes and behaviour. It colors how we see and experience life. During prayer, we must allow ourselves to go back into that memory to feel and express our emotions. See yourself as that child. Tell the other person how they made you feel. Express your anger by yelling or hitting a pillow or crying if sad until there aren't any tears left to cry. Ask Jesus where He was at that moment and allow Him to heal the hurt that comes with the memory and to replace any still-believed lies with the truth. Jesus will give you a picture in your mind that will act as a healing ointment for your mind and heart. When I did this, I saw a picture of God's tears washing over me from heaven above and He gave me a Scripture that says He weeps when we weep and collects our tears in a bottle. God really does care about you! Tell Him to take the hurt and pour in His healing power and peace instead. Will you come to Jesus and allow Him to heal your inner child? Don't allow the sting from others' words or actions continue to mold the way you see yourself any longer! The picture of your future doesn't have to be framed by your past. There isn't anything that others have said or done to you that God can't heal. Give God a chance to change your future by letting Him redeem your past! He promises in Isaiah 61 to give you beauty for ashes and the oil of joy instead of mourning. He loves you and wants you to enjoy your life to the fullest!

Permitting your inner child to forgive is a crucial step that you must take to experience complete healing. Some people have great difficulty with this because they think that by forgiving the other person, they're letting their offender off the hook. They believe that by staying angry they're serving revenge and punishing the other person for what they've done, while in retrospect, the only person they're punishing is themselves. Forgiveness is an active choice or decision you make in your mind that releases you from a prison, a place of constant torture in your mind. Forgiving an offender doesn't justify what they've done. They are still accountable before God. This allows God to work on your behalf by putting Him in control to make things right. Trust me, forgiving is for your sake! Matthew 6:14–15 says, *"For if you forgive men when they sin against you, your heavenly Father will also forgive you. But if you do not forgive men their sins, your Father will not forgive your sins."* Yes, you may find this difficult. You may even have to forgive them many times over as instructed in Matthew 18:21, but eventually your feelings will line up with your decision, as you are obedient to God's Word and pray for those who have hurt or persecuted you.

"After Job had prayed for his friends, the Lord made him prosperous again and gave him twice as much as he had before." (Job 42:10)

Job was a man familiar to great suffering. One day he was the wealthiest and most prosperous man in the land of Uz and the next he lost everything, including his ten children. In great mourning, he cut himself with broken pottery and sat in the ashes. At first, his friends were sympathetic and came to sit with him, saying nothing for seven days. As time went on, they began to argue and insult him relentlessly, saying he must have sinned against the Lord for such trouble to happen. Job continued to have the right attitude and remained faithful, never cursing God or his friends. His walk was blameless and upright out of his love for the Lord. Job did what was right by pressing past the emotional pain his friends had caused him and prayed for them. In doing so, God blessed him two–fold for the trouble he endured.

We've all experienced some sort of pain at the hands of others. If you'd like to turn your situation around, pray for those who have hurt you! Remember that remaining blameless means watching your tongue. Don't pray for someone and then turn around and gossip about them. That would be like tying your prayers up in knots. Give the situation to God and allow Him to work on your behalf.

I have to admit, I struggled with sharing my story in fear that it wasn't honouring others. However, God clearly showed me that we're to honour Him by telling others our story when it is done with a pure heart (Psalm 107:2). If we're telling to devalue another person, then that's wrong. We are to acknowledge what God has done for us by saying, "yes this happened, but look what God has done for me and how He has healed me. We aren't honouring our parents by bottling up our feelings, hiding them, and then acting like nothing ever happened.

We need to learn to honour ourselves by being true to ourselves. In return, this is honouring God as well. Then be sure to take your issues to God to be healed. Don't brush matters off and pretend they're no big deal. They are! If something crushes your spirit and makes you sad, you can be sure it hurts God's heart too. Journaling is a great way to connect with your true feelings; it connects what is going on in your head to your heart. It even brings relief. Again, I want to emphasize, if you feel hurt, sad, angry, etc, say so. Write out your feelings on paper. This will reveal your spirit's belief system and will help you recognize unhealthy patterns. Ask God to heal these areas and retrain the way you think. God will heal your thoughts and feelings as you forgive. He can't change the past, but He can change your future by healing your pain.

Sometimes, we can't even see our own bitterness until others point this out.[2] Even then, sometimes we can't see it because the enemy has blinded us spiritually. We give him access through our sins of unforgiveness. It takes God's grace to open our eyes. We must bind the enemy, in Jesus' name and loose the truth in, in Jesus' name by praying these very words (Matthew 16:19). It is the Holy Spirit who opens our eyes to the truth. God plants seeds of truth in our hearts and waters them until they grow big enough for us to see. It is only with God's help that we can recognize the lies of the enemy and see the truth. When we finally recognize this, we're then able to deal with the situation appropriately by giving it to God. There will be times when people hurt or anger you and when they do, it's important to confront them, rather than let these issues fester. If we don't get things out in the open and express ourselves, it's likely that we will become angry, bitter, and then resentful (Matthew 18:21–35).[3]

Studies show that unresolved issues can cause sickness! Dr. Carolyn Leaf, author of "Who Switched Off My Brain?" educates the public about how toxic emotions cause approximately 87% of sickness. What I understood from Dr. Leaf's book and hearing her speak is that our brains form thorny trees like pathways where negative thinking patterns have developed through wounding. Negative or toxic emotions release toxic chemicals. Over time, shadows develop on the brain and cause the body to break down where these shadows correspond in relation to the body. Certain parts of the brain control certain organs. Cancer cells or tumours will actually stop growing when these issues are dealt with. The brain can repair these pathways through steps of forgiveness and by altering our thinking patterns within four days by thinking positive thoughts.[4]

Many people who are bitter become spiteful and want to take revenge. To experience true healing, we must first recognize our feelings, learn to express them and then give them to God.[5] We also need to take the next step to forgive and release each wrong and hurt, so we can enjoy the freedom that comes from God's forgiveness (see Matt 18:21–25).[6]

Scores of people stuff issues down inside their hearts and forget about them. I did, thinking it was the "Christian thing" to do. By doing this, we can delay our own healing and hurt others and ourselves in the process.[7] Signs of unresolved problems will spring up later as anger flare–ups, depression or sickness. Sometimes people form addictions such as shopping, sex, food, drugs and alcohol, etc., in an attempt to cover their pain or comfort themselves. Individuals may become anorexic or bulimic as a means to find some type of control in their lives.

Sometimes we take offense to things that others say because of our past wounding and judgments we have made in those situations, depending on how we expect to be treated. We each have a root system in which we receive from our surroundings, nurture from God, others, nature and ourselves.[8] Studies have shown that we receive our root system in the first six years of life.[9]Our root system, which is our spirit, learns either to receive goodness or not. A bitterroot causes someone to drink harm, regardless of how it was meant to be taken, whether in action or in word. John and Paula Sandford explain bitterroot expectancy in their video, "Healing Life's Hurts", as a psychological device within us that defiles others by projecting signals to others of the way we expect to be treated.[10] For example: Perhaps a child feels one sibling is favoured over them and in result their expectation causes the parent to show the other sibling extra special treatment. It may also color the way we see or hear things. Someone may give a person a compliment about how nice they look that day and instead, they take it as an insult, thinking: *"What was wrong with the way I looked yesterday?"* This is how bitterroots can defile. According to the Nelson Canadian Dictionary, defile means: "1. To make filthy or dirty; pollute. 2. To debase the pureness or excellence of; corrupt."[11] These bitterroots cause one's words or intentions to be debased, rather than taken for their true intention and value!

God began to reveal to me all the bitterroot judgments and ungodly beliefs I had made. I didn't realize that when someone hurt me, I actually made an ungodly belief and judged that the person would always treat me in a hurtful way. For it says in Matthew 9:29b, *"According to your faith will it be done to you."* Whatever we believe happens in our lives. I always believed I would be mistreated and, in the process, I was. That's why it is so important that we are aware of what we are thinking and choose to think on the positive side of circumstances. This is done by guarding our hearts with faith, hope, and love.

We need to know the truth in God's Word about ourselves and believe it as truth! We also need to reject all the lies the enemy tries to tell us. Philippians 4:8 tells us to think on whatever is true, noble, right, pure, lovely, admirable, anything that is excellent and of good report. If it's not positive, discard it!

Because of the rejection I endured as a child and the bitterroots I had developed, it didn't matter what people said or did to encourage me. I was unable to receive the good or positive from it. My brokenness had become my new truth. I took on guilt and shame and thought I wasn't worthy when others did something nice. I was skeptical with everyone and assumed they wanted something from me!

Bitterroot judgments and expectations operate on the law of sowing and reaping. When someone has hurt us, we tend to make a judgment, expecting them to treat us a certain way.[12]When we have sin that we have not confessed and repented of, whether as a child or an adult, we later reap from the judgments we have made.[13] Have you ever wondered why certain things keep happening to you? We sin when we judge, and end up doing the same things we judge others for. We need to be so careful because, in times of pain, we tend to judge those who have hurt us, without even realizing it (see Matthew 7:1–2; Hosea 8:7a; Galatians 6:7).

Seeds of rejection were planted at a young age because of being abandoned by my father. I became bitter because of unforgiveness, which in turn formed a root system that caused me to expect to be rejected by my father and others. I put great time and effort into pleasing him and others, to gain attention and acceptance, yet he seemed only to notice and affirm others. This just added to my anger and frustration and wore me out in the process. There were times my father did bless me, but all I could focus on were the times he blessed others. People who are hurting often hurt others in the process. In times of hurt, we make inner vows that act as walls to prevent others from hurting us again. Even if we aren't aware of this, our subconscious still remembers and acts on them. This is why people do the strangest things. If we are unaware of the inner vows we have made, the truth is only a simple prayer away.

all the time? Eventually, people get worn out feeling they can never add up and they move on to other relationships where they can relate better. Perhaps you feel as if no one ever listens to you. This can form an ungodly expectation that causes others not to listen and often creates a vow in your own heart to block out others. Are there certain hurts in your life that happen over and over again? Below are a few questions that may bring some situations to mind:

- Have you been rejected and refuse to allow others into your heart by forming walls of self protection? Are you self-reliant, distant or a perfectionist?

- Have you failed at something in the past and vowed never to try again?

- Were you ridiculed for crying as a child? Have you vowed not to show emotion?

- Do you always think of yourself as a victim? Do you think everyone is always out to get you, that life challenges will never get easier?

- Were you harshly disciplined as a child and as a result avoid disciplining your own?

It doesn't matter what vow you have made, there is a simple prayer you can pray to break the effects of negative beliefs and change any inner vows into healthy expectations. Ask the Lord to reveal to you the areas where you suffer with bitterness, anger, and resentment, along with what vows you have made. Get a paper and pen to write down the issues and the names of those involved. This will provide an easy reference while praying the healing prayers below. As you sit quietly, God will bring issues to mind. He may reveal these judgments and vows through your circumstances as the week progresses, so keep a notepad handy. Note: Bitterroot judgments, expectations, and inner-vows are the sins we commit when others hurt or wrong us. Misunderstandings can also result from misperception. To experience full freedom, we must ask for forgiveness as well as forgive others for what they've done.

Dear Heavenly Father,

I give You permission to dismantle every lie and replace it with the truth. Bring to my mind all bitterroot judgments, expectations, and inner vows that I have made to confess and repent of them, that I may enjoy healing in my life. In Jesus' name I pray. Amen.

Negative Beliefs

Dear Heavenly Father,

Please forgive me for forming judgments and negative beliefs towards You, others, myself, and even institutions. Please forgive me for judging _____ (name), for _____ (specific judgment). I choose to forgive, release, and bless _____ (name), for their involvement in forming these negative beliefs and myself for believing these lies. I renounce my old reactions to my past in Jesus' name and choose to respond the way God wants me to. Grant me the faith, strength, and discernment to believe the truth. In Jesus' name I pray. Amen.

Renouncing Inner Vows

Dear Heavenly Father,

I acknowledge and ask forgiveness of my sin of vowing that _____. I forgive, release, and bless _____ (names), for hurting me. Please forgive me and dismantle all the ungodly inner vows I have made. Lead me by Your Holy Spirit to be and do all that You've called me to. In Jesus' name, I renounce the inner vow that _____ (be spe-

cific). I forgive myself for making this vow and _____ (name those involved) for their involvement. I renounce all bitterroot judgments, expectations, and vows in the name of Jesus and ask You to uproot them. I declare that I'm blessed and no longer bound by them. I now choose to be led by the power of Your Holy Spirit to follow Your Word. In Jesus' name I pray. Amen.

Find out what the Bible says about your situation and meditate on that truth! We need to know the truth of God's Word so we can recognize the lies Satan tries to implant in our minds.

God began to open doors for me to speak and share my testimony. As I prepared my message for one particular church, I felt God press upon my heart to share about my abuse. At that point, I wasn't really comfortable with it. I struggled with the thought until God gave me a vision of a beautiful, young, blonde lady who was tormented by unforgiveness and hatred. She had been sexually abused by someone in authority over her as a teen. I knew right then that God had a divine purpose in which He would redeem the suffering I had endured. My calling was to help others. After the service, many people approached me with similar stories and expressed how God opened their spiritual hearts and eyes about how they needed to forgive and let go of the injustices done to them. They allowed God to remove the bitterness, anger, and resentment, as well as let go of the self–pity they were wallowing in. As I walked across the parking lot to leave, I heard a female voice call me.

"Nancy, can I have a minute of your time?" She asked, as she gently grabbed my elbow. I quickly turned my head to see who was talking to me. Amazed, I stood staring into the face of the very young lady I'd had the vision of!

Standing next to her van, she poured her heart out to me for almost an hour. She wasn't sure if she could forgive the man who violated her and caused her so much pain. She suffered from bitterness, anger, resentment, shame, and self-hatred. This, I believe, was the beginning of her healing journey. Thank God for His grace! She has since received prayer counselling and is well on her way to freedom. If you're at the same point as this young lady and aren't quite sure if you can ever forgive, I believe that if you ask God to help you forgive, He will bring about a change in your heart until you are able to reach the next step. I've heard numerous people say, "If we don't forgive, it's like drinking poison and hoping the other person will die." We are hurting ourselves by holding on to unforgiveness. I understand all about wanting justice! We must keep in mind that we reap what we sow, and if we want mercy, we have to give it! Are there people in your life that you need to forgive? Have you blamed God for the negative things that have happened in your life, not realizing that His plans are only for your good and not for your harm (Jeremiah 29:11)? Do you blame yourself for past mistakes or things gone wrong? If you would like to experience the freedom that forgiveness has to offer, please say the following prayer.

Prayers of Forgiveness

Dear Heavenly Father,

Thank You for sending Jesus to die for my sins; I realize to be forgiven I must first forgive. Please give me the strength to let go of the injustices made against me, to be merciful, that I may obtain mercy. I choose to forgive _____ (name) for_____ (be specific). I release and bless those who have hurt me so that I may receive a blessing. Please be my vindicator by working in their hearts and draw them into repentance. I ask you to forgive me for my ungodly attitude, words, bitterness, anger, and resentment (etc). Forgive me for judging _____ (name) for _____ (be specific) and therefore allowing a place for the enemy to wreak havoc in my life. I renounce all bitterroot judgments and expectations and ask You to release me from the reaping and the sowing of the judgments I have made in these areas. In Jesus' name I pray. Amen.

Soul Attachments

We are created by God to be in relationships, first with Him and then with others. Our souls bond in the spiritual realm with one another by ties. These ties act as roots that either feed or disperse positive or negative spiritual energy to or from our souls. For example: when people say or do positive things to us, this creates healthy soul attachments, but when negative events or words take place, a negative spiritual soul attachment is created. This happens in abusive, violent, controlling, dominating, manipulating or fear-based relationships. God warns us, in the Bible, to choose our friends wisely that we may have healthy connections because our souls knit together with others, when we are in relationships. In 1 Samuel 18:1 it says, *"After David had finished talking with Saul, Jonathan became one in spirit with David, and he loved him as himself."* David had a healthy soul tie with King Saul's son Jonathon. Genesis 15:18a shows us that we can also have a soul tie with God: *"On that day the Lord made covenant with Abram and said..."*

God created each of us with our own body, soul, and spirit. Our soul consists of our mind, will, and emotions. Our body is our physical container that houses all three and is physically affected when either our soul and or spirit is broken. Symptoms manifest as a way of telling us something's wrong. Your "spirit", the real "you", never sleeps. We are connected to God by our spirit; when our spirit is broken, that connection we have with Him becomes blocked. It was God's intention for a man and woman to come together after marriage, not before. Their bodies fit together as one, as an act of worship and a symbol of their love.

This act not only joins them together in body but also in spirit. That is why God said the two shall become one (Mark 10:8). Sex is a gift from God to bring a husband and wife together in unity (relational). God created everything good, including sex. Everything we do God's way is a form of worship to Him. Anything we do outside of God's will is worship to the devil. This opens a door in our lives for the demonic. Sex outside of marriage can damage a person's spirit.

Take a woman, for example. Sex connects a woman emotionally to a man. Every woman needs to feel protected by her man. When they come together, a spiritual bond is created. If that relationship ends, she feels betrayed. Men are also vulnerable, but tend to be more logical and were created with the instinct to protect. When the relationship ends, he is wounded by having his sense of purpose crushed. Would people consent to this if they knew it also wounded their spirit? The world's view is twisted from God's view and order. They don't know or understand the things of God because they don't see or recognize the consequences for their actions due to spiritual blindness. They feed on instant gratification, think it's normal and many times don't consider how decisions will affect their spirits! When sex happens outside the covenant of marriage, it can cause division. The wounded parts of a person's spirit inhibit the spiritual flow to properly allow the couple to give and receive within the relationships, including their relationship with God.

When people have sex outside of marriage, unhealthy soul ties bond people together. Their soul binds together with every sexual partner they've ever had. I Corinthians 6:16 validates this point. It says, *"Do you not know that he who unites himself with a prostitute is one with her in body? For it is said, "The two will become one flesh."* Doing things outside of Gods plan opens a person's life up to the curse, rather than the blessing. God created the act of sex to signify the marriage covenant. Technically, that means every person someone has had sex with is their spouse in God's eyes. Picture yourself on your wedding day. The minister pronounces you husband and wife and you've just kissed the man of your dreams. You're trying to walk down the aisle but you're having difficulty because everyone you've ever slept with is linked to your arm and everyone they've been intimate with is linked to theirs. But that's not all, on your other arm, your spouse is dragging alongside everyone he's ever slept with and they're linked to other people as well. Did you realize that a parade (of spiritual attachments) packed itself for your honeymoon? This bondage will hinder your soul and marriage until you ask God to cut off each attachment.

Some people believe that if they marry the person they've had sex with, then it makes everything okay. This is a deception from Satan that robs a couple from experiencing the joy and completeness of being one. Sex before marriage is sin and until it is confessed and repented of, it will affect and hinder the blessings in their lives, whether they're married or not. Humans were created as spiritual beings to have spiritual connection with God; our sin hinders that connection. When we repent of our sin, that connection is restored and healed. Our unconfessed sin gives Satan legal right and access into our lives and the lives of our children until we break that bond by confessing and repenting of our sin. Jesus can heal our spirit if we confess, repent, and receive this forgiveness. Once we find healing for our mind, will, and emotions, our body will heal as well. It is important to remember what Christ has already done for us on Calvary.

Say the prayer below for each attachment you need to sever. After you do, you will feel lighter and have more freedom in the bedroom! Trust me, it works! This is effective with abuse situations or any type of previous relationships.

Dear Heavenly Father,

Please forgive me for my part in forming unhealthy soul attachments. Please forgive me of my sin of fornication/adultery _____ (be specific). Lord, cut all ungodly soul attachments with _____ (name). Please remove anything unholy that came into my spirit through this attachment and bring restoration. In Jesus' name I pray. Amen.

Note: God will sever a soul attachment when we ask. Remember God created people with free will. He doesn't control them or us in how we'll handle or react regarding future confrontations.

Soul Attachment Prayer for Abuse, rape etc.

Dear Heavenly Father,

Please forgive me for holding bitterness, anger and resentment towards _____ (name) for _____ (be specific). By the power of Your Holy Spirit, I forgive and release _____ (name) for _____ (be specific). Lord, cut all ungodly soul attachments with _____ (name). Please remove anything unholy that came into my spirit through this attachment and bring restoration. In Jesus' name I pray. Amen.

Rejection

Because our spirit always perceives and never sleeps, the wounds of rejection can damage a child's spirit even while in the womb. We are given our spirit by God at the moment of conception. Research reveals that when the egg and sperm come together at conception, a spark ignites.[15] Studies have also proven that the unborn fetus can sense outside sources of stress.[16] They are also calmed by relaxing music and recognize and respond to their parent's voice.[17] God's Word promises that even in times of rejection, He will always be there for us (*Psalm 27:10*)!

There are countless people suffering on the inside because of rejection for many reasons. Life has turned into a vicious cycle of broken people hurting others as a result. You may not have been an unwanted child, but everyone has suffered some form of rejection at one time. Have you allowed that rejection to wound your spirit? Has it coloured the way you see yourself, controlled and shaped your life? Have your created self–protective walls? We act out of these depending on what's in us.

Jesus wants to heal your spirit and make your life whole. Are you ready to take that step? If so, take your hurts to Him. God already knows, but you need to get it off your chest for your own sake. Start by telling Him who hurt you and what they did. Acknowledge how you feel, tell Him your deepest hurts by expressing your full emotions. Do you feel betrayed, angry, sad, rejected, unloved, unworthy or dirty? Let it all out! Facing the pain will bring healing! Once you feel the full release, it's important to confess and repent of your own anger, bitterness, and/or resentment to enjoy complete freedom. Jesus revealed during His ministry that a person's physical condition is often a result of their spiritual condition. If a person's emotions are healed (their innermost being), God promises in Psalm 103:1–3 that their physical body will also be healed. Sit quietly, breathe deep slow breaths, and invite the Holy Spirit to fill you. Enjoy the calm serenity as you feel His presence.

My Prayer for Those Rejected in Spirit

In Jesus' name, I bless and call forth your spirit to be healed, that you may be and do all that God created you to be. Holy Spirit, please open this person's eyes and ears that all lies would be exposed and removed. By Your grace and mercy reveal and restore truth to this person. Help them to receive Your love and accept themselves as you do. Father, please heal their innermost being, so they may enjoy complete healing in their body, mind, and soul, in Jesus' name I pray. Amen.

You have been created for such a time as this. Know that you are loved and accepted. Walk in your gifts and talents. Hold your head up high for you have been chosen as a child of the Most High God. Seek and accept Him and He will grant you the desires of your heart.

Back to My Story

After speaking at the church that day in June, our family went to a friend's house for a visit and a swim. I had some abdominal cramping and ended up passing what looked like a dime size tumour. It was a white, rubbery, tube-shaped mass that looked like fat, with purple spider veins running through it. Although I didn't save it, my oncologist said its description sounded accurate. I believe the Lord blessed me for my obedience that day!

Do You Feel Alone?

As I attended the majority of my appointments alone, quite often I experienced an ache deep in my heart as I sat waiting. My eyes roamed through the crowded waiting room feeling sorry for myself to see most people accompanied by their spouse, mother, father or friend. It wasn't that I didn't have any offers; I did. I didn't want to inconvenience anyone or be a burden, especially my husband with his work schedule. I didn't see myself as important enough to ask! I had to remind myself constantly that I wasn't alone and that I was loved. Satan knows our sore spots and will dig in them any chance he can get. We have to remember to take the negative thoughts and lies captive and to cast them down and choose to think about the truth in God's Word according to our situation (2 Corinthians 10:3–5). The truth is I saw myself as a bother and a hindrance. I didn't feel worthy or valuable enough to ask others of their time. I also didn't like the feeling that I owed anyone anything and had a very hard time receiving. I really had no reason to feel blue about being there alone, because it was my choice. Then one day I met a girl named JoAnne at one of my appointments. She immediately initiated a conversation and asked questions about my diagnosis, which is a very common occurrence in an oncologist office. Although we shared a similar diagnosis, she was very bitter and angry toward God. She was a pretty girl, approximately the same age and build as me, with a dark, tanned complexion. The plain black t-shirt, black pants, and black handkerchief she wore on her head to cover the loss of her hair, reflected the anger she felt within. Have you ever heard of a God moment? Well, let me tell you, I don't think it was a coincidence that we had the last two appointments of the day! We had all the privacy and freedom needed to talk openly and honestly. Her husband and two aunts came to support her because she was having such a difficult time with her situation. Her mom had died in a car accident half-way through her treatment and she was angry with God for taking her mother during a time when she felt she needed her the most. She was unable to see any good in her situation. The very blessings that sat beside her, a faithful husband and two adoring aunts who loved JoAnne with a mother's love, had banded together and committed themselves to walking through this journey alongside her, each step of the way. Their love for her was very evident. Her family expressed their gratitude towards me for shining some light on her path, as I pointed out the truth from God's Word about His love for her and how blessed she was that her aunts had stepped in to take her mother's place. Yes, I agree that it doesn't take away the pain of her loss or replace her mother, but it does certainly help fill a void. God is in the business of restoring what has been lost or stolen by the enemy. From that moment on, I decided to allow others into my heart and to receive the kind offers from them gratefully. People wouldn't ask to be part of our lives if they didn't want to be, or if they didn't care. Just because several people have hurt me in the past, doesn't mean that everyone has ulterior motives. From then on, I decided to stomp out all the negative thoughts in my mind and choose to dwell on the positive ones! I'm no longer willing to lose out on wonderful friendships and I'm trusting God to be my vindicator, when necessary.

God Hasn't Forgotten You!

Are you bitter, like JoAnne was, thinking that God has forgotten about you? He hasn't! God has always been there for you. Perhaps you just haven't realized it! God never promised that life would be perfect. As a matter of fact, He told us there would be hard times but that He would carry us through each step of the way! Jesus is God in a body; He knew exactly what it was like to face suffering and loss. God Himself had to hand over His only child and watch Him suffer for our sake for a greater purpose. It grieved Him to have to do that. Yet, He joyfully did it for us. Sometimes we don't understand why things happen. We may never know or understand while we're on this earth; however, I do know this: God loves you and will see you through.

There are many examples in the Bible that God always remembers His people and acts on their behalf. In Genesis 7, we read how God warns Noah about the great flood that would destroy the earth because of the wickedness of the people. Noah wasn't perfect, but God still considered him to be righteous because of his heart towards God. God, in His goodness, showed Noah and his family favour by telling Noah to build an ark. In Genesis 8:1, we're reminded that God remembered Noah and the animals by sending a wind over the earth to make the waters recede. Once the water dried up, they were able to leave the ark and start over on the earth. They had thankful hearts and showed God honour and respect by making an altar to worship Him.

God delivered the Israelite slaves from the hand of Pharaoh after hearing their groaning (Exodus 6:5–6). God acted on their behalf by redeeming them and making them His own people. Let me remind you that God is still the same yesterday, today, and forever. This proves that He is faithful and still acts on our behalf today. Countless women each month are brokenhearted to find they're once again not pregnant. Millions of dollars are spent on fertility drugs and procedures each year, yet many are unsuccessful. Scores of young women who undergo chemotherapy worry about the chance of permanent menopausal effects and wonder whether they'll ever know the joys of motherhood. If this is a matter of concern, you may find hope in Genesis 30. Rachel desperately wanted a baby, but couldn't conceive! Jacob, her husband, was also married to her sister Leah, who had several sons. Rachel was jealous of her sister and cried out to God. Genesis 30:22 says, *"Then God remembered Rachel; he listened to her and opened her womb."* God blessed her with a son named Joseph. This is only one of many examples of God remembering His children.

In Psalm 68:5, God promises to be a father to the fatherless and a defender of the widows. All throughout life's journey, God has placed solid godly male figures along my path to act and guide as stable father figures, including the man I married. God heard and remembered my prayers, even as a young child. When my dad was gone, several families took us under their wings, acting as angels on earth and showed us God's love. When I was nine, my family couldn't celebrate Christmas in the traditional manner, because there wasn't any money for food, not to mention gifts. On Christmas Eve, there was a huge snowstorm, but that didn't stop God's love! The Lord put it on the hearts of members of our church to collect an offering for our family. Fancy wrapped parcels and boxes of food were delivered to our doorstep. Several days later, my dad came knocking on our door after being gone for seven long years. This put an immediate stop to the abuse I was suffering and brought provision for our unmet needs. We have a wonderful Heavenly Father that we can depend on. All we need to do is ask and have child-like faith.

"Which of you, if his son asks for bread, will give him a stone? Or if he asks for a fish, will give him a snake? If you, then, though you are evil, know how to give good gifts to your children, how much more will your Father in heaven give good gifts to those who ask him!" (Matthew 7:9–11)

When I was sick, God provided for my every need and showed me His true character by sending me love beyond belief through a husband who stood by me, children who inspired me to live, love, play and laugh, friends, family, and even strangers who prayed, sent cards, gave words of encouragement, flowers, gifts, food, and helping hands. God protected me through numerous surgeries, eight rounds of chemo, twenty-five rounds of radiation, nine months of Herceptin treatment, and reconstruction. Through these difficult times, God showed me how loved and valuable I was and am. There is no way on earth that I could ever return all the kind gestures bestowed upon me and I have learned to receive and accept these acts of kindness as they were intended to be, gifts!

In the past, I spent far too much time listening to the negative voice in my head that told me I was ugly, unloved, stupid, and unwanted! Do you believe the lies that ring in your head? That's exactly what they are, lies! God reminded me through Beth Moore that according to Ephesians 1:3–8, we are loved, blessed, chosen, accepted, adopted, forgiven, and redeemed.[18] Knowing these truths can put a whole new perspective on things for you. If we can look at situations in a positive manner and realize that we're in God's hands, it opens up the heavens to allow blessings to flow into our lives. Are you able to take the negative situations in your life and find the positive aspects within them? Ask God to help you have a new outlook. Being thankful has a lot to do with being able to see God's goodness.

Even if you do find yourself alone, you never really are, because God promises to always be with you. Just as God acts on behalf of those rejected in spirit, He also touches the lives of the widows and orphans by calling His people to care and meet their needs. I believe single mothers fall under the same category. If you yourself are in a health crisis, and would like God to help: God promises to protect and deliver those in times of trouble, who have looked after the needs of the widows and orphans (Psalm 41:1–4). Do what you can to help others and see what God does for you!

It's Not a Loss

In Romans 8, Paul reminds us that the glory believers will experience in eternity will far outweigh the suffering endured here on earth. God has an amazing reward. We can also experience the joy of redemption here on earth. God wants to bless us even on earth for the trouble we face. Many times we are called to go through things so that we will have compassion and help others around us. It is within these circumstances that we mature and grow. These places remind us to be thankful after we've reached our promised land. God can take our messy pasts and redeem them to bring meaning and purpose. I work in several youth ministries. My background helps me relate and connect with kids that are often misunderstood or rejected. I have compassion for single parents as well, because I watched my mother struggle. I know what it feels like to be hungry and not to have fashionable clothes. In other words, God has given me insight that the average person may not have, along with a sense about certain situations, without the need of the spoken word.

"But God sent me ahead of you to preserve for you a remnant on earth and to save your lives by a great deliverance." (Genesis 45:7)

God's plans are always good! I believe that just as God used the sufferings of Joseph to save the lives of those during the famine, He has also saved and sent me out to share my testimony to save, heal, and deliver countless lives that otherwise may have been lost as a result of sickness. What Satan means for our harm, God wants to use for our good. Regardless of the trials Joseph faced, God brought about great prosperity to him. (See Romans 8:28 & Jeremiah 29:11.)

The seven years my mother spent as a single mother also gave her a heart of compassion for the hungry, hurting, and needy. She later served in the community as the Coordinator of a local Food Bank for five years, demonstrating God's love and goodness to those in need. My children are very blessed because they've never lacked anything. For this reason, I've taken them to the food bank to stock shelves, so they could see the other side. These services weren't available when we were younger, but God always provided.

A few years ago, my mom remarried a wonderful man named Percy. He really loves her! He makes her laugh and enjoys taking her on trips, which is something she never got to do with dad. He never really felt comfortable travelling and that's okay. My Dad chooses to lead a quiet life at home with his two dogs, and is quite happy. Our family gets together on all the holidays now and everyone gets along. Mom and Percy even give Dad a ride!

Back in the summer of 2006, when I injured my hip and back during the dog attack, I was fortunate enough to have partial insurance coverage for my physiotherapy treatments and chiropractor appointments. God also helped me deal with and face my fear of dogs. I learned that it is God's love that squeezes out the fear in our lives, as we trust Him.

During chemo, God blessed us in an amazing way. One of Rob's friends from work gave us an above-ground swimming pool. How incredible is that?! It provided endless entertainment for the boys and painless exercise for me all at the same time. There are so many more examples I could give you. I hope that with the ones I have, you can see the goodness of God. Try taking the negative situations in your life and rearrange your thoughts with a positive twist. It's amazing how a positive attitude can change your outlook and bring joy! Are you able to find the positive aspects in your circumstances? Is there some way you can take what you've learned to help others? God promises to redeem our situations and bring good out of the bad (Isaiah 61:1–3), when we focus on His goodness.

Have You Forgotten God?

"Be careful to follow every command I am giving you today, so that you may live and increase and may enter and possess the land that the Lord promised on oath to your forefathers." (Deuteronomy 8:1)

It's easy to forget what God has done when you start thinking negatively. Even though God delivered the Israelites out of slavery from the Egyptians by performing great miracles, and led them to the Promised Land, they continued to rebel, complain, and give into their fleshly desires. Psalm 106 clearly paints a picture of what happens when we forget what God has done for us or go against the wisdom He has provided for our protection. When the Israelites were out in the desert, they quickly forgot all the things the Lord had done for them. In doing so, they incurred diseases, plagues, oppression, and death. God delivered them over and over and yet they continued to fall into sin and destruction. The people prayed: *"Remember me, O Lord, when you show favor to your people, come to my aid when you save them, that I may enjoy the prosperity of your chosen ones, that I may share in the joy of your nation and join your inheritance in giving praise."* (Psalm 106:4–5)

"But he took note of their distress when he heard their cry; for their sake he remembered his covenant and out of his great love he relented." (Psalm 106:44–45)

God is so good! Sometimes we cause many of our own problems by the choices we make and yet God will come to our aid when we turn to Him. He's a faithful, compassionate God. I took my eyes off God's goodness for a time and slipped into a negative thinking pattern. My thoughts were consumed with everything I couldn't eat, all the pain I'd endured, and the disappointment I felt toward certain people. It didn't take long before I started having health issues again.

We need to trust God and refuse to be offended with people or life's circumstances. When we do, God blesses our circumstances and eventually turns them around for our benefit as He did with Joseph. Joseph knew how much God truly loved Him. This was the key that kept him from becoming bitter. Knowing God's love is also a major step leading to inner healing. Although some people have been taught this truth their whole lives, they still haven't grasped this concept with their hearts because it's head knowledge that needs to get down into their heart through revelation! If you're serious about wanting inner healing, find every Scripture you can about God's love. Read it, memorize it, and write it out until it becomes firmly rooted into your heart. Ecclesiastes 3 declares that there is a time for everything, including your healing! I believe today is the day! Are you ready?

Dear Heavenly Father,

Thank You for Your love; may a true revelation of this ignite in my heart. Please forgive me for the times I've not recognized Your goodness because my eyes were clouded by negativity. Forgive me for my rebellion. Remember me and show me Your favour. Please come to my aid. May I enjoy the prosperity of Your chosen ones and experience Your joy as I give You praise (Psalm 106:4–5). In Jesus' name I pray. Amen.

(Scriptures of Love: John 3:16; Romans 5:5; Romans 5:8; Romans 8:38; Psalm 145:13b; Jeremiah 33:11b; 1 John 4:19.)

Facing the Facts

"Then you will know the truth, and the truth will set you free." (John 8:32)

Many people don't want to face the truth of their past because it is painful. They make excuses and reason away their dysfunctional behaviour and blame their circumstances on their past. Blaming your past only hinders your healing and holds you back from enjoying your future. Face it! When you press past the pain, there's amazing freedom and peace that comes. I believe this is the next step to inner healing. It starts when you rid yourself of old thinking patterns, such as victim mentality. Ask God for grace to see things differently and come to a place of understanding so you can press past the anger, bitterness, resentment and hate. Don't get discouraged, healing is a process. I like to compare it to an onion because it has many layers.

Trust and believe in God to work everything out in your situation for good. Increase God's power in your situation by agreeing with His plans for your life. When you complain about your situation, you are putting your life in agreement with what the Devil wants. Learn what God's Word says about you and your situations. Then watch your thoughts and choose to have faith. God wants to restore your soul.

Remember to love and respect yourself. If you're not able to treat yourself as well as you treat others, you've got some work to do. God never intended for you to be a doormat. Learn to speak up for yourself and deal with issues when they arise. You'll be healthier because of it!

Generational Sins and Curses

Our sins and the sins of our ancestors not only negatively affect our lives, they can affect the lives of our children and their descendants if we don't put a stop to them (Deuteronomy 5:8). Our sins, when unconfessed, along with weaknesses visit down through the generations. For the Bible says, *"The Lord, the Lord, the compassionate and gracious God, slow to anger, abounding in love and faithfulness, maintaining love to thousands, and forgiving wickedness, rebellion and sin. Yet he does not leave the guilty unpunished; he punishes the children and their children for the sin of the fathers to the third and fourth generation."* (Exodus 34:6b, 7)

Sins can pass down through the family line just like genetics do. Confessing and repenting of the effects of the sins of our ancestors can break the chains that bind family strongholds. Unconfessed sin opens a door to the demonic. It allows Satan access into our lives. Do you have a family history with problems such as alcohol, drug abuse, fornication, depression, suicide, illnesses and disease, witchcraft, lying, etc? Do you want to put a stop to generational sins and curses?

Pray and ask God to reveal the sins of your ancestors, so that the truth will set you free. Talk to any living relatives and ask them questions about your family history. Reassure them that your intention isn't to point fingers and blame. They may want to leave the past well alone and not divulge any old skeletons. Sin lives in and likes the darkness where it can stay hidden and hold power over you. When it's brought out into the light it no longer has the same hold. We need to identify our generational roots, so they can be cut off at the initial source and be forgiven. Even if they're unwilling to share, the Lord can reveal these things through prayer. By forgiving your relatives for the effects that their sin has had on you and asking God's forgiveness, those roots can no longer bind you. In 2 Chronicles 7:14, God promises: *"if my people, who are called by* *my name, will humble themselves and pray and seek my face and turn from their wicked ways, then will I hear from heaven and will forgive their sin and will heal their land."*Are there certain sins you struggle with? Be honest with yourself. Truth is the light that comes in and exposes the darkness, allowing the healing power of God to move. Be sure to keep short accounts with God. When you slip up, be quick to repent. Once God has revealed the sins of your ancestors, and your own sins, pray the following prayer.

Dear Heavenly Father,

I forgive and release my ancestors, parents and myself for the sin of _____ (be specific and thorough). I forgive them for passing these sins and curses down to me. Please forgive me for the sins of _____ (be specific). I repent of them now. Break off any effects their sin has had on me. By the power of Jesus' name and His precious blood I break the curse of _____ (be specific) off of my life and ask for Your protection from these sins and curses. I place the cross of Jesus between the sins and curses of my ancestors and myself. May the freedom Christ died to give me flow down from the heavens upon me, from this day forward. In Jesus' name I pray. Amen.

Note: You may also like to use the soul tie prayer for God to cut off any ungodly attachment. When you confess and repent of your sins, the legal hold of Satan breaks. However, Satan knows the weaknesses in your family line and confession won't stop him from tempting or targeting your kids! Also remember that when we judge, we also repeat the same sin pattern. Be careful to judge the sin and not people. We have free will and have full right to be angry. But that unforgiveness is exactly what put the unforgiving master in jail where he was tormented. Instead, let's learn from our mistakes and make better choices from this point. How often do you do things your own way and then get mad at

God because you suffer the consequences? Remember, it's often our free will that put us in our place!

I'm sure sexual immorality has touched almost every generation. Even in ancient times, it was rampant. Sodom and Gomorrah were destroyed for this reason. Many people of Samaria and Judah worshipped Baal, a false god that incorporated the worship of the sexual anatomy. The people sacrificed their children to the idols for food and practiced fornication, prostitution, rebellion, and adultery. They also committed adultery with their idols through masturbation and desecrated the sacredness of the House of God, practicing profanity there. People still worship the false god of Baal today; some worship knowingly, while others do so out of ignorance.

Because our society has become so desensitized, many are unaware of what is and isn't sin. Anyone who commits sexual sins, sins against their own body. God views this as wickedness. I'm not telling you this to make you feel condemned. God wants to bring restoration to your life. The devil is the one who always tries to condemn us, while God reveals our sin to draw us closer, through repentance. As discussed before, God created sex as an intimate means to communicate love to one another as a married couple. Sex is from God and it is good! God intentionally wired each one of us with sexual desires so that we would be attracted to our marriage partner and want to reproduce to have a family. This is another gift from God! He also created sex to help our immune system and to give us pleasure. Many people, both male and female, view sex as dirty. This likely stems either from past abusive sexual experiences or from the remarks that parents made because they were uncomfortable about the subject. It weighs on the heart, subconsciously hindering them from enjoying this gift from God. The sin of immoral sex is what makes us feel dirty. And it definitely isn't wrong when we enjoy it according to God's plan for our lives. Listed below are sexual sins to confess and repent if necessary. Find a trusted Christian counsellor where you can receive prayer and experience freedom and healing. This can also provide needed accountability where there is addiction. If you're questioning certain items listed or you're not quite sure how you feel, read the Scriptures below to bring clarity regarding what sexual immorality is and how God sees it. They will also give needed strength and renewal of mind when needed.

(References: Jude 6–7; 2 Peter 2; Genesis 19:1–29; Ezekiel 16:48–50; Ezekiel 23:18; Genesis 19:30–38; Genesis 35:22; Genesis 49:3–4; 1 Chronicles 5:1; Numbers 25:1–10; Judges 19; Ezekiel 23:1–10, 11–49; Proverbs 5:15–19; Proverbs 6:24–26; Romans 1:20–32; 1 Corinthians 5:1–13; 1 Cor. 6:13, 18–20; 1 Thessalonians 4:3–5; Revelation 2:19–25; Leviticus 18:22, 20:1; Gen. 19:5–8; Judges 19:22–24; Judges 16–1; Deuteronomy 22:5.)

Remember God gives us guidelines so that we may live in health, blessing, and prosperity. I pray that God would heal and restore your sexual life (without stumbling blocks) the way He intended it to be.

"There must not be even a hint of sexual immorality, or of any kind of impurity." (Ephesians 5:3)

Sexual Sins

- Abuse—sexual mistreatment, cruelty or violence.

- Adultery

- Bestiality—sexual relations with an animal.

- Fondling, caressing outside of marriage is considered the same as prostitution in God's eyes. Many teenagers think that as long as they aren't having intercourse, then what they're doing doesn't classify as sex, but it is! Oral sex included.

- Oral Sex—Kissing, fondling, and caressing is more than acceptable when married, but take note that semen wasn't meant to be released into the mouth or swallowed. Some healing ministries believe that this act allows unclean spirits to enter, from what they've witnessed during deliverance ministry. And it is thought to be the cause of many women's throat and stomach problems.

- Fornication—During Bible times, when a man and woman made love, they were considered married. That was their wedding ceremony. They were legally bound as husband and wife before God. Times may have changed, but God's view hasn't! Sleeping with someone is the same as marrying them in His eyes. If the relationship breaks up and one or both move on to another relationship, adultery is committed. Even though they may not be bound by our legal system, they're tied to a spiritual one. An engagement ring is a symbol of betrothal, not a marriage certificate. Fornication is the cause of many sexually transmitted diseases.

- Homosexuality—same sex relations.

- Incest—sex within a family.

- Lust—unquenchable desire for more.

- Masturbation—used as a means to bring self-comfort. An obsessive act that has a spirit of lust attached, often using fantasy and or pornography, causing guilt and self-condemnation.

- Pornography—the use of media to display naked people.

- Prostitution—selling one's body.

- Rape—sex without consent.

- Sadism—inflicting punishment during sex.

- Sodomy—anal copulation with same or opposite sex or with an animal. God created the anus for output only! This tissue is sensitive and can easily tear, causing damage. AIDS is believed to be the curse originating from this sin.

- Transvestism—someone who dresses in the opposite sex's clothing to arouse sexual desire.

- Voyeurism—the compulsion to watch people sexually.

- Exhibitionism—exposing sexual organs to shock others or have them watch sexual acts.

- Perverse, crude, sexual talk (Ephesians 4:29).

If you have fallen into any of the sins listed, please pray the following prayer as well as the generational sin prayer previous to break the yolk of family bondage. Confession, repentance and forgiveness close the door to any legal right the enemy may have. We also need to keep our children in constant prayer and bring them up in the teaching of the Lord to guide them!

Dear Heavenly Father,

I ask You to forgive me for my sexual sins of _____ (name your past and present sexual sins) and wash me clean. Thank You that when I confess my sins, You are faithful and just to cleanse and forgive me from all my sin and unrighteousness (1 John 1:9) I place the cross of Jesus between these sins and myself and may Your free-

dom and liberty wash down on me like rain, setting me free from all guilt, shame, and condemnation. Jesus, I make You Lord over my life. Please bless me with the strength to walk in purity, holiness, and integrity in my body, mind, and spirit. I ask You to heal, restore, and bring balance to this area of my life according to Your Word. Remove all lustful desires from my heart and deliver me from temptation. In Jesus' name I pray. Amen.

In my family, there was also a history of Freemasonry. Both my great grandparents on my father's side and my mother's father were Free Masons. I learned the following information from Elle–Elle Ministries: Freemasonry is a world–renowned secret society that elevates men through their achievements and they're bound by powerful oaths and penalties. If members reveal their secrets, the oaths they've sworn open the door for curses to be passed down through their family blood line. As a result, many unexplained deaths and or health problems have occurred. Many may see this as genetics, but how do you explain freak accidences, all of the same nature that end with similar results? I've heard of a family that has experienced three generations of mishaps involving a blow to the head that resulted in the loss of sight in the eye. But until someone within the family recognizes the truth and renounces the oaths and curses, the enemy will continue to prey on this lineage. Freemason beliefs and ceremonies are based on Hinduism, Kabbalism, and Rosicrucianism, with pagan religions of Egypt and Greek Mythology. They exclude true teachings of Christ and forbid prayers raised up in the name of Jesus. Any type of worship we submit to, either knowingly or unknowingly, places us under that spiritual authority (e.g. Yoga places a person under the authority of the kundalini serpent). Free Masons inadvertently have the façade of being Christian–like because of their good works, but their rituals mimic those of witchcraft ceremonies and the floors in their Masonic temples have a five–point star (pentagram).

During the swearing–in ceremony, a hood–wink is placed over their heads and they declare spiritual blindness. It's not until they've reached the highest levels in this society that the truth regarding their worship is revealed! They worship Lucifer. Albert Pike, the founder of The Masonic, wrote a book called "Morals and Dogma". In it, he wrote, "The dunces of Christians who once opposed witchcraft have done a great disservice to mankind." This man clearly disliked Christians and their beliefs. His goal was to entrap good Christian men into spiritual bondage that hindered them from truly serving God and having spiritual insight from Him. They have also created other branches called Shiners, Amaranth, DeMo-lay, Scottish Rite, York Rite, etc., and other organizations to include women and children such as the Rebecca's, Eastern Stars, Job's Daugh-ters, Rainbow Girls, etc. Because of time and space, I'm unable to go into great depth; however, I feel that you'd benefit by researching Kent Sy-mington's website through Christian Restoration Ireland. The informa-tion is truly fascinating and enlightening! What's in your past that needs to be broken? Don't be afraid! Your freedom is around the corner.[19]

Lordship Prayer

Dear Jesus,

I realize that to become completely whole I must place You first and make You Lord over my entire life and being. I invite You now into my heart and life to become my Saviour, Redeemer, Deliverer, and Lord over my entire life. I make You Lord over my mind, will, emotions, attitudes, decisions, reactions, physical body, spirit, my fam-ily and relationships, my sexuality and its expression, my work and good deeds, my possessions and needs, my finances, and even the manner and time of my death. In Jesus' name I pray. Amen.

Prayers: adapted from Mark & Patti Virkler's workbook, "Prayers that Heal the Heart." Used with permission.

Lordship prayer adapted from Elle Elle Healing Ministry Notes.

---

[1] Jones, AJ. *Finding Father: The Father Heart Series/6-Disc Set*; (Toronto, ON: Catalyst Home International, 2006), (www.CATALYSTHOME.ORG).

[2] Arterburn, Stephen. Stoop, David. *The Spiritual Renewal Bible, Spiritual Disciplines Devotionals and Profiles*, "Speak the Truth", Key 3, Exposing Our Buried Sins", *New Living Translation*. (Wheaton Illinois: Tyndale House, 1998), p.1288.

[3] Ibid.

[4] Leaf, Dr. Carolyn. *Who Switched of My Brain? Controlling toxic thoughts and emotions*. (South Africa: Switch On Your Brain, 2007).

[5] Arterburn, Stephen. Stoop, David. *The Spiritual Renewal Bible, Spiritual Disciplines Devotionals and Profiles*, "Speak the Truth", Key 3, Exposing Our Buried Sins", *New Living Translation*. (Wheaton Illinois: Tyndale House, 1998), p.1288.

[6] Ibid.

[7] Ibid.

[8] Toronto Airport Christian Fellowship Pastors Conference Notes, January 2002.

[9] Arnott, Carol. Sandford, John & Paula. "*Healing Life's Hurts Bitter Root Judgments and Expectancy" Vol. 1* (VHS), (Toronto: Toronto Airport Christian Fellowship Conference).

[10] Ibid.

[11] Nelson. *ITP Nelson Canadian Dictionary of the English language. An Encyclopedic Reference* (Scarborough, ON: International Thompson

Publishing, Nelson; A division of Thompson Canada Limited, 1997), p. 363.

[12] Arnott, Carol. Sandford, John and Paula. *"Healing Life's Hurts Bitter Root Judgments and Expectancy" Vol. 1* (VHS), (Toronto: Toronto Airport Christian Fellowship Conference).

[13] Ibid.

[14] Virkler, Mark & Patti. *Prayers That Heal The Heart Workbook* (Elma, N.Y.: Communication With God Ministries, 2001). Used with permission.

[15] "About Carol Agneesens." *Pacific School for Biodynamic Integration.* 27 Oct. 2010 (http://wwwbiodynamicsschool.com/ignition.html).

[16] "Can your stress affect an unborn baby?"*Helium.* 27 Oct. 2010 (www.helium.com/.../842352-can-your-stress-affect-an-unborn-baby).

[17] "How to bond with your unborn baby on MedicineNet.com?" *Medicine Net.com.* 27 Oct. 2010 (http://www.medicinenet.com›...›women's healthaz.list). "Prenatal Music, Reading, Voices & Sounds for your Unborn Baby in Utero." *Promoting Literacy*: Prenatal Bonding with Your Unborn Baby Through Books. 27 Oct. 2010 (http://www.earlymoments.com/.../Prenatal-Child-Development-Tips/).

[18] Moore, Beth. *Believing God* (Nashville, TN: Life Way Press, 2004).

[19] Ellel Ellel Ministries. *"The Christian Response to Freemasonry"* CD's, (Westport, ON: Ellel Ellel Ministries, Canada, 2007), (info.ontario@ellelministries.org). Website: (www.ellelministries.org/canada).

Chapter Ten
Don't Give Up!

When you pass through the waters, I will be with you;
and when you pass through the rivers, they will not sweep over you.

Isaiah 43:2a

Has life got you down? We all face seasons in life that hold different ranges of difficulty. At times it seems as if we are able to tackle the world regardless of the magnitude of a problem and at other times, we feel as if we can't possibly continue even when facing a minute challenge. Do the troubled waters seem deeper than what you feel you can wade through? Are you at a point now where everything in you wants to give up? At this point you may have endured a great amount of pain and you likely don't want to ever see another needle or have another test performed in your life, if you can help it. Perhaps your emotions are stirring uncontrollably within you. Maybe you're tired of it all, tired of getting bad news.

Well, I've got great news! Today is a new day! Our feelings are so fickle, they tend to change moment by moment and so can your situation. This morning, as I waited with Spencer for his school bus to arrive, I noticed that it was an incredibly gorgeous spring day. The sun was shining, the snow was beginning to melt and there was a soft warm breeze. I could hardly wait to go for my morning walk and breathe the fresh air into my lungs.

Before I left the house I put some laundry in the washer and did a few odd chores. The moment I zipped up my jacket and set my foot out the door the wind picked up with great force and snow and sleet started pounding down from the heavens. I stood at the door and debated whether or not I should head out. I could wait until the squall stopped and go at a later time, but I was concerned that I might miss it altogether. Knowing the value of exercise, I put on my head warmer and brave face and ventured out into the great Canadian blizzard! I may have been getting a workout but I sure wasn't experiencing the same warm, fuzzy feelings as earlier. But sometimes a girl has to do what a girl has to do!

Five minutes after I returned home, the wind and snow had completely died down, the sun had returned and I could hear the birds chirping. Go figure! It's Canada, what can I say? You can't always depend on the weather.

Like the weather, we should never rely on our feelings to make decisions. Our feelings are not always founded on fact, but are based on our flesh which has the tendency to change at any given moment. Our flesh tends to be flimsy and weak. We need to set our minds on doing those things that are best for us. Stop putting things off. Your positive decisions today will bring about a better tomorrow. We all struggle with wanting to give up from time to time when faced with challenges. But nothing of great value was ever accomplished by just wishing!

Have you set goals for yourself that contribute to enjoying a happier, healthier lifestyle? Are you filled with determination to do what you can to help yourself or are you like the millions of others who give up after a short time because they encounter some sort of difficulty? Perhaps you need to eat right, to exercise more or to cut out smoking? The benefits will far outweigh the grief felt. Keep up the good work and recruit family and friends for added support. Remember the old saying "misery loves company." Well, who said you had to be miserable? It's all in the way you view things! If you perceive these goals as dreadful tasks, then they will be just that. If you take the same goals and see them as positive ways to improve your life, then you will enjoy the journey and gain much from the experience. You will reap the benefits from your efforts and it will do your body good. The hard work will pay off in the long run. It takes time to see the benefits, so don't be discouraged! It took time for your body to deteriorate so it only makes sense that it will take some time to strengthen and build it back up again.

Make a decision and stick with it! When you form new habits it can be difficult at first. Remember the reasons you decided to make certain changes in your lifestyle in the first place. Always start out slowly and increase as you gain strength, to be sure not to over–exert yourself. The better shape you are in, the healthier you will feel and be. Always make sure you have your doctor's permission. Setting attainable goals for yourself will help you stick with it. The sooner you start, the better off you'll be.

The choices we make today will affect us tomorrow. If you feed your body junk, that's what it will be. We have all heard the consequences that result from making poor health choices, yet how many people continue to ignore the warnings! Forming healthy habits now will benefit your body later. You will live longer, have more energy, and generally feel better physically and emotionally.

The Bible encourages us to build our lives on the Rock which is Jesus Christ as He is the great Corner Stone. When you build on a solid foundation, the structure is strong and durable and can withstand the storms of life when they come, no matter how hard or furious.

Let's look at the parable about the two men who each built themselves a house. The first man built his house on rock, which offers a solid foundation that is not easily moved or destroyed. When the storm came, the house stayed intact. The second builder built his house on the sand. This was foolish because sand is easily tossed to and fro by the wind and is unstable and ever–sinking. When the rain came, the house built on sand collapsed because it lacked a solid foundation. The storm was too much for the house.

Will you make Jesus your rock? Whatever your life challenges may be at this time, God promises that you will not be drowned by the waters of life. You may also be enduring a health crisis or perhaps you are reading this book because you have a family member who is suffering and you're trying to make sense of it all. No matter what has brought you down, God promises that He will bring you through. Please, never give up hope! God wants to lead you through the troubled waters in your life, to victory's shore!

Giving up is the easy way out. You owe it to yourself to press past these feelings and any obstacles you may encounter, to fight for your life. You're worth it! Whatever your situation, find meaning and purpose to carry on.

Take a moment to think about the future you'd like to have and the things you'd like to accomplish in your life, that you haven't had a chance to do yet. If you focus on your goals, this will help you continue forward and give you something positive to live for. Think about the things you'd like to do with your family and friends once you've finished treatment. Perhaps you could plan a trip. Laugh and have some fun planning it. It doesn't hurt to dream a little. If money is an issue, find inexpensive ways for a get–away, like spending time at the beach, park, theatre, museum or local zoo. Planning the future is good and it's something to look forward to, but remember to take moments each day to build lasting memories that will also aid in pulling each individual involved through this dark time. Get out your photographs and reminisce about old times to give yourself some strength and determination.

It's important to keep a positive mindset. If you don't, negative thinking will defeat you! A very wise person once said to me that, "You set the direction of your life by your thoughts." In other words, if you think you can do something, you probably will! If you think you can't, you won't! Part of persevering is keeping up a good attitude even when things around you seem bleak. Having faith and hope, even in the midst of trouble, is possible when we remember that there isn't one situation that God can't handle! (See Mark 10:27b.)

God's power is mighty when we exercise our faith. Are you someone who is always expecting the good in every situation or do you always see the negative? Do you think that if you don't hope for something good, then you won't be disappointed when something bad happens? If this is the case, you need to shake off that mentality. You'll get exactly that because you're using faith in the negative!

I remember the horrible experience I had with my first chemo treatment and how my emotions began to stir within me as the day approached to receive my second dose. This was a pivotal moment for me. I could easily have been consumed with self-pity. I could have dreaded it to the point where I would have lost all my joy in anticipation of the treatment; however, instead I chose to have hope.

I had hope that the new medications would make me more comfortable for the next treatment. I decided to expect the best to happen. As things turned out, my second chemo treatment went much smoother than the first, by a long shot. By yielding to this choice, I was able to go about enjoying life with my family even though I knew the treatment was coming. It wasn't the medication or the doctor that I placed my trust in, but God. His Word promises that those who put their trust in Him will not be put to shame (Psalm 25:3).

What is hope? The Canadian Dictionary explains hope as: to wish for something with expectation of its fulfillment, to have confidence and trust.[1] Hebrews 11:1 says, *"Now faith is being sure of what we hope for and certain of what we do not see."* That was the Scripture my Bible was open to when my brother-in-law, Tim, took my picture for this book. The Lord had spoken to him about photographing me at a specific time. Apparently the world needed to see my bald head in all its glory. Out of obedience to God, Tim asked me one day if I'd be willing to have this done. He had no idea why, but he had a strong sense that he needed to do this. At that point, I hadn't said anything to anyone about the strong desire stirring inside me about writing this book. I just knew in my heart it was something God was calling me to do. God had put a picture in my mind of exactly what the front cover should look like and Tim presented the same layout without me saying a word. Once again, that is God! The Bible compares those who trust in the Lord like those who rise up on wings like eagles.

"But those who hope in the Lord will renew their strength. They will soar on wings like eagles: they will run and not grow weary, they will walk and not be faint." (Isaiah 40:31)

Life is an occasion we need to rise up to. The eagle is a majestic bird that uses thermal currents to rise up above perilous storms and soars with very little effort. We too, like the eagle, can soar above the storms in life as we place our trust in God. He will give us the inner strength to continue on. It is when we put matters into God's hands that the burden becomes light and we can fly with ease, no matter what the circumstances look like in the natural. We can use the obstacles placed in front of us to rise above the storm as we rest in God's arms of love.

One night during a time when I was having an extremely hard time getting my mind off my circumstances, I dreamt I was sitting in the back pew to distance myself from those who had hurt me. The room was dark, yet I recognized the faces of those around me. The minister spoke directly to me, encouraging me to rise above my circumstances. I tried to get up off the pew, but the weight of my troubles hindered my ability to stand. Then Gloria Copland, a spirit-filled Bible teacher from the States, came to where I was sitting and laid her hands on me. As she prayed, my eyes focused in on the cross at the front of the church. As they fixed to the cross, my heart diverged away from my problems and onto Christ, reminding me that He has already conquered my problems on Calvary. As I let go of all the turmoil, my body lifted up off the seat and floated around the room above all the people. From the moment I chose to trust God, the dark room illuminated.

This chapter evolved from a very difficult time where several facets in life were creating a great amount of pressure. It took the strength of the Lord to persevere. At times we know what we should do, yet we feel like giving up because our flesh is weak. I pray that God in His goodness ministers to you in this book the way He ministered to me during this time. The truths can be applied to any situation, not only to those fighting physical ailments.

Obstacles

Self-Pity

When you sink into the self-pity mode, you are allowing yourself to become a victim. It causes everything you say and do to be framed with the "I am a victim" mentality.

Maybe I have to ask you the same question that Jesus asked the invalid at the pool of Bethesda. "Do you want to get well?" The pool of Bethesda was a place where crowds of sick people would come to wait for the pool waters to be stirred by an angel of the Lord. The first one into the pool would be cured of whatever disease they had. When Jesus saw the man lying there, He asked him if he wanted to get well. The man told Him he had no one to help him into the pool (John 5:1–7). This man spent his whole life lying by a pool waiting for his miracle because he was full of excuses for why he couldn't get healed. I have no one to put me in the pool. It's too hard. No one will help me. If he wanted it that badly, he could have found a way. Miracles don't happen with this kind of passive attitude.

Are there excuses in your life that are holding you back? You need to get honest with yourself. Do you want to get well? Do you really want to see your situation change? Then you need to stop wallowing in self-pity and move forward. I can be blunt because I took a trip there myself for a short time! Feeling sorry for yourself only drags you and the others around you down. What's better, attention because you're sick or freedom because you're well? You need to press past feeling sorry for yourself, let go of that victim mentality and get your mind set in victory mode.

Jesus didn't even reply to the invalid's sad story, He replied, *"Get up! Pick up your mat and walk."* (John 5:8). The man was cured instantly. If you really want to see your circumstances change, you need to change your attitude, stop making excuses, get up, and move on.

Many people only focus on the things they don't like about their lives, rather than concentrating on the positive aspects. If we concentrate too heavily on the negative points, they become magnified. The mole hills become mountains, making us overwhelmed, uptight, and discouraged. Complaining about our situation only feeds the negative. I realize there are times when we need to reflect on situations, working through things in our minds; this is all part of life, but it isn't healthy to let yourself become totally consumed with the negative. Each day contains something to be thankful for. Remember, there is always someone else worse off than you! Are you ready to pick–up your mat and walk?

Grief

It's quite normal and even healthy to grieve for a period of time. You've been through hell and back and let's face it; it's changed your whole life! You probably wish you could turn back the time! Your body will never be the same, it looks and feels different and may even still hurt! Not to mention many of your relationships have been altered. Yes, there's a grieving process each one of us needs to go through. You may have gotten angry with God and the world and then that very anger turned into a great sadness. Crying is a good release as it helps us let go of all the bottled up emotions we carry inside. But then there comes a time when our crying needs to stop. Don't let life's disappointments keep you down.

During Bible times, in Israel, the law only allowed people to grieve for 30 days after the death of a loved one (Deuteronomy 34). God even encouraged Samuel to stop grieving after the alotted period of time and move forward with life after the death of King Saul (1 Samuel 16:35). He did this by telling Samuel to get up and go anoint David son of Jessie to be King.

This example shows that it is healthy to express your emotions but there is also a healthy time period involved. Be kind to yourself and acknowledge your feelings and take time to lament. Grieving is a natural process but it also should only be for a season. If you stay in despair long enough you will get caught in its pit. Have your time of mourning and then choose to move forward by learning from your experience. At least take what good you can out of it. Satan wants to hold you back by keeping you in your pain. God wants to heal your pain so you can enjoy your life to its fullest. He has a good plan for you!

Anger

When we have been through a traumatic experience, there are normal stages one's emotions go through. Often people will experience denial, shock, anger, resolution, confusion, numbness and frustration.[2] After denial and shock dissipate; anger is often the next stage in the cycle experienced during grief.[3] This is a natural response to situations gone wrong. God designed us to have this reaction to equip us to face problems that need solving. It's very healthy to feel anger, but it is unhealthy to stay that way!

Are you angry with your doctor because he misdiagnosed you or missed something obvious all together? Perhaps your anger is directed at the overloaded health care system that made you wait for needed treatment? One of the main reasons doctors go to school for seven years is to make a difference in this world and help; they don't deliberately set out to hurt anyone! We live in an imperfect world where mistakes can happen to good people. Sadly, sickness is on the rise and we are in great need of doctors. I believe this could be the main reason for slip-ups; they can only do so much. Don't kid yourself. I'm sure they have their own guilt to wrestle with! Choose to forgive them and let God work in their lives on your behalf.

Do you think God has let you down by allowing negative circumstances to happen in your life or the life of a loved one? Do you question why some people can go around abusing their bodies and get away with it, while others, who live healthy lifestyles, can't. It's a natural reaction to see this as unfair. Do you feel like you're being punished and wonder why bad things happen to good people? We live in a fallen world because of the sin of Adam and Eve. When the Israelites came into the Promised Land, the Lord set before the people life and death. He revealed the behaviour that would bring life and the behaviour that would bring about sicknesses and death (Deuteronomy 30:19). Then He told them to choose life! It's not God's will for anyone to be sick! Satan is the one that uses the "open" door of sin to put sickness on people! Jesus came to demolish the dark works of the enemy, and give us a good life (John 10:10). Jesus broke off the curse of sin and death by dying on the cross. If we choose to live by the Law, thinking it's our righteous acts that get us to heaven, we then fall under the Law which is impossible to keep and therefore open ourselves up to these curses. However, if we have a relationship with God and are led by God's Spirit, we live in freedom and are not bound by the Law. We do uplift it because we want to do what's right because we love the Lord. We enjoy our freedom at a great cost so it's important for us not to take advantage of this by living by our old sinful nature. This proves that God wants what's best for His children because He is good! One of the greatest desires every parent has for his or her children is for them to be healthy and happy. You wouldn't want your child to be sick and neither does your Heavenly Father. If you want to get mad at someone, get mad at the devil and all he stands for.

Are you being held captive by your own guilt and anger? Do you torture yourself with questions like, "What if I had done this, or what if I hadn't done that?" This anger you are feeling is not helping your health in any way. As a matter of fact, it's like a toxic poison that eats you from the inside out and will destroy you if you continue! Be gentle with yourself, you're human! Humans make mistakes but they can also learn from them. You can enjoy freedom from anger by choosing to forgive and move on, for your own sake. God wants to do a new thing in you, but unless you let go of the past, you won't be able to move ahead. Use the valuable lessons from this experience to help others and overcome evil with good!

Depression

If grief is not dealt with, it can turn into depression. When a person is suffering from depression, it is as though something has literally sucked the life out of them, leaving them sapped of all energy and strength. What is it in their life that has had such an impact? Depression is often a result of suppressed issues such as anger turned inward or constant focus on negative things that don't seem to change. Have you ever gone to bed angry and woken up depressed? You probably found yourself angrier than when you went to bed! I've learned through experience that the longer you suppress anger, the larger it grows. I try to sort out and deal with my anger before I go to sleep because I don't like living in a black hole.

Depression has many symptoms that vary with the individual.[4] Some cases are more severe than others. Warning signs may range from poor concentration to inability to make decisions, change in appetite, inappropriate guilt, or feelings of unworthiness, low self-esteem, fatigue, insomnia, oversleeping, and thoughts of suicide or death.[5] It is quite common for sufferers to withdraw from others.[6] The enemy loves to get people alone where he can oppress their minds and make them believe their circumstances are hopeless. This is a lie the enemy uses to destroy lives.

For years, the devil would attack me on Mother's Day, reminding me of all the situations I'd failed at with my kids and ways I had let myself down. A few years ago, I sat alone in church with tears streaming down my cheeks, unable to sing along with the beautiful music that usually lifted my spirit. Even though it was Mother's Day, it had started off like any other day. There was no breakfast in bed, card or flowers. Instead, I cooked my family breakfast, did the dishes and then argued with them about coming to church with me. My mind flooded with thoughts and feelings about how I wasn't valued. I longed for them to share my faith. Then, as I sat in church contemplating ending my life, the Lord sent me a timely message not to give up. He opened my eyes to see the truth. I had believed lies that caused me to form ungodly expectations about how my family would treat me. From that moment, I made a decision to see the good in my family, not to compare them to others and not to base my worth on what others do or don't do for me. We often set ourselves up by having high expectations that we expect others to fulfill, without letting them in on our secret! Men are not mind readers! Big deal if I had to make breakfast, do all the dishes and then go to church alone. I had a family, food, dishes to eat on, and a caring body of believers to share my faith with. I actually came home, made lunch and did all the dishes again. Not to be taken advantage of, but to send the devil a clear message. It's stupid when you think about the whole thing. Why go through all the trouble to survive cancer and then turn around and consider giving up like that? I prayed and released my family and myself from the expectations that only God can fulfill and placed my desires and concerns in God's hands. God has promised me that the good work He has begun in my family, He will bring to completion before He returns (Philippians 1:6). God has helped me realize that my family does have their own faith in Him and that each relationship with Him is uniquely developed and expressed in its own way. I haven't thought about ending my life again. It's crazy, the pressure we put ourselves under. Life, in general, can bring you down if you continually stare at the things you dislike. Being positive and focusing on the things you can be thankful for will help you keep your head up even when things aren't ideal. I'm thankful I can draw my strength from the Lord. God offers us happiness even in the midst of our trials. It's wonderful to know that we're never alone and that He's always there to help.

Thankfully, a lot has changed since that day! I actually look forward to Mother's Day now. My family truly goes out of their way to make my day really special. They still don't bring me breakfast in bed, but that's okay! They do, however, fill my life with amazing love and joy and show me their appreciation in many other ways. Even better than I'd ever imagined, and they mean the world to me! They always loved me. I just wasn't able to see it because I didn't love myself!

In the winter months, many people are affected by the lack of sunlight. God has given us other natural remedies to help release our feel-good hormones, such as exercise, vitamin D, and dark chocolate (in balance). These are all meant to give you a healthy boost.

If you struggle with depression, don't worry, you are not alone. Roughly 18.8 million American adults are diagnosed with depressive disorder each year.[7] Sometimes people need a little medical help for a little while. That's ok. There are some people who refuse to go to counselling because of their pride. They think that it's embarrassing and is a sign of weakness.

Both sickness and depression are directly related to unresolved issues.[8] Years back, news reports shared studies that women who suppress their feeling do damage to their hearts! It's important to lay down our pride and get help. Learn to express yourself and release those bottled up toxic feelings you've held in for so long! Your say in life matters!

It's great to have friends to talk to but this is not always the best idea. Professionals are trained to give specific wisdom and insight needed for particular situations. It is important to receive unbiased opinions that are open and honest. It keeps the pressure off those who may find it hard to cope. Friends that find it hard to cope will often not allow you to talk, by blurting out only the answers they want to hear or avoid you! Rather than having to work through resentment, it's best to choose someone disconnected from your circumstances. Weigh your options wisely and remember God is always there to listen!

"I waited patiently for the Lord; he turned to me and heard my cry. He lifted me out of the slimy pit, out of the mud and mire; he set my feet on a rock and gave me a firm place to stand. He put a new song in my mouth, a hymn of praise to our God. Many will see and fear and put their trust in the Lord." (Psalm 40:1–3)

Guarding Your Thoughts

Are you guarding your thoughts as discussed in Chapter 7? Remember to discard the negative thoughts and replace them with positive ones. This is achieved one thought at a time. Pray if you need to. God will give you the strength. If you have health issues, visualize yourself completely well and doing the things you love best. Proverbs 29:18a, (The Amplified Bible) reminds us that where there is no vision, the people perish. To succeed at something, we must first envision our goal in our minds. The thoughts we have today will determine our tomorrow. We must have determination! Have you ever wanted something so strongly that you could almost taste it? That's what I'm talking about. Once you have that vision, you'll be able to speak the positive into your situation. Remember this: If you tell yourself you'll never be able to do something, you'll never succeed. Our mindset is directly connected to our hearts. When you tell yourself something often enough, you'll end up believing it. What you think in your heart will follow through in your actions. What goes in will come out! Matthew 12:34b says, "For out of the abundance of the heart the mouth speaks." What you believe in your heart comes out of your mouth and right back into your ears. Your words are powerful (Proverbs 21:18). Your thoughts have a direct impact on how you feel about yourself and your situation, which then impacts what you say, how you behave, and then determines what habits you form. Do you need to reprogram your thinking so that what comes out of your mouth will benefit your future? If so, this can be done by renewing your mind daily from the Word of God! (Romans 1&2)

Envision Yourself Happy and Healthy

Our minds hold great suggestive power! As a child, I felt I didn't receive the attention I craved unless I wasn't feeling good or was hurt. At night when I lay in bed, I imagined myself getting in terrible accidents or becoming ill so that my mother would pay attention to me. Do you think it's just a coincidence that I ended up in the circumstances I did? We have to be very careful where we allow our minds to travel.

At bedtime, I often meditate on healing Scriptures, imagine myself healthy and strong, and end with a prayer of thanksgiving for my healing. I always drift off into a peaceful sleep when I do this. Prayer and Scripture both contain power to heal.

Positive thinking sets our course because it influences how we feel, which affects what we say and shapes our behaviour. Many professionals and athletes use this method to overcome obstacles and succeed.

Run Your Race

"Therefore, since we are surrounded by such a great cloud of witnesses, let us throw off everything that hinders and the sin that so easily entangles, and let us run with perseverance the race marked out for us. Let us fix our eyes on Jesus, the author and perfecter of our faith, who for the joy set before him endured the cross, scorning its shame, and sat down at the right hand of the throne of God. Consider him who endured such opposition from sinful men, so that you will not grow weary and lose heart." (Hebrews 12:1–3)

We all have a race to run! God promises a wonderful prize in the end for all who are faithful. To win, you must hurdle every hindrance and continue forward until you've attained your prize. When you fall down, get back up and keep moving. Try to learn from your mistakes and celebrate each success. Follow the directions God gives you and stay focused on your goal. Staring at the obstacles will cause you to stumble with discouragement.

What is hindering you today from running your race? Sinful habits and negative mindsets will entangle you and hold you back. As we look to Jesus, these hindrances will fall away. He suffered, beyond belief, for each one of us and conquered the enemy so we could enjoy our lives. Make a choice to let go of all the negative thinking, self pity, victim mentality, anxiety, doubt, unbelief, fear, pride, anger, bitterness, and resentment and move forward to enjoy your life to its fullest. You no longer have to drag these chains around. Jesus is waiting to carry your burdens and help you across the finish line.

Dear Heavenly Father,

I ask that You would pour out Your grace upon me and enable me to persevere through this dark time. Please break off any self–pity, negative thinking and fear and fill me with hope, faith, and determination to continue on. Help me to see the good in every situation and put the wisdom and knowledge You've given me into practice. May Your presence be tangible and real to me. Help me to place my trust in You and to rise up above this situation, as if on eagle's wings, so that I will not grow weary or lose heart, in Jesus' name I pray. Amen.

(Perseverance Scriptures: Hebrews 6:12; Hebrews 10:23, 35–36; Hebrews 12:1; Romans 5:3–5; 1 Thessalonians 5:16–18; James 1:2–4.)

---

[1] Nelson. *ITP Nelson Canadian Dictionary of the English language, An Encyclopedic Reference* (Scarborough, ON: International Thompson

Publishing, Nelson; A division of Thompson Canada Limited, 1997), p. 655.

[2] "Knowledge of the Grief Process." *Hospice.* 27 Oct. 2010 (www.http://hospicenet.org/html/knowledge.html).

[3] Ibid.

[4] Zahnwit, Tina & Dyson,Wanda. *Why I Jumped* (Grand Rapids, MI: Fleming H. Revell, a division of Baker Publishing Group, 2006), p. 219.

[5] Ibid, p. 218.

[6] Ibid.

[7] Zahnwit, Tina & Dyson,Wanda. *Why I Jumped* (Grand Rapids, MI: Fleming H. Revell, A division of Baker Publishing Group, 2006), p. 219.

[8] Leaf, Dr. Carolyn. *Who Switched of My Brain? Controlling toxic thoughts and emotions* (South Africa: Switch On Your Brain, 2007).

Chapter Eleven
Managing Stress

You will keep in perfect peace him whose mind is steadfast,
because he trusts in you.

Isaiah 26:3

Running a house with three boys can be a challenge! Keeping up with the laundry, meals, housework and homework can be a feat in itself. When you add doctor's appointments, volunteering, music lessons, art classes, tutoring, and six trips to the hockey rink into the mix, life can get quite hectic. With that said, I've had to learn firsthand how to combat stress by prioritizing and organizing life, so it doesn't get the best of me. We all have our fair share of stressors and as you can imagine, being ill doesn't help. The purpose of this chapter is to give you a closer look at what happens to our bodies during times of pressure and nervous tension, and offer some effective tools to help reduce your stress, thus helping you to attain a happier, healthier life style.

If you're anything like me, you can only tolerate a certain amount before things start to rattle your chain, especially when responsibilities pile up and time is of the essence. This is when circumstances tend to weigh me down. When I lose my sense of control, I start to panic and feel as if I'm being suffocated.

Tips for Reducing Stress

It's important to know your trigger points. Once you've identified them, ask yourself a very important question. Why does this circumstance upset me so much? Stress is usually always rooted in a fear of some type,[1] most commonly from a childhood experience. When you're aware of your fear, you're then able to put the situation into perspective and deal with your own unhealthy habitual behaviours that causes you to react and feel the way you do. With this addressed, you're then able to deal with the situation at hand in a more logical way without getting upset. Some steps to help you through are: 1. Acknowledge and address your feelings. 2. Express your feeling in a healthy way. 3. Choose not to feel guilty about expressing them. Often we worry about how other people will react once we've revealed our feelings. Don't allow your mind to go there. That's between them and God. Let people own their own issues. 4. Pray and choose to have peace even when they don't agree. God will take care of it, you don't need their approval.

Here's an example you can probably relate to. Like many, I enjoy having a clean house. As you may recall, there was a time when I was obsessive about it because I feared that not keeping things perfect would result in my being rejected. I gained approval and acceptance through perfectionism. Even after I'd given up my perfectionist lifestyle, I'd get upset and angry when my family would come in and make a mess after I'd worked really hard to clean and tidy the house. Then I'd feel guilty about speaking up. My family would leave things around for me to pick up and throw their coats on the floor in front of the hook because they didn't feel like hanging them up. What a vicious cycle. On one hand, I gained a sense of purpose through accomplishment, yet it also made me feel devalued, unappreciated and disrespected when I had to pick up after them. But the problem wasn't all them. A huge part of it was me! For years, I'd catered to everyone, wanting their approval. I'd trained my family and others to treat me that way. First I needed to let them know that the rules had changed. Second, when they didn't follow through with my expectations, I needed to speak up and make sure they picked up, instead of doing everything myself and then resenting them for it. This greatly reduced my stress. Besides, everyone needs to do their part. The stress in this situation all rooted from my childhood issues and fear of not being accepted and valued as a person. Take the necessary time to recognize and address your fears to reduce your stress.

I learned the following information from Dr. Don Colbert: Scientific studies directly link stress to sickness and disease because it elevates the cortisol levels within your body. Cortisol is the chemical our brain produces when we are under stress. It's common knowledge that stress suppresses the immune system. It is the job of our immune system to keep us healthy by destroying cancer cells. We can try to elude stress, but it's inevitable in this world, therefore we need to learn how to deal with stress by reducing it as much as possible and by finding ways to de–stress when it can't be avoided. Sleep is a very important to our immune system and helps raise our stress tolerance. When we are sleeping between the hours of twelve midnight and three a.m., the pituitary gland in our brain produces a chemical called melatonin which prevents cancer cell growth. Cortisol also depletes our bodies of the necessary melatonin which keeps our emotional reflux centre in our brain strong. If this deteriorates it causes the organs to begin breaking down and become cancerous by sending wrong messages. It's plain and simple. Stress has the ability to kill! It raises the cortisol and produces an acidic environment within your body and produces free radical cells. These cells damage the healthy cells and can eventually cause sickness if stress stays at a constant high. According to Dr. Colbert, at least seventy-five percent of doctor appointments are related to stress.[2]

God has given us natural methods to combat stress before it combats us. There is an endless list of the symptoms stress can cause. In the past, I have experienced shortness of breath, heart palpitations, tightness in the chest, depression, headaches, insomnia, stomach upset, and even irritable bowel. When I was sixteen, I suffered from a bleeding ulcer because I was a chronic worrier and later in life developed acid reflux due to stress. I didn't know how to deal properly with the stress that resulted from arising negative circumstances. Even when everything was going well, I still worried about trivial things. I worried about what I looked like, what to wear, what people thought of me, whether someone would think I was smart or not; you name it I worried about it! And it all stemmed from the fear of rejection. I was so afraid of being abandoned again that I walked in fear all the time.

Worry is a Waste of Time

Worrying doesn't change anything! It does however, prevent change and cause more stress and anxiety. This allows an open door for the devil to wreak havoc. Decide today to give all concerns to God because He cares about you (1 Peter 5:7). He doesn't want you to be anxious about anything (read Matthew 6:25–34). God is more than capable to take care of your problems. Somehow, some way, He'll take care of all the details. Trust Him with each step and He will guide you on the path of peace. Learn to relax and enjoy!

My friend, Michelyne, has a favourite saying "Let go, let God." There's great advice in that little statement. If you find yourself worrying about something, say a little prayer and let it go. If you catch yourself worrying, tell yourself, "No, I'm not going to worry about that. I trust that God is taking care of things right now. I may not be able to see what's going on, but I trust God is working on my behalf behind the scenes."

Michelyne also has a God box. This isn't a place where you keep God and let Him out on Sunday mornings or for the moments you need Him. This box is used to put prayer notes in to God. It has the same purpose as a prayer journal. A spot you then may look back at as a reminder that you've already given your request to God and that He is looking after things. This is a great way for children to grasp the idea. A private place they can keep their concerns and later return to see how God has answered their prayers.

I have a friend that was suffering from such bad anxiety attacks from stress that she was blacking out. God showed her a way to overcome this problem by envisioning the attack as if it were a light bulb turned on. She then envisioned herself turning off the light bulb by a switch, placing herself in control and she verbally told her body to switch off the stress. By using this technique and working through her issues with prayer, she was able to overcome this problem.

Surround Yourself with Positive People

God blesses us with our family and gives us a choice in whom we pick for friends. Do yourself a favour and choose wisely! Sheila Wray Gregoire often starts her inspirational speeches with a joke about choosing our girlfriends like we would a good bra; giving the advice that we should keep the supportive ones and put the saggy ones to rest! Although we shouldn't just discard people because they're unsupportive, there is some truth to what she's saying. We need to take a good look at our relationships and perhaps remove ourselves from the unhealthy ones. Even if it's just for a time until you learn how to properly deal with them. If so...step back for direction, take action God's way and leave the results to Him. Take some time to evaluate your relationships. Are they one-sided? Do you have any friends that seem to be interested or concerned only with themselves? Do they only call when they want something? A relationship should go both ways, that's what makes it a relationship! God gives us the grace and love to give to others in return, but if you're the only one giving all the time, there's a problem. Your relationship is out of balance. God didn't create you to be a doormat! There are people who'll walk all over you if you'll let them. Ask God what His will is for each situation. Certain relationships will wear you out if you're not careful. Always pray and only do what God tells you to do. Sometimes certain friendships are only for a season. When He says it's time to move on, you need to listen. Satan will use guilt or whatever he can to steal your joy and keep you stressed. Is there someone in your life that is very negative? People who are extremely negative all the time can be very draining. In this case, we need to shake the sand off our boots the way the disciples did after the truth was rejected as a means to letting go of the negative energy and moving on. For this reason take these people in small doses and make sure you spend time with the Lord to get re-energized. The Bible warns us that whoever we surround ourselves with we take the risk of becoming like them also. (See Proverbs 22:24–25; Deuteronomy 20:8b; Proverbs 13:20.)

Do the people you hang around with gossip about other people? What makes you think they are not talking about you? Do you not want God's best for your life? Surrounding yourself with positive people will lift your spirits and help you keep a positive mind set. This type of relationship will provide the support and fulfillment you desire. Don't forget to be a good friend in return. It's wonderful to be able to share the gifts and talents God has given you with others. That's what friendship is all about!

Caution: Sometimes we place expectations on people who were never equipped or meant to fulfill certain needs. It's very important to look to God for your needs to be met and not to people! He'll put the correct people in your life at the right time, and remember not to get upset when it's not who you think it should be! It's time to put God in charge of your relationships!

Sometimes people don't really think about what they are saying and are only trying to make conversation. It amazed me, how many people would start a conversation by telling me of all their friends or relatives that had, or died of, cancer. You can't avoid this; there will be times when people are negative or bad news is given. When this happens, learn to guard yourself by taking control of your thoughts.

Find a Good Support Group

When people have a strong support system they cope much better under stressful situations and as a result are happier and healthier.[3] There are many different types of support groups available designed to relate to specific needs. This could give you an outlet to share openly certain concerns that you may be unable to discuss with those close to you. Bonding with others in similar situations often increases your strength and wisdom, while providing an outlet of fun to take your mind off your situation. People are there for the sole purpose to discuss and answer any questions you may have or to lend an ear when you need to talk. This also takes the pressure off your loved ones who may find it overwhelming or difficult to discuss. Some people don't like the thought of sharing with complete strangers, while others may prefer this. Find an outlet you're comfortable with!

Walking with a friend not only decreases stress, it will motivate, energize, and give you a chance to catch up. People tend to hibernate when feeling down. You may not feel like getting out, but you'll most likely feel better afterwards. Expand your horizons and try a new hobby like painting, pottery, quilting, sketching, and knitting, mosaic glass artwork or playing an instrument. Do it alone or take a friend, the choice is yours.

Relaxation Techniques

(Make sure you have your doctor's approval before trying these exercises.)

- It's very important that you learn how to relax. Start by finding a quiet place to sit and close your eyes.

- Take a deep breath in through your nose and hold it for five seconds. Slowly exhale out of your mouth. Repeat this technique several times.

- Shrug your shoulders up and hold this position for 5 seconds. Now slowly let your shoulders down and allow them to relax.

- Practice your breathing technique again.

- Stretch your arms straight out front, shoulder height as far as you can for five seconds. Let your arms fall down by your sides.

- Hold your arms out to the sides, stretching them as far as possible for five seconds, and then let them relax.

- Stretch your arms up and hold them for five seconds and then relax.

- Repeat your breathing exercise.

- Push your legs, pressing your feet down to the ground as hard as you can for five seconds.

- Let your legs, feet, and toes relax. They should feel loose and warm.

- Allow your whole body to become limp.

- Open your eyes, and slowly stand. Shake your arms, now your legs.

- Breathe in one more time through your nose, hold five seconds and release through your mouth.[4]

Other Ideas: Get adequate sleep, have a cup of chamomile tea, enjoy a foot soak in Epson salts, take a hot shower or relaxing bath with lavender oil, enjoy light exercise, watch a funny movie, do deep breathing and stretching, have massage therapy (discretion needed, read Chapter 14 to learn more) and be honest by expressing your true feelings.

I have tried all of these relaxation methods and have found them to be very beneficial, although prayer, meditation on the Lord and His Word, and "hiding in the secret place" are my favourites. They have proven themselves to be the most calming, and effective, in my life. You're probably wondering what on earth is "hiding in the secret place?" I know it sounds like the familiar childhood game called "hide and seek." Although what I'm referring to is a form of escape, it's not a game! What kind of grown woman hides in a secret place, you might ask? A smart one, I believe! Have you ever heard of a prayer closet? The closet may provide the necessary privacy one might desire, but you don't have to literally stuff your body into this small space, though I know a few people that do. Any quiet place you can rest that doesn't have any distraction is great. Prayer allows us to express and share our emotions with God in a positive manner without having to worry about being judged or interrupted. This is a perfect way to let go of the issues that are troubling you. One of my biggest problems in life is that I'd like to fix the entire world. I think it's because of the way I'm wired; I would love to be everyone's hero, repairing everyone's hurts and meeting all their needs, but unfortunately the job's too big for just me. After a while you get worn out from the added emotional load strapped to your back along with your own. It becomes overwhelming. When we learn to take on only the responsibilities that God asks us to and stop feeling guilty for the things we don't, it's very freeing. As I previously discussed, there isn't any reward for doing the things we're not meant to do and if we don't allow others to use their gifts, we're also robbing them of their reward.

Prayer

"Do not be anxious about anything, but in everything, by prayer and petition, with thanksgiving, present your requests to God. And the peace of God, which transcends all understanding, will guard your hearts and your minds in Christ Jesus." (Philippians 4:6–7)

Prayer is a wonderful way to relieve stress and it has the ability to changes our lives. Many people wonder why we need to pray when God is Sovereign. The answer to this question is found in Genesis, in the very beginning, when God created man. God chose to work through man, giving him free will as a means to build a relationship with us. When God created the earth, He gave man (us) authority and dominion over all of "the earth." If we don't pray, God's hands are tied, per se, until we release our concerns to Him through faith–filled prayer. We limit God with our pride and unbelief. Therefore, He sits back and waits, because of the rights He has given us, until we humble ourselves, stand up in faith, and ask. In other words, although God is all powerful, He's a gentleman and doesn't take action until He has been given the authority by man through prayer and words. I do believe He often sends messages of intervention. Yet our hearts need to be open and willing to recognize the signs.

Can you see why prayer is so important! When we pray, we're giving God the right to work His miracles. If bad things happen in this earth, it is only because of the choices we've made! Man, not God, took prayer out of our schools and governments and then we wonder why the world is such a mess! If we want to see our circumstances change, we need to get praying and include His powerful Scripture.

Even though man sometimes gives Satan access to their (God–given) authority through sin, Jesus took the authority back from Satan when He died on the cross. This made Jesus the highest authority. Therefore Satan can't keep the legal right held by sin over our heads when we've truly repented. Jesus is Lord over all! When we accept Christ as Lord and Saviour (through relationship), we're made joint heirs along with Christ and are given the rights to operate within His authority. This gives us the freedom to ask the Father whatever we want. We can trust that we'll receive whatever we ask for when we remain in constant relationship with Him. Which means abiding in love at all times. It is then that we become in tune with God's heart and know His will for our lives (John 15:7–11). This gives confidence in prayer. God has given believers in Christ the authority to come to Him, asking whatever they want in Jesus' name. All we have to do is trust and believe.

You can rest assured that God in His Sovereignty and goodness will only grant those things that are in your best interest. He has a special plan for each one of us and always does His best to guide us where we need to be at every given time. God also has an overall plan for the world. Satan is furious because he knows his time is running short! Most of what has been prophesied in the Old Testament has already come to pass. Revelation, which is the last book in the Bible, proclaims God's victory! Yes, God wins and saves all His faithful followers while Satan and his demons burn in the pit of hell.

The Bible tells us to pray without ceasing. This means we are to bring our requests to God throughout the day when they come to mind. You don't have to be in a certain position or place. This can be done anywhere at any time! Starting and ending your day with prayer is also important.

"Come to me, all you who are weary and burdened, and I will give you rest. Take my yoke upon you and learn from me, for I am gentle and humble in heart, and you will find rest for your souls. For my yoke is easy and my burden is light." (Matthew 11:28–30)

These are Jesus' words for those weary from the burdens of life. God never intended for us to take on any stress. When we take on responsibilities of others that were never meant to be ours, we get burnt out. You may have a personality similar to mine. Here's a new little twist for you to think about. Sometimes there are things God wants a person to learn in a situation, but if we are always running to fix everyone's problems for them, they'll never learn the valuable lesson intended. That's why it's always important to pray for God's direction, even when it comes to doing something nice for someone. We aren't the world's savour! Does this new perspective give you a little freedom?

I believe it is very important to be an emotional support for others and pray for them when they're on your heart. Pray and do what He asks and leave the remainder in God's capable hands. Have you ever considered that God has someone else for the job other than you? He knows what's best for everyone in the situation. If we think we are the only one that can do the job, then we have a problem with pride. Jesus wants us to come to Him when we're tired and stressed. His loving arms are where we'll find peace.

Jesus also experienced overwhelming times of pressure and grief. It didn't seem to matter where Jesus was, people always looked to Him to meet their needs; even at the most inconvenient moments. At the time of His first cousin's death, Jesus got into a boat to be alone for a while. The people followed Him anyway and met Him at shore the minute He landed. Many people would likely get frustrated by this but Jesus had a soft heart for the people and healed their sick and later performed a great miracle by feeding the five thousand people with five loaves and two fish because they were hungry.

"After he had dismissed them, he went up on a mountain side by himself to pray. When evening came he was there alone." (Matthew 14:23)

When life's demands begin to overwhelm you and you feel emotionally spent, take the opportunity, as Jesus did, to find a quiet place to spend time with the Father. Jesus knows what it's like to hurt and grieve. Are you in the need of strength or guidance? Do you need to be refreshed physically and spiritually? Our Heavenly Father wants to hear from you. He understands and knows you better than anyone else does. He wants to carry your burdens and soothe your heart. The Bible tells us to come to Him like a little child. If we will acknowledge God in everything, choose to pray and trust Him with a thankful heart instead of being worried, anxious or upset, God will grant us peace and direction as promised in Philippians 4:6–7 and Proverbs 3:5–6. God doesn't want us to carry those things. If we want our prayers to be answered, we need to pray with authority with the right motives and keep from strife (James 4:2, 3). If we are asking out of greed, or if we're envious or jealous, we will not receive it. God won't give us anything that's out of His will so we don't have to worry. Trust Him to know what's best. Just pray. When we come to God, we are seen through what Jesus did for us on the cross, so come boldly before His throne! He wants you to come. Our faith only works when we treat others with love. If you want your prayers to be answered, you need to choose to love others regardless of their behaviour. Pray for them. Love is more than just talk, it's taking action. Keep your mouth from gossip, grumbling, fault finding, slander, and criticism. As said before, our prayers will not be heard if we're behaving this way or if we're holding unforgiveness. It is the righteous man who activates God's power through prayer of faith and receives what he asks for. So have faith, walk in love, and ask with the right motive. When we concentrate on treating others right and are obedient to God's direction, He'll grant us the desires of our heart. Chasing them isn't necessary. Matthew 7:7 tells us to ask repeatedly until we receive our requests. James 1:8 reminds us to focus on being positive to connect into God's power. This means we must look past what we see with our natural eye and be certain about what we hope for. It's those who believe, who find rest in God (Hebrews 4). Make Him your shelter and oasis today. Cast your cares on Him instead of letting your circumstances get to you, by praying a simple prayer and trusting Him to give you the answers you need or the solutions to the problems you face.

Heavenly Father,

I'm thankful that You care about me and my life with all its details, large and small. I bring my burdens to You and lay them at Your feet. Please take them; they're too heavy for me to carry. Help me to rest in You. Please protect me from the negative effects of stress. Fill me with Your Holy Spirit to give me the physical, emotional, and spiritual strength I need to carry on. In Jesus' name I pray. Amen.

Finding the Secret Place

Have you ever experienced being in the very presence of God? God is omnipresent, which means He is everywhere, all the time (Psalm 139), but there are different levels of His tangible presence that we can experience. When I've spent time in the "Secret Place" I've experienced greater amounts of comfort and felt more refreshed from being saturated in the Lord's presence than through any technique I've implemented. Stretching exercises and deep breathing practices all have their practical benefits, but "hiding in the secret place" fills us with joy (Psalms 16:11), gives us needed strength, protects us from the damage that comes from oppositional words (Psalm 31:20; Isaiah 54:17), and also provides an additional source of needed protection.

"He who dwells in the shelter of the Most High will rest in the shadow of the Almighty. I will say of the Lord, "He is my refuge and my fortress, my God, in whom I trust." (Psalm 91:1–2)

Earlier in this book, you learned that praise opens the door to God's presence. When we worship God, His presence intensifies and becomes tangible. Sit in a quiet place and invite the Holy Spirit to come. Praise God for all His wonderful attributes, and allow yourself to express your heart to God by casting all your burdens on Him. As you do, you'll experience a great release that is accompanied by an amazing sense of well–being. Some people find it easier to incorporate soft worship music into this time. As God's glory falls down on you, your body may experience various sensations. Your head may feel as if it's swirling, your body might tingle, feel chilled, get covered in goose bumps or feel thick. Not everyone will always experience God's presence the same way. Experience God firsthand and bask in His glory. There is life and healing in His presence. Prayer and meditation on the Word can both be done in the secret place. The secret place is nothing other than spending time alone with God.

During the exodus of the Israelites from Egypt, Moses refused to go unless the presence of God followed them, because he knew the importance of God's presence in their lives. For this purpose, the priests carried the Ark of the Covenant, containing God's presence, to lead them each step of the way. They were guided by a cloud during the day and a pillar of fire by night. They weren't to move or stay unless directed by the Lord.

Years later, after the tribes had reached their destination of their Promised Land, God had King Solomon build a tabernacle in Jerusalem to house the Ark of the Covenant. The Tabernacle was made up of three rooms.[5] The outer court was where the priests performed sacrifices.[6] This was enclosed with a fence and had only one way of access through one gate.[7] Like the gate, Jesus is our only way of access to the Father. And now because of what Jesus did on the cross, we can come boldly before God's thrown. In other words, when we present ourselves before God, we are actually presenting ourselves through what Jesus did. This is one of the reasons why Christians pray in Jesus' name.

The second room in the Tabernacle was called the Holy Place.[8] This is where the congregation gathered to worship.[9] We're no longer bound by the walls of a church to worship God. This can be done anywhere by opening our hearts up to Him. However, it's still important to gather together as a body of believers to gain strength in unity. Unfortunately, many people have stopped going to church because they're offended by God or others. Some people use the excuse that Christians are hypocrites. But you know what? We're all hypocrites in one form or another. Think about it! How many times have you told someone not to do something, and then turned around and did it yourself? That's exactly what a hypocrite does. Church is the best place for us; it's one method God uses to clean us up. If we were perfect, we'd already be in Heaven!

The Holy of Holies was the innermost court where the priest entered once a year to make atonement for their sins.[10] Because of God's holiness, the priest always entered this place of communion and adoration using a cloud of incense to dim their sinful presence from Him.[11] The priest always wore a gown that had bells on the bottom portion of the robe, with a rope wrapped around his waist in case he made a mistake and died. If the bells stopped ringing, the people knew to drag him out by the rope. Even though God remains the same, we are able to come into His presence without fear because of the shed blood of Christ. Jesus is sitting on the mercy seat and is our High Priest. There is no longer the need for sacrifice because Jesus is and was the only perfect sacrifice. We may now come boldly before the Father's throne because Jesus' blood removes the sight of our sin from God's eyes. When you accept Jesus as your Saviour, God sees you through the blood of Jesus. We don't need to go through a priest to have relations with God. We can now come boldly to the throne of grace (Hebrews 4, 8, 9, 10). I don't see anything wrong with religions practicing confession because confession breaks the power of darkness off of sin. However, I see no need to do penance because Jesus already received the punishment for our sins.

Some people feel like they cannot approach God because of the things they have done in their past. Even the greatest of saints have sinned (Romans 3:23). There isn't one sin that God isn't able to forgive. Again for emphasis, God very much wants you to come to Him. He created you along with mankind for the purpose of relationship. He has made relationship possible through the acceptance of Jesus.

Daily quiet time with God helped me experience amazing peace as I read my Bible and prayed for my circumstances to change and improve.

There's an amazing difference to the amount of stress I can tolerate when challenges surface and I've had my devotional time with God.

Meditating on Scripture

Meditating on Scripture can be done during quiet time with God, as well as throughout the day. God's Word is alive, active, energizing, and has the power available to change your circumstances, along with the ability to keep your mind strong. Meditating on positive thoughts will decrease your stress, release your feel-good hormones and may boost your immune system.

Worship Music

Listening to praise music throughout the day is something else I've always done to lift my spirits. It fills me with joy, especially if I'm feeling down. During my journey with cancer, this helped keep me focused on God's ability to save me, rather than the grim details or the messages my body was sending.

Journaling

Writing in a journal helped me sort out my feelings, particularly when I felt confused. It gave me a chance to vent without saying the wrong thing to someone and made it easier to find a solution. Divide the page in half and write the things that trouble you on one side, with a positive outlook written on the other for each negative statement. This can give you an entirely different perspective. This exercise helped me to identify mixed feelings, bring clarity, and see the good in each situation, and contributed to healing my emotions when I'd taken offence. I also prayed and asked God to help me work through the issues. I forgave and blessed those who'd upset me and asked God to open their eyes and work in their hearts. This freed me from resentment and gave me the peace I needed to enjoy my life. Journaling is also a great way to record memories. I love reading about the things my boys have said or done. It amazes me how much I've forgotten. Sometimes things may not seem so funny, but there'll come a day when you might just laugh.

Bringing my concerns to God always gives me an amazing peace. He created the whole world and is well able to take care of more than a few minor details. The Scripture about God measuring the waters out in His hands has brought me such comfort, knowing that His ability to save is far greater than any little problem we have (Isaiah 40:12). He is well able to do above and beyond what we hope for and imagine (Ephesians 3:20).

If you're having a hard time seeing the bright side of life, try writing out a list of things you're thankful for. This sets your mind on what's important and helps start your day out right. There are many things we all can be thankful for, life being the first; salvation, forgiveness, God's mercy, and His grace, to name a few more.

Christian Prayer Counselling

Stress is a physical reaction to negative toxic thoughts.[12] These thoughts cause physical damage to your body because they cause the wrong chemicals to be released by your brain.[13] Dr. Carolyn Leaf says that by walking through repentance and forgiveness, the negative pattern (thorn like memory trees) in the brain can be reversed.[14] Going to a Christian counsellor is a great way to find healing from past hurts and issues. Sharing your deepest feelings, hurts, and even sins with a trained professional who has a godly perspective is essential for your true healing. Countless people have spent millions of dollars on secular counselling, yet haven't experienced true healing. Bringing God into the picture is the missing component. Christian counsellors will deal with issues from a godly perspective and pray for healing and change in your life. Consider the great power available through prayer.

The Power of Suggestion

Words are powerful! They have the ability to encourage or discourage. They hold tremendous power over the way we act and think! Why not speak positive affirmations and confessions about your situation, in addition to confessing God's promises from the Bible? It may save your life!

- I will conquer this sickness because I can do all things with Christ's help (Philippians 4:13).

- I'm not always going to be sick because God's Word says by Jesus' stripes I am healed (1 Peter 2:24).

- I will eat and enjoy the things that bring health to my body because God satisfies my mouth with good things and gives me the strength to exercise (Psalm 103:5).

- I have the faith I need to overcome. God has given me the measure of faith I need and will lead me into triumph (Romans 12:3; 2 Corinthians 2:14).

- God will provide all my needs according to His riches in glory (Philippians 4:19).

- God gives me the wisdom I need when I ask (James 1:5).

Transform Your Thought Life

There is an upside to every card being dealt to us in life. It depends on us as individuals as to whether we are going to flip the card over and play the game of life with joy and anticipation of winning the game or whether we're going to stare at the ugly side and wallow in defeat. The choice is up to you! Jesus, even though He had to face the cross, remembered the joy its outcome would bring to our lives. This gave Him the strength to carry on (Hebrews 12:2). This advice could be applied to everyday living; it's not only for those who happen to be struggling with medical issues. Perhaps you have a difficult marriage or child, or you're not happy with your circumstances at work. Thinking positively and reframing your thoughts can change your entire outlook on the world around you. Problems can become magnified if we concentrate on them too much. Get God's perspective and put them in their rightful place.

Much of our stress is caused from wrong thinking. The journey to positive thinking begins with recognizing when we're thinking negatively. Many times we don't even pay attention to what we are thinking about. When we identify a negative thought in our minds, we're then able to discard it. Many times people assume the worst in a situation in fear of being disappointed with the end result. What would it hurt to look at the bright side of things? Wouldn't it be better to hope for even a little something good than to receive a whole lot of bad!

Many people worry about what other people are thinking. We should never assume what others are thinking. Body language can say a lot about a person, but we should never presume something is our fault when someone is grumpy or cold. We can get so caught up in our little world that we believe it's always about us, when it's not. Everyone has issues in life and the world doesn't always revolve around us and our situation. Don't allow your feelings to rule over a situation. Our feelings can change at any given time and just because you feel a certain way, doesn't mean that's the way things really are. Stop trying to take ownership for every little thing that happens. If you're concerned that you have offended someone, by all means go speak to them and straighten things out, rather than worrying. If you have hurt them you can do your part by apologizing and continue on. Either way, you will gain peace. And remember, you're only responsible for your reaction in a situation. If they choose not to forgive you, the matter is now between them and God.

It's your choice! No one else can choose your thoughts for you. Paul gave instruction to the church to think on things that are good, noble, and of good report. (Philippians 4:8) Are you thinking that seems impossible in the situation you're in right now? I understand how hard it is. God doesn't ask us to do the impossible! He only expects and asks us to do that which is within our reach. He's the miracle worker, not us. Deuteronomy 30:11 says, *"Now what I am commanding you today is not too difficult for you or beyond your reach."* If you can change the way you think, you'll automatically change the way you feel and speak. This will bring blessing in your situation. Just as God called those things into Abram's life, by giving him the name Abraham which meant "father of many nations", at a time when Abraham had not yet received a child, God asks us to speak the positive into our own situation. The Bible refers to this as *calling things that are not as though they were* in Romans 4:17. Let me clarify. I am not telling you to go around lying about your situation to people; that's not what this Scripture is talking about. When you're home alone doing laundry or walking on your treadmill, I want you to speak the positive over your situation. It may seem a little odd when your circumstances are pointing one direction and you are speaking the opposite! If you're out and someone asks how you're doing, you could reply, "right now the Dr. says... and .... But I believe God is going to heal me! You may feel like people are going to think you're nuts! You can't afford to worry about what people think right now! Take the Scriptures that apply to your situation and meditate on them, quote them, pray them. This will transform your thinking and change your circumstances over time! If you need to remind yourself of the power that comes from God's Word, go back and read Chapter 3.

As I've said before, the journey to positive thinking begins with recognizing when we're thinking negatively. Pay attention to what you're thinking about. Identify the negative thoughts and discard them. Believe in the best. Ask for God's help to be positive if you're having trouble.

Learn to Laugh

Laughter is a wonderful kind of medicine. It's inexpensive, there is no pain involved, unless you laugh so hard it makes your ribs hurt, and it doesn't taste bad. *Speaking of pain, did you know that laughter can actually raise your pain threshold? It also has the ability to boost your immune system, reduces stress, lowers blood pressure, reduces food cravings, exercises the heart, and reduces muscle tension, as well as lifts your spirit! Laughter takes your mind off stressful issues and helps relieve negative emotions.*[15] Let's face it, sometimes life is hard and we all could use a good laugh. I purposely bought my son "Mr. Bean" movies for Christmas to help lighten things up around the house. Since this is a breast cancer story, I figured a good bra joke was in order. It's been revolving around the internet for years. Please don't be offended, it's all meant in good fun. It's called, "What religion is your bra?"

> A man walked into the ladies department of a Macy's and shyly walked up to the woman behind the counter and said, "I'd like to buy a bra for my wife."
>
> "What type of bra?"Asked the clerk
>
> "Type?" inquires the man, "There's more than one type?"
>
> "Look around," said the sales lady, as she showed a sea of bras in every shape, size, color, and material

imaginable. "Actually, even with all of this variety, there are really only four types of bras to choose from." Relieved, the man asked about the types.

The sales lady replied; "There are the Catholic, the Salvation Army, the Presbyterian, and the Baptist types.

"Which one would you prefer?" Now totally befuddled, the man asked about the differences between them. The sales lady responded,

"It is all really quite simple...The Catholic type supports the masses; The Salvation Army type lifts the fallen; The Presbyterian type keeps them staunch and upright; and The Baptist type makes mountains out of mole hills."

Here's another joke: What do you call a mastectomy bra? Answer: Holders of False Idols.

I won't put a religion on this one. You'll have to figure it out for yourself. Remember, it's all for fun.

Have you ever wondered why A, B, C, D, DD, E, F, G, and H are the letters used to define bra sizes? If you have wondered why, but couldn't figure out what the letters stood for, it is about time you became informed. (A) Almost Boobs..., (B) Barely there....(C) Can't Complain...(D) Dang...!, (DD) Double dang...!, (E) Enormous...!, (F) Fake..., (G) Get a Reduction..., (H) Help me, I've fallen and I can't get up...! They forgot the German bra, Holtzemfromfloppen.[16]

After my surgery I was unable to wear a bra with prosthesis for at least eight weeks. Apparently it wasn't very noticeable, or so I've been told. But when friends would come to visit, sometimes I would lose my balance (from low blood pressure). I often joked and blamed it on being lopsided, to lighten the mood. When they saw me having fun with the situation, it gave them a sense of relief and permission to relax and enjoy themselves. It's your choice! You can laugh or cry, but I'd rather laugh and have a good time. It's such a great way to reduce stress.

I developed a very serious mindset growing up. After getting sick, I asked God to give me a sense of humour and I have to admit, I have come a long way! Life is short enough as it is, so you might as well enjoy the journey. No one else can do that for you!

Live Each Day As If It's Your Last

Living each day as if it were your last is not an excuse to spend money negligently. It is, however, a means to live without regret; to spend time building positive memories with friends and family. To leave a legacy behind that one can be proud of. Imagine how you could alter someone's day by giving them a hug, a warm smile or a few sincere words of affirmation. What can you do today that will make a difference in someone else's life? It's not about how long we live, but what we do with our lives while we're here! Take the time to write your loved ones a letter of endearment and include funny stories and fond memories. It's wonderful to reminisce. Don't be afraid to allow yourself to be vulnerable; people like it when you're real! You may even have a good laugh or cry that will boost your immune system at the same time! People need to hear that you care. Don't just assume they know. Many people wait until a loved one's funeral to express this. By then it's too late!

How will others remember you? Are you gracious to those around you? Will they think you're generous or stingy, humorous and carefree or grumpy, uptight and serious? Will they say you were kind, compassionate, and loving or would they choose the words mean, cold hearted or distant to describe your nature? If today was your last day on earth, how would you treat it differently?[17] Would you be a little nicer to those around you? We should live our lives that way every day! Today is a new opportunity to start your life over and do things differently. Are there any loose ends you need to tie up? Do you have relationships that need to be mended? Is there someone you need to ask to forgive you or bestow forgiveness upon? Today is the day to approach your relationships differently.

In life, we're not always going to make the right choices or say the right things. However, if you apologize when you do, it shows humility and helps restore lost respect. When you don't feel good, don't use that as an excuse to behave badly. Excuses are copouts! Warn others ahead of time, so they will understand and perhaps give you a little space. Get alone for a few minutes to collect your thoughts until you can handle the commotion. Draw your strength from God. He planted self-control within you and it is your responsibility to act on it.

Learn to let go of past mistakes. Don't give them control over you. Value the time you have and what you've done that's positive. Cut out the meaningless things that steal your time away and enjoy the little things in life. Eat better! Exercise in balance. Celebrate life and survivorship! Be your own advocate and listen to your intuition.

Finances

Finances can become a huge burden during times of treatment. Many are unable to work due to sickness and sometimes the extra expenses can drain your savings account. This can be quite a concern when not all needed treatment is covered by our health care system or insurance companies. During treatment, free rides to and from appointments are offered through the Cancer Society. If you prefer to drive yourself, receipts for parking and mileage can be saved for income tax purposes, but you must have parking stubs to claim your mileage. Be aware that amounts must exceed 3% of your income to be claimable. Help is offered through Trillium for uncovered medical expenses. Still, you must qualify within a certain tax bracket to utilize this service. They use a sliding scale with which they require proof of income (tax stub) from the previous year. Community Care Access Centers (CCAS) provide limited free services and discounted rates for people, yet have long waiting lists and are only able to provide a few hours a week because of cut-backs in funding, unless you're paying for private care. Hospice (a non-profit organization) offers free support that depends on donations from outside sources.

People in a higher tax bracket may feel they're being penalized for being sick when they've worked just as hard as others. It doesn't matter what category you fall into, if you're God's child, He promises to make the injustices in your life right! Bring your needs to Him and watch Him provide.

"I will repay you for the years the locusts have eaten." (Joel 2:25a)

"Instead of their shame my people will receive a double portion, and instead of disgrace they will rejoice in their inheritance; and so they will inherit a double portion in their land, and everlasting joy will be theirs. For I, the Lord, love justice; I hate robbery and iniquity. In my faithfulness I will reward them and make an everlasting covenant with them." (Isaiah 61:7, 8)

If you make Jesus your Lord and put your trust in Him, God promises to repay you double for the hardships you've endured. He will redeem, deliver, and restore the places of devastation that the troubles in life have devoured.

God wants to be your provider! During the writing of this book, money happened to be really tight, due to some unforeseen events. I desperately needed an editor for my book but didn't have the money to pay one. One morning I prayed in desperation, asking the Lord to provide. I knew He was able. I just didn't know how He was going to do it. The pressure from obstacles seemed to come from every angle. That morning while out for my walk, I bumped into Jacquie, an old friend, walking her golden doodle. She mentioned she had finished some courses to start a freelance editing business in her spare time. I hugged her in excitement and told her I'd let her know if I needed her services. Could she be the one? I wondered. Still I let the thought go because I really didn't have the money to pay her. In the meantime, the Lord revealed to me in prayer who I should ask to proofread and several weeks later my three proofreaders, Cindy, Wanda, and my mom, stepped up to the plate after giving it prayerful consideration. One day, at "Mom's Time Out", I requested prayer that God would give me clear direction for my book and meet my needs for an editor. My friend Suzanne, approached me afterwards and expressed that she strongly felt I should consider our mutual friend, Jacquie. I told her I'd love to use her but explained my financial situation and asked her to keep the matter private. One week later, as I sat at my computer, wondering what I was going to do, I heard tapping at my kitchen door. When I opened the door I was surprised to see Jacquie standing with a huge grin on her face.

"I just stopped by to ask if it would it be alright if I edited your book for free?"

For a moment I just stared back with my mouth open wide. I was speechless and stunned with amazement. Finally I stuttered back "Yes. Yes! Of course you can! Thank you, thank you so much! You have no idea what an answer to prayer this is!"

As soon as she left, I ran to the phone to call Suzanne and tell her the news. She laughed hysterically and reassured me that she had kept my confidence.

I serve an amazing God! You see, God has no limitations. He promises in Philippians 4:19 that He will meet all of our needs according to His glorious riches. God's riches consist of everything in this earth as well as those in Heaven (Psalm 24:1). I also desperately needed some new pants, but didn't have the extra money for that either. I brought my need before the Lord in prayer and left it in His hands. The moment I'd get the urge to shop, I'd feel the Lord telling me to watch my money. God nudged me to give away the pants I had that were too big as seed for my own harvest. Even though I wasn't using them anymore, my mind questioned whether that was a good idea. The fact that I may need them again kept popping up in my thoughts. Our natural instinct, when we're experiencing lack, is to hoard. Despite this uncertainty, I decided to trust God, knowing that if I needed bigger pants down the road, He would provide. Two weeks later a friend dropped off a huge bag full of gorgeous pants, capris, and shorts that she no longer needed. I was amazed! Every pair fit beautifully! This is only a few examples of what God has done. I relied on Him to fulfill a need and He blessed me far above and beyond what I'd hoped or imagined! God desires to demonstrate His grace, goodness, and power to you also.

Looking to God to provide isn't an excuse to live outside what you can afford. God expects us to be good stewards of our money. We need to find balance and live within our means. Use wisdom instead of being motivated by feelings. An extra outfit may not seem like it'll break the bank at the moment, but it may if some unexpected bills come in.

Many people try to keep up with everyone else by purchasing all the latest and greatest items. But have you ever thought that perhaps they may be drowning in debt? Jesus warns us about coveting in Luke 12:15 and reminds us that a man's life doesn't consist of the abundance of his possessions. Make a future plan by creating a budget now and do your best to stay within your limits. Find the joy in being content with what you have. The disciple Paul was familiar with both plenty and lack (Philippians 4:11–12). He discovered the secret to being content in whatever circumstance he faced by remaining in the joy that came as a result of his relationship with Jesus. God wants His children to be blessed with nice things but He doesn't want us to go into debt to have them. If we do, it makes us a servant to the lender. God wants us to prosper His way. Many experts recommend saving money each month, spending some, and giving some. Nobody seems to have trouble spending it. However, the saving and giving can be a challenge for some.[18]

For those in a situation of lack, there are numerous things you can do to cut costs. It feels good to buy brand new merchandise, but it isn't always practical or the best choice for our environment. Hanging laundry will cut down on gas or hydro. Although turning down the heat and wearing a sweater and slippers in the winter months is often a method people use to save money, it's probably not wise during treatment. Staying warm should be a priority. You don't want to put your health at risk by catching a cold. Unfortunately, eating healthy costs more, but buying cheaper, processed food (if you can call it that) really isn't an option. Good nutrition should be your focus. You need to take good care of your body.

Search for the sales in flyers, make meal plans, and buy groceries accordingly, so there's no waste. You may contact manufacturers and ask for coupons for your favourite healthy products or visit websites and print out coupons offered online. Websites reveal what goes on sale at certain times of the year. Track how many weeks your favourite items go on sale and buy the amount you'll need until it goes on sale again. Products usually go on sale every four weeks and remain for a certain period of time. Many stores offer shoppers loyalty cards as well.[19]

Please remember to put your health first!

"The blessing of the Lord brings wealth and he adds no trouble to it." (Proverbs 10:22)

Protection and blessing are linked to obedience. For this reason, God asked me to tithe a certain amount a month to a healing ministry to sow seed for my own healing. When we give an offering to the Lord (whatever way He asks) it releases a blessing from Heaven. If something is bound on earth it is bound in Heaven until it is loosed on earth (Matthew 16:19). This is done by giving. Because I'm a stay–home mom and didn't have the extra money, I wasn't quite sure how I was going to do this. Yet God faithfully provided even this. For the first while, I began finding money in puddles next to my parked car or people would hand me money at speaking engagements that covered the amount the Lord asked me to send. You see, God asks us to tithe ten percent of our earnings so that we will be blessed. He owns the world and everything in it (Psalm 24:1), so it's not like He really needs our money. He asks us to give for our benefit. As we discussed before, the world is created on a foundational law of reaping and sowing. Luke 6:38 says, "Give, and it will be given to you. A good measure, pressed down, shaken together and running over, will be poured into your lap. For with the measure you use, it will be measured to you." When we give tithes and offerings to the Lord which belong to Him in the first place (Malachi 3:8), He blesses the remainder of our money to go farther than it would have before (2 Corinthians 9:10) by rebuking Satan the devourer. (Malachi 3:10–11)

This is the only principle God tells us to test Him in. If we will be faithful to God by following this principle, God promises to open the floodgates of heaven to pour out a blessing so big that we'll be unable to contain its volume. He wants to bless us with more than enough. There have been a few times I've forgotten to tithe. When I did, my husband's overtime often dropped, appliances broke or something happened that would take any extra money away. But worst of all, health issues would pop up. Tithing is like Heaven's insurance policy. Only you don't have to fight for a return in your investment! God gladly pays up. (2 Corinthians 9:10)

In the past, I allowed fear to hinder my obedience in giving. I looked at the state of the economy rather than at my Heavenly Father's bank account. But when I finally got hold of these truths and chose to walk in faith instead of fear, my financial circumstances began to change. The more I allowed myself to be led by the Holy Spirit, the less my flesh dictated to me.

God has already provided for your need. Isaiah 53:5 says, "... *the punishment that brought us peace was upon him and by his wounds we are healed.*" Well, the word "peace" translates to "prosperity" from the Hebrew language to English,[20, 21] which means what Jesus did on the cross was done so that we may prosper in all things. When Jesus said it was finished at the cross, He was also referring to our financial blessing. Jesus completely fulfilled His call and defeated the enemy. That defeat meant the enemy had lost his dominion over everything in the believer's life according to their faith! Why not unwrap this gift with your faith? If you have a financial problem, inspect the condition of your faith. That's what God works with! If your faith is in good condition, check your love walk! But don't forget, you have to plant financial seed to reap a financial harvest! See Psalm 34:10b, Romans 8:32 and Philippians 4:19. We'll explore this a little more in the next chapter.

Prioritize Your Tasks

Often cutting down on stress means taking a new approach to the way we do things.[22] One of the most helpful tips I've learned is to make a list of things I need to do according to importance and mark them off once accomplished. This keeps me from becoming overwhelmed and helps remove pressure by allowing me to see my accomplishments. Don't focus on what hasn't been done yet. Take each situation one step at a time and stop trying to pack so much into your day. It's not healthy to be running on adrenalin all the time; it may even become a danger zone. Rushing all the time can add stress to your life. Slow down a little and allow yourself more time.[23] This will make the tasks you do more enjoyable. Try not to over–commit yourself either.[24] Pray about everything and only say "yes" when God leads you. Otherwise, you may find yourself worn out! Just because something seems good, doesn't mean it's in your best interest. Often when we over–commit it's because we don't know how to say no, are compelled by a sense of guilt, or we have a problem with pride![25] Do you think you're the only one that can do the job right? Ask God to re-veal the reasons why you do certain things. If you are prideful, ask for forgiveness and allow others to help when God directs. If you struggle with control, put God in charge. If you're motivated by guilt, deal with the root cause and let it go. Be sure to accept truth in situations to bring peace and refuse to give place to lying thoughts. Whatever it is, ask God for the strength to change and follow His guidance. If we're doing too much, we're often less efficient. It's easy to get stressed when you're tired. When you find a good balance, you'll be more productive and much happier in the process.

Simplify Life

Often it's the simple things in life that bring the most joy. When we complicate our lives and plans, we just add stress.[26] Take each day one step at a time and try simplifying things. For many years, I planned everything I did with perfection. If the planning didn't exhaust me, fulfilling my goal did and in the process I was too busy to enjoy what I was doing.

The story of Mary and Martha, in Luke 10, provides a wonderful example of this. Jesus had come for a simple visit with the girls. Mary, knowing what mattered, chose to spend time developing her relationship with Jesus, while Martha decided to complicate the visit by preparing a fancy meal. Instead of enjoying his companionship, she occupied herself with unnecessary tasks and became frustrated and angry with Mary for not adhering to her plans. Jesus just wanted to spend time with them. How often do you overcomplicate life when a simple plan would suffice?

Learn to be flexible with people and events; not everything is going to work out the way you plan. I can't tell you how many times a drink has spilt on the floor just after I'd mopped it and company was about to arrive. I've learned that if I can't change my circumstances, I need to change my approach in how I deal with them. Choosing to be happy and saying out loud, "I can be happy even though this or that has happened," will change your attitude and affect your emotions in a positive way. Learn to be merciful. Instead of getting angry, learn to pick your battles wisely before your battles get the best of you!

Do you feel tired and stuck? Take a good look around your house. Do you have unnecessary clutter lying around? Are your closets stuffed with clothes that you never wear? Start by decluttering your home.[27] Have some fun with it. Go through your possessions and give away to charity anything that you don't need or wear.[28] You'll feel better for it and someone else will benefit. As a result, when our home is well-organized, our thoughts tend to be also.

Helping Your Kids Cope

Just as external pressures have the ability to cause us stress, kids can easily get stressed too! Keeping with regular routines around the house as much as possible will help give them a sense of security and comfort. Keeping the lines of communication open by sharing only the necessary details is important. Children often overhear parents talking. It's better if they hear information coming from you. Be sure to use wisdom here. Too many facts could frighten and overwhelm them. Please don't make promises you can't keep, but do reassure them with words of affirmation. Let them know that God is always with them no matter what happens. Writing letters of fond memories and endearments to your children will bless them with keepsakes for a lifetime and boost their spirits. Using humour whenever possible, helps keep the atmosphere positive. Be sure to apply healthy boundaries and ask others to respect them. When people are sick, ask them to stay home. Remember to honour yourself by honouring the boundaries you make. If you don't regard yourself, no one else will either. Your children will likely need extra attention at this time. Be sure to make yourself available to answer all questions or to comfort them when they're afraid. The phone and outsiders may have to wait. It's easy to lose sight of their needs when much of the focus is on you.

Kids tend to act out when stressed. Try to concentrate on the important issues. When you comment on every little issue, you'll likely break their spirit. Learn to pray and let issues go. If you're stressed, they'll feed off it. Rely on God and do your best to remain stable. Teachers or coaches need to be informed during times of distress so they can keep an eye on them and provide the necessary compassion and understanding. Implementing these tips will also cut down dramatically on their stress, which will in turn help eliminate yours.

We often get frustrated with others because of their choices. If we would take the time to understand why other people do the things they do, this would greatly reduce our stress. When issues come up with your kids, take the time to talk to them about why they did what they did, instead of throwing out advice or jumping down their throats. If you can put yourself in their shoes for a moment and relate to them on their level of thinking, you may have a better chance of getting them to see your point or at least listening to you when the time is right. Try this with others as well. When you find out where people are coming from, the things they do will likely irritate you less.

In conclusion to this chapter, I would like to encourage you to find balance in everything you do. I believe it's an important key that will help you truly enjoy your life. This can be a challenge for those with a personality similar to mine, who do everything with an "all or nothing" philosophy. Don't forget to get your rest, eat properly, drink sufficient amounts of pure water, use the necessary steps to reduce your stress, and exercise regularly. Do what you can and leave the rest in God's hands. It doesn't matter what's going on in your life, Jesus will be right there beside you through it all.

---

[1] Leaf, Dr. Caroline. *Who Switched of My Brain?* (South Africa: Switch On Your Brain, 2007).

[2] Colbert, Don, MD. *The Seven Pillars of Health* (Lake Mary, Florida: Siloam, 2007).

[3] Cloud, Dr. Henry, *The Secret Things of God* (New York, NY: Howard Books A Division of Simon & Schuster, Inc., 2007).

[4] Garland, E. Jane, M.D., F.R.C.P. (C), Clark, Sandra L., PhD. *Taming Worry Dragons: A Manual for Children, Parents, and other Coaches* (Vancouver B.C.: Children's & Women's Health Centre of British Columbia, November 1995, Revised November 2000), p 36, 37.

[5] The Tabernacle—Introduction. The Bible Study Page. 05 February 2010 (http://thebiblestudypage.com/taber_intro.shtml)

[6] The Tabernacle—The Ark and Mercy Seat. The Bible Study Page. 05 February 2010 (http://thebiblestudypage.com/taber_ark_mercy.shtml)

[7] The Tabernacle—The Fence and the Outer Court. The Bible Study Page. 05 February 2010 (http://www.the biblestudypage.com/taber_fence.shtm)

[8] The Tabernacle—Introduction. The Bible Study Page. 05 February 2010 (http://thebiblestudypage.com/taber_intro.shtml)

9 The Tabernacle—Introduction. The Bible Study Page. 05 February 2010 (http://thebiblestudypage.com/taber_intro.shtml)

[10] The Tabernacle—The Ark and Mercy Seat. The Bible Study Page. 05 February 2010 (http://thebiblestudypage.com/taber_ark_mercy.shtml)

[11] The Tabernacle—The Ark and Mercy Seat. The Bible Study Page. 05 February 2010 (http://thebiblestudypage.com/taber_ark_mercy.shtml)

[12] Leaf, Dr. Caroline. *Who Switched off My Brain?* (South Africa: Switch On Your Brain, 2007).

[13] Ibid.

[14] Ibid.

[15] Colbert, Don, MD. *The Seven Pillars of Health* (Lake Mary, Florida: Siloam, 2007). Referenced from: Bayer, Rich. PhD, *"Benefits of Happiness,"* Upper Bay Counseling and Support Services, Inc., April 11, 2005). (http://www.upperbay.org/benefits_of_happiness.htm).

[16] "What Religion is Your Bra? - A Joke." *Thrifty fun.* 2 Nov. 2010 (http://thriftyfun.com/tfl17523517.tip.html).

[17] Carlson, Richard PH.D. *Don't Sweat the Small Stuff.* (New York, New York: Hyperion, 1997).

[18] Finance Resource: Meyer, Joyce *"How to handle your finances"* CD Set. (Fenton, MO: Joyce Meyer Ministries). Referenced from: Katz, Robert W., CPA with Katz, Jamie. *Money Came by the House the Other Day* (Sanford, FL: DC Press, 2006).

[19] "Money Saving Queen.com."*The Power of coupons by Sara Roe.* 2 Nov. 2010 (www.money savingqueen.com).

[20] Goodrick Edward W., Kohlenbergen III John R. *The NIV Exhaustive Concordance* (Grand Rapids, Michigan: Zondervan, 1990), p.1637.

[21] "Shalom." Wikipedia: The Free Encylopedia.19 January 2010 (http://en.wikipedia.org/wiki/Shalom).

[22] Meyer, Joyce. *100 Ways to Simplify Your Life* (New York, NY: Faith Words, 2008).

[23] Ibid.

[24] Ibid.

[25] Ibid.

[26] Ibid.

[27] Ibid.

[28] Ibid.

Chapter Twelve
Entering Your Promised Land

The Lord had said to Abram, "Leave your country, your people and your father's household and go to the land I will show you. I will make you into a great nation and I will bless you; I will make your name great, and you will be a blessing. I will bless those who bless you, and whoever curses you I will curse; and all peoples on earth will be blessed through you."

Genesis 12:1–3

God promised Abram that he would become the father of many nations if he would leave his family and go to a new land, a land that was lush and prosperous. By faith, Abram set out at the age of 75 with his wife Sarai and his nephew, Lot, for the land of Canaan, a place he had not seen through his natural eyes, but through the eyes of faith. This is an amazing account of how God can take a situation that appears impossible to the mind of man and turn it around and do something great.

"Jesus replied, "What is impossible with men is possible with God." (Luke 18:27)

What is your desired Promised Land? Is it a place in life that holds promise of no sickness and disease in your body, or perhaps for a loved one, a safe environment for your children, peaceful relationships, satisfying job, or a special accomplishment that will fill a specific dream or purpose? Whatever it may be, God wants you to have and enjoy a good life and has placed those special desires into your heart for a purpose. First you must attain the faith and hope needed to reach your Promised Land. We all have specific hopes and dreams for our lives; for some, past disappointments have left them fearful and afraid to hope. As a result, they guard themselves with a cold front and secretly hide their desires deep within the recesses of their hearts. However, faith and hope are the keys that God uses to work within your situation and these must be activated to receive.

Are you facing difficulties that seem impossible to overcome in the natural? When your flesh feels weak, your mind will want to follow. This is when it is important to look at God and what He can do, instead of your circumstances. He is bigger than any problem we may encounter. I have found that as I keep my eyes on my goal, rather than the obstacles I face, they lose their magnitude. Think of your obstacles as stepping stones that build character.[1] This will enable you to keep a positive mindset.

Has God given you a specific promise from His Word or spoken one directly into your heart? Meditating on these promises will increase your faith and give you the hope to endure when opposition comes. Seek God. Ask Him for the promise He has for your life, if you haven't yet received one. At times, well-meaning people can bring discouragement. You must leave behind the opinions of others, along with doubt, unbelief and the lack of your own ability, to press forward toward your goal. God will help you in your weaknesses. Be obedient to what God tells you and put your cares in His hands. As you do, your faith and trust will develop.

"For no matter how many promises God has made, they are "Yes" in Christ. And so through him the "Amen" is spoken by us to the glory of God." (2 Corinthians 1:20)

God is not asking us to leave our families, although we must let go of self-destructive habits, such as self-pity, excuses, and other old mindsets, to reach the abundant life God has for us. Let go of the past. A victim mentality will keep you in a pit of despair. We cannot fulfill our destiny by staring at the obstacles or having a passive attitude. To reach our destination we must proceed forward expecting a miracle by having faith and hope.

God is able and does perform miracles, although we are still responsible for doing our part as well. God knows our personality. We often have to go through the pain of a circumstance so that we won't fall back into our old destructive habits that put us in that situation in the first place. Some people wait around doing nothing when they should be taking action. If you are in need of physical healing, do your part by taking care of your body, drinking lots of pure water, getting the proper sleep and rest, exercising, and eating right. If you're in financial trouble, do what you can to get out of debt. If there are things you know you should do, then you're obligated to do them. God offers us the promises that will bring about change, but we must take action by following His direction to receive them. If you're not sure what to do, ask God!

When someone wants to go to university, they prepare by taking high school classes that relate to their desired field. Before they even graduate, they work to save for tuition and look around at different schools to which they can apply. They don't just sit around and wait for the universities to come to them. No, they take action! God wants us to step out in faith to do what's possible and as we do, God will step in and perform the impossible! God is calling you to rise up and take action (Isaiah 61:1). What steps do you need to take towards receiving your goal?

Following God's Plan

When Abram was 99, the Lord appeared to him to make a covenant with him, saying; *"As for me, this is my covenant with you: You will be the father of many nations. No longer will you be called Abram: your name will be Abraham, for I have made you a father of many nations. I will make you very fruitful; I will make nations of you, and kings will come from you. I will establish my covenant as an everlasting covenant between me and you and your descendants after you for the generations to come, to be your God and the God of your descendants after you. The whole land of Canaan, where you are now an alien, I will give as an everlasting possession to you and your descendants after you; and I will be their God."* (Genesis 17:4–8)

God also changed Sarai's name to Sarah. Sarah began to reason regarding the promise. God wanted to bless Abraham and Sarah with a child in His timing. This was not happening soon enough for Sarah so she took the matter into her own hands and gave her handmaiden to her husband, thinking that God must have needed an avenue other than through her womb to fulfill the promise. Abraham listened to Sarah's reasoning and followed her plan. It wasn't God's!

Oh, if they had only trusted God with their hearts! Choosing our own way over God's direction can cause enormous grief! When Sarah's handmaiden, Hagar, became pregnant, she became very resentful toward Sarah. Can't say I blame her. Expected to lay with a man out of duty, one she obviously wasn't in love with. Although her path was laid out for her, any dreams or desires she may have had for her own life were over. Sarah became bitter herself, faced by the constant reminder of her inability to provide her husband with a desired child. In her pain, Sarah mistreated Hagar. Distraught, Hagar fled to the desert. God, in His compassion, sent an angel to meet with her. The angel told her that if she would go back and submit to her mistress, her descendants would greatly increase. The angel shared that she was going to have a son and instructed her to name him Ishmael. In addition, the angel advised her of his future stubborn and wild disposition that would cause him to be in opposition towards everyone (Genesis 16:9–12). In obedience, she returned and had the child as instructed.

How many times has God given us specific directions with the intention to bless us and we've done things our own way out of doubt, lack of desire, or impatience? In spite of their mistake, God heard Abraham's cry and made Ishmael the father of 12 rulers. God's covenant promise was still established through the womb of Sarah, but was delayed 13 years. God is able and willing to redeem the messes we've made. Don't beat yourself up. Face the situation. Take ownership and do what's right. It's not too late. Often we still have to deal with the repercussions of our bad choices. We see this as we look at the descendants of Ishmael. It was through them that the Karan (this is the Arabic religious rulebook which is their equivalent to our Bible) was developed (they persecute Christians) and there's still tension between the Arabs and the Jews today. Abraham and Sarah made a serious mistake. Nevertheless, when God makes a promise He follows through because He is a God of His Word!

"Because of the Lord'S great love we are not consumed, for his compassions never fail. They are new every morning; great is your faithfulness." (Lamentations 3:22, 23)

God told Abraham to circumcise himself and his descendants after him for all generations as a sign of this covenant and that Sarah would bear him a son, to be named Isaac. God sometimes asks us to remove things from our lives as a sign of obedience, dedication, and love for Him; things that bring harm to our body, mind, and spirit.

"Without weakening in his faith, he faced the fact that his body was as good as dead—since he was about a hundred years old—and that Sarah's womb was also

dead. Yet he did not waver through unbelief regarding the promise of God, but was strengthened in his faith and gave glory to God, being fully persuaded that God had power to do what he had promised." (Romans 4:19–21)

The world would have laughed as they did at Noah when he built the ark. Both Sarah and Abraham laughed knowing how unusual the circumstances were. Many things we're called to believe, in faith, don't make sense in the natural. How could they possibly become the parents of many nations when their bodies were as good as dead? Yet he chose to believe the impossible because he knew nothing was too hard for the Lord!

When doubt and unbelief try to creep their way into your mind, do as Abraham must have done, and strengthen yourself with encouragement. Faith is not based on logic or the reasoning of man. The world bases their beliefs on what they see with their eyes, but faith's foundation is based on believing what you cannot see. God asks us to reason with Him (Isaiah 1:18) by trusting Him with our whole heart and not leaning on our own understanding (Proverbs 3:5). Remind yourself of all the times God has pulled you through difficulties and focus on what God has promised rather than on what the circumstances look like or what people say.

"*Against all hope, Abraham in hope believed and so became the father of many nations, just as it had been said to him, "So shall your offspring be.*" (Romans 4:18)

Believing is the key. Abraham believed and as a result, he received. It was what brought the promise of God into his life. Faith is what connected him to God's plan in the spiritual realm and brought it forth into reality (Romans 5:2). Faith is not based on what we see with our eyes, but what we view with our hearts; the desires we hope for in our lives. God wants us to act in faith; it pleases Him! It is those who believe that receive their promise. Our faith is activated by love, when we choose to love others in spite of their weaknesses and failures. Our faith has the ability to move the mountains in our lives. It is out of our love for God that we want to obey His Word and then are filled with the faith to follow through.

Today, people think believing means to acknowledge something as real, but in fact believing means "trusting and obeying".[2] Satan believes God exists but He isn't living in the Promised Land or going to Heaven! Believing God means trusting and obeying what He asks of us! Trust is built through experience! As you experience God for who He really is, you'll quickly learn that you can trust His character. And when you do, you'll automatically want to obey Him in return.

Reminding God of His Promises

In Luke 18, we are reminded in a parable told by Jesus to pray without ceasing. A widow continually came to the town judge requesting justice. Although he didn't care about people or fear God, he eventually gave her what she wanted because he knew she would keep coming back. (See Luke 18:6, 7, 8.)

Sometimes people don't understand why they need to ask God for things, especially if He's already promised them in His Word. As said before, God chooses to work with us because He wants to have a relationship with us. It clearly states in James 4:2 that we do not have because we do not ask! When we pray, it's important to remind God of His promises because it clearly states in His Word that He watches over the earth to perform His Word. God is faithful! When we remind Him of His promises, He remembers and acts on what He has promised.

Don't give up; be tenacious. God promises that if we persevere and don't give up, when we have done the will of God, we will receive what He has promised (Hebrews 10:36). Be patient and believe until your answer comes (vs. 36, 38). If your trusting God for healing, believe until your symptoms disappear. It takes time! Stay in the Word and be consistent with reading, meditating, and confessing the promises regarding your situation; this will keep the doubt out of your heart!

"Ask and it will be given to you; seek and you will find; knock and the door will be opened to you. For everyone who asks receives; he who seeks finds; and to him who knocks, the door will be opened." (Matthew 7:7, 8)

Prayer is the answer to many of our troubles (see James 5:13–16). It is an amazing way to connect with God and tell Him what we need. He already knows, but He wants to hear it from you. Talking to Him is one way to build on your relationship. It's up to you. He gave us free will because He didn't want puppets or robots for children. He desires for us to approach Him the way a little child would come to their earthly parents with hope and expectation. Perhaps you find this difficult because your earthly father is unapproachable. God's not like that. God's not angry with you. He loves you and wants you to come to Him. Set the fear aside and come to Him. He's waiting with open arms. Experience the Father's love He has for you. Go to Him expecting in faith, it is the key to answered prayer.

The righteous have power-packed prayers that make things happen. Accepting Jesus as our Saviour is the only act that makes us righteous in God's eyes. Maintaining a clear conscience by following God's direction and confessing and repenting when He reveals sin in our lives will open the door to receiving your requests. Don't stress about not being perfect, that's God's job. Just come before Him with a pure, believing heart and watch your circumstances change!

If doubt pops into your head when you pray, immediately remind yourself that all things are possible with God. It only takes faith the size of a mustard seed to move mountains (Matthew 17:20) and we've all been given a measure of it.

In previous chapters, we discussed how our emotional wounding has the ability to cause sickness. Holding on to offense, bitterness, anger, and resentment is an ungodly response, and is sin. Sin can hinder our prayers (Mark 11:25, 26; Proverbs 15:29). In James 5:16 it shares that something incredible happens when we're able to open up to a trusted confidant and share our downfalls. There is a strength that comes with accountability. Sin no longer has the ability to hold its dark grip over you because you're taking back the authority God originally gave you, instead of allowing Satan to hold it. It is very important to follow up with prayer to complete the necessary healing process and to guard your heart and mind with peace. This works with any type of sin.

"Now faith is being sure of what we hope for and certain of what we do not see." (Hebrews 11:1)

"Let us hold unswervingly to the hope we profess, for he who promised is faithful." (Hebrews 10:23)

God is faithful indeed. Still, we do have a responsibility to keep faith. When we follow through with our part, God is able to do His. Remember God is sovereign; He is more than capable to fulfill a plan, except He chooses to work with us and through us and will not force Himself on anyone because He is a gentleman.

"It is written: 'I believed; therefore I have spoken.' With that same spirit of faith we also believe and therefore speak...So we fix our eyes not on what is seen, but on what is unseen. For what is seen is temporary, but what is unseen is eternal." (2 Corinthians 4:13, 18)

The ability to believe is attained through hearing the Word. You can always tell what someone believes in their heart by what comes out of their mouth. Perform your own faith check by listening to what you're saying. If your words are wavering with doubt and unbelief, get in the Word and study the promises until you feel strong. You'll know because your attitude will be positive as well! Staying in the Word will keep you that way. Matthew 17:20 tells us...*"if you have faith as small as a mustard seed, you can say to this mountain, 'Move from here to there' and it will move. Nothing will be impossible for you."* Line your words up with what the Bible says about your situation. If you want healing, pray Scripture and make positive confessions saying "I am healed in Jesus' name," with belief that you have received it!

Consistency is the key to receiving the desired result.[3] This can be difficult at times. Especially when symptoms crop up and people are asking how you are. But we need to stop speaking symptoms and sickness, because we get what we say.

Therefore your reply could be," I believe God has healed me" or "I believe God is healing me." But you do need to truly believe this in your heart for it to actually happen. I've had people ask how I am and then repeatedly ask me again because I didn't say what their flesh was dying to hear! They'd say, "No, how are you really?" I don't even think I looked bad! Change the subject if you need too. We need to listen to the Words of God, act on what His Word says and then stand firm believing that we have received the promise (Romans 10:9–11; Hebrews 10:38). Faith is a powerful spiritual force that will change your circumstances as you align your words and attitude with what God says in His Word. It is the ability to believe what God says over what the natural looks like.

Read Mark 11:22–26. Obedience is a major key to receiving what we ask. When we are obedient to God's commands, we can ask what we want and we will receive it. This is held by a simple condition of believing (trusting and obeying) in Jesus and requesting within God's will. This is learned by reading His Word. First John 3:21–23 reveals this truth... *"Dear friends, if our hearts do not condemn us, we have confidence before God and receive from him anything we ask, because we obey his commands and do what pleases him. And this is his command: to believe in the name of his Son, Jesus Christ, and to love one another as he commanded us."*

Proverbs 21:21 says, *"He who pursues righteousness and love finds life, prosperity and honour."* Therefore if we want to prosper, we must follow through with God's Word and be obedient. Health and blessing both come from being obedient (Proverbs 4:20–22).

The Lord hears and acts on behalf of those who have a heart for the poor (see Proverbs 21:13). In Acts chapter 10, we learn of a Roman Centurion named Cornelius, a devout man of God who often prayed and gave generously to those in need. One day an angel of the Lord appeared to him in a vision and replied... *"Your prayers and gifts to the poor have come up as a remembrance before God."* If we're charitable towards the destitute, God promises to also meet our needs.

"Blessed is he who has regard for the weak; the Lord delivers him in times of trouble. The Lord will protect him and preserve his life; he will bless him in the land and not surrender him to the desire of his foes. The Lord will sustain him on his sickbed and restore him from his bed of illness." (Psalms 41:1–3)

Do you think to bless others? Are you battling with an illness? God promises to remember you when you remember those who are less fortunate. The Bible states that when we give to the poor, it is as if we are lending to God and we will be blessed for it. The poor can be found everywhere. What can you do to make a difference? Blessing comes as a direct result of allowing God into your finances.

Plan of Action: Increase your faith by reading the Word. Obey the Word. Focus on your goal rather than on what hasn't happened. Confess and repent of sins. Love. Pray and believe you've received it! Speak the Word over your life and wait patiently. Tithe and bless the poor.

Called to Believe

We receive the blessing of God by believing Him, not through our righteousness. I hope you clearly understand that we do not get to Heaven by our deeds, it is not something we can earn; it is only through faith in Jesus Christ our Lord. It's a good thing because we're not perfect. Righteousness came through believing. Abraham was considered righteous because of his faith; he certainly didn't do everything right. On earth, people get paid according to their hard work. In Heaven, we're recognized for our faith. It is the only thing that presents us as righteous before the Father.

It's not a matter of our righteousness that we possess our "Promised Land." For it says in Deuteronomy 9:4b, 5a... "No, it is on account of the wickedness of these nations that the Lord is going to drive them out before you. It is not because of your righteousness or your integrity that you are going in to take possession of their land ..." When someone bases their salvation on following the law of the Ten Commandments, they are tied to a curse that opens their lives to misfortune.

"All who rely on observing the law are under a curse, for it is written: 'Cursed is everyone who does not continue to do everything written in the Book of the Law.'" (Galatians 3:10)

Although our salvation is not attained by following the Law, we are still called to uplift it. This doesn't mean we're still bound to perform sacrifices, rituals or ceremonies.[4] The Ten Commandments were given to the Israelites during the Old Testament times to show them right from wrong (Exodus 20:1–17). They were commanded to teach them to the forthcoming generations. God needed to give His children guidelines to live by. And we are still called to teach them to our children. Read Exodus 20:1–17.

"The Ten Commandments" (Read Exodus 20:1–21)

Our world was created on a foundation of Laws. Take gravity for instance. What goes up must come down! When you throw a ball up into the air, this force causes the ball to come back down. If you read Deuteronomy, you'll see there were repercussions for disobedience. We can clearly see that God never wanted His children to choose the wrong path and reap destruction because He set before them the blessings and curses and told them to choose the path leading to life (Deuteronomy 30:15)! Again we're offered free choice. They had to reap what they sowed. If they chose the right path, they received the blessing and if they chose the wrong path, they suffered the consequences by their own choices; opening their lives up to sickness, disease, and lack, through the curse of the Law. However, God in His goodness sent Jesus to die on the cross to take the curse of sin upon Himself, so we would be able to live under Gods' grace through faith. Jesus didn't abolish the Law when He died on the cross but rather fulfilled it so that we might live in freedom (Matthew 5:17). We receive this blessing of freedom by faith.

"Christ redeemed us from the curse of the law by becoming a curse for us, for it is written: "Cursed is everyone who is hung on a tree." He redeemed us in order that the blessing given to Abraham might come to the Gentiles through Christ Jesus, so that by faith we might receive the promise of the Spirit." (Galatians 3:13, 14)

When we live under the Law, within our own ability to earn salvation, we live outside of God's grace. Living by the Law is all about people trying to earn righteousness. This is what God meant when He spoke of those who worship Him in vain because they honour Him with their lips, but have hearts that are far from Him (Matthew 15:8). Salvation is not based on us living by the rules God has set. We receive salvation through accepting Christ as our saviour with our faith, and having a relationship with Him. That's it! Grace is about what God has done. God gave us Jesus to free us from the curse. This grace is received when we invite Jesus into our lives. We are so blessed to live in the age of grace.

"Blessed are they whose transgressions are forgiven, whose sins are covered. Blessed is the man whose sin the Lord will never count against him." (Romans 4:7–8)

Did you hear that? When we make Jesus the Lord over our lives, God takes our sins and remembers them no more (Isaiah 43:25). What an awesome gift! He considers us righteous in His eyes not because of our works, but because we believe Him. This isn't something you can earn! It has to be taken by faith. And when we do, we follow through with obedience.

Satan loves to lie to people and make them feel as if there is no hope for them. It doesn't matter what you have done in your past! It is forgiven and forgotten. What a deal. All you have to do is truly believe in your heart that Jesus is the Son of God, that He died for your sins and was raised from the dead and that He is in Heaven sitting on the throne of God. Confess it with your mouth and you will be saved (Romans 10:8–10). When you invite Jesus into your heart the Word says you become a new creation on the inside. That is where the term "born again" comes from because it resembles a new birth. Obviously you don't return to your mother's womb, but you do get a chance to start anew, this time as a baby Christian. God changes you from the inside out and eventually you'll see its fruits. Picture yourself wearing dirty rags for a moment. That's what we look like spiritually to God before we accept Christ. After we do, God takes those filthy clothes off of us and replaces them with the 'Robe of Righteousness', which means that from that point on, God sees you through what Jesus did instead of your sin. There is a basic salvation prayer at the back of the book.

We receive God's Holy Spirit by faith, not by living by rules (Galatians 3:2, 3). He wants each one of us to welcome Him into our lives by faith.

This is how we're justified. Faith is what made Abraham righteous in God's eyes (Galatians 3:6). Those who believe are considered descendants of Abraham and receive the same blessing by faith (John 8:31–41; Galatians 2:7, 9).

In Galatians 5:3, 4 we see that those who don't live by the leading of the Holy Spirit cut themselves off from the Lord and are obligated to live by the whole Law and in the process remove themselves from God's grace. We are filled with the Holy Spirit as we believe in Jesus as the Scripture states (John 7:38). To live by the Spirit we just simply ask the Holy Spirit to come into our lives to guide and direct us. He will give you a clear sense of what to do. It is important to be obedient to what He shows you because when we obey the direction of the Holy Spirit we are not under the Old Testament Law (Galatians 5:18).

Christ's death on the cross ended the continuous sacrifice of animals to cover the sins of man. The shedding of Jesus' blood enables us to worship in God's presence. He was perfect and therefore sacrifices were no longer necessary. He made His followers perfect in the eyes of God forever (Hebrews 10:14). Forever! When God looks at His children He sees us through Jesus. It's as if He wears "Jesus contact lenses" in His eyes.

The Holy Spirit also testifies to us about this. First He says:

"This is the covenant I will make with them after that time, says the Lord. I will put my laws in their hearts, and I will write them on their minds." Then He adds: "Their sins and lawless acts I will remember no more." And where these have been forgiven, there is no longer any sacrifice for sin." (Hebrews 10:15–18)

God will always direct us to the path of righteousness which leads to love, joy, peace, patience, kindness, goodness, faithfulness, gentleness, and self-control (see Galatians 5:22). These are the fruits of the Spirit.

The Holy Spirit will only guide in the ways that line up with these characteristics; if they don't line up then you can be certain it's not God.

Living by God's grace doesn't mean we live a free-for-all life style! The carnal ways of the world lead to death. It's necessary to renew your mind with the Word of God; this transforms your mind and crucifies our sinful nature. This will give you the necessary strength to say no to the things of the flesh and the wisdom to know God's perfect will (Romans 12:2). Those who live by faith will automatically want to obey God out of their love for Him. And when we screw up, there is grace to catch us, as we forgive and show mercy to others. Be careful. Some will try to justify this freedom in Christ to fit the lifestyle they want. This is a dangerous game to play. We are not to misuse our freedom in Christ to give into our fleshly nature or the immoral pleasures of this world. We are, however, to serve one another in love (Galatians 5:13).

"*The acts of the sinful nature are obvious: sexual immorality, impurity and debauchery; idolatry and witchcraft; hatred, discord, jealousy, fits of rage, selfish ambition, dissensions, factions and envy; drunkenness, orgies, and the like. I warn you, as I did before, that those who live like this will not inherit the kingdom of God.*" (Galatians 5:19)

We learn in Romans 8:7, 8 that the carnal mind of a sinful man is hostile to God and can't and will not submit to God's Law because he is controlled by his own sinful nature.[5] The Spirit and human fleshly nature are in opposition with one another. Death is a result of following the sinful lusts of the flesh, but God promises that those who obey the Spirit of God will enjoy eternal life. Jesus defeated Satan on the cross and then took back the keys of death and hell, along with the authority Satan stole through deception, and gave them back to us. Satan is only able to gain this authority back through sin. He uses sin as access to put sickness and disease on people or open the door to poverty and lack. We strip Satan of this legal right when we confess and repent of our sins.

As Christians we have the authority over the enemy (Matthew 16:19). God has given His children these keys to improve our lives. Learn how to use them and don't be afraid to walk in the authority Jesus died to give you.

Before returning to Heaven to intercede on our behalf, Jesus left us His Spirit to give us everything we need and more. If you need guidance, comfort, encouragement, and strength, Jesus is waiting to advocate and intercede on your behalf.

Jesus was tempted in every way known to man, yet He didn't sin (Hebrews 4:15).

In First Corinthians 10:13, God provides us hope that we may not fall under defeat as well for it says; *"No temptation has seized you except what is common to man. And God is faithful; he will not let you be tempted beyond what you can bear. But when you are tempted, he will also provide a way out so that you can stand up under it."*

Satan is the tempter. God doesn't tempt us but He will, however, use trials to test and develop our faith (James 1:12–15; 1 Timothy 3:9–10; Hebrews 11:17). Our faith is built up when we read or hear the Word of God, while our patience only develops under trial. According to the Canadian Dictionary, patience is the capacity to endure hardship, difficulty or inconvenience without complaint; it emphasizes calmness, self control, and the willingness or ability to tolerate delay.[6]

Patience and faith work hand–in–hand.[7] Patience holds your hope up so that your faith will not waver and fall. If you lose your patience, you'll lose your faith, which brings forth your promise in the spiritual realm.[8] Hebrews 6:12 encourages us as it speaks this truth, *"We do not want you to become lazy, but to imitate those who through faith and patience inherit what has been promised."* You must persevere! (James 1:2–4)

Obeying God's Commands

"Jesus replied: 'Love the Lord your God with all your heart and with all your soul and with all your mind. This is the first and greatest commandment. And the second is like it: Love your neighbor as yourself.' All the Law and the Prophets hang on these two commandments." (Matthew 22:37–40)

When we choose to love God, completely submitting to His direction, including loving our neighbour as ourself, the entire Law is summed up and sustained.[9] God's grace doesn't remove the Law. It gives us the power of the Holy Spirit to walk in love and enables us to bear the fruit of the Spirit that protects us from the curse of the Law. In many facets, choosing to walk in love with others shields us from being entrapped into a large number of sins. (Read John 15:9–10; 1 John 3:24; John 13:34.)

We are called to follow Christ's example of love. He loved to the highest degree when He laid down His life for us (1 John 2:7, 8). This didn't remove the foundation of the Law, but magnified the height of love's degree.[10] Jesus often quoted from the Old Testament which displays its continued existence.[11] Deuteronomy 6:5 tells us to... "Love God with all our heart, mind and soul," this encases four of the first Ten Commandments. It is also quoted in Matthew 22:37 along with an additional command in verse 39, telling us to "love our neighbour as our self." This new command covers the remainder of the Ten Commandments and establishes its importance. Therefore we must continue to be obedient and uphold the Law by imitating Jesus' love for others.[12] Many times we lack loving others out of our own selfishness and jealousy.

Our flesh fears for its own needs to be met and makes the decision to withhold. But our flesh doesn't have a mind to know that when we give, we actually receive. The principle of reaping and sowing also works with love. God is love and when we choose to walk in love with others, we are filled with God's love in return, which is His Holy Spirit. His Spirit also empowers us and when we walk in love with others, it activates our faith.

There are many people in this world who believe they're better than others and treat them as such. Our world would be a much better place if we could all treat each other the way we would like to be treated instead of judging and looking down at them. Wouldn't it be wonderful if everyone was thought of equally? Let's start a revolution of love and discipline ourselves by choosing to love others in spite of their differences.

If each one of us would make this decision to do what they could, it would change the world. Don't be someone who makes excuses thinking, "What can one person do?" You never know until you try. Your shining light may inspire multiple people who in return could inspire many more, until we have a revolution of love on our hands! We can make a difference, one act of love at a time.[13]

Let's take another look at what love is like so we can live by God's example;

"Love is patient, love is kind. It does not envy, it does not boast, it is not proud. It is not rude, it is not self-seeking, it is not easily angered, it keeps no record of wrongs. Love does not delight in evil but rejoices with the truth. It always protects, always trusts, always hopes, always perseveres. Love never fails..." (1 Corinthians 13:4-8a)

Could you replace the word 'love', as it is written in the above verses for your name or do you fall short from such character?[14] If so, are you willing to allow God to work in your life and make you more like Him? The next time you're in the check-out line at the grocery store and the person behind you has only a few items, let them go first. Give someone who looks grumpy or sad a smile. It may be the very thing that saves their life! These things only take a few minutes of your time and make you feel so good on the inside. You may change someone's outlook on life!

We learn the importance of love as we read 1 Corinthians Chapter 13. It tells us that we can receive and operate in all the gifts and abilities recognized by both God and man, give everything away to the poor and be a martyr in our faith, but unless we operate with a loving heart everything done on earth will have been in vain. These good deeds will be of no value. God compares such a person to a resounding gong or clanging cymbal. Does that resound in your ears? It struck me. If we don't love others we're comparable to this echoing annoyance. Clanging cymbals are extremely grating to the ears unless they're mixed with music. Likewise, our good works will appear the same to God unless they're mixed with love. I know one thing! I want to please my Father because He's been so good to me. How do you feel? When Jesus returns to the earth all things as we know it will have passed away and the only things that will remain standing are faith, hope, and love. Even in this, God emphasized love as the most important.

The Old Testament law demanded that the woman caught in an adulterous relationship be stoned to death. We're now under a new covenant of grace with God. He wrote the law on our hearts, the new law says we must love the one caught in sin and forgive them their trespasses rather than stone them because we too are not without sin.

Therefore we need to live at peace with everyone, including those who are hard to love. Often the characteristics that grate us in others are traits we don't like in ourselves. With God's help we can accept each other and grow to love even the unlovely. I believe that everyone that comes into our lives has been placed there by God for a specific reason; either to teach us something or to be taught by us. Perhaps both! If we could view all our relationships with this perspective, it might be easier to co-exist with those that challenge you. Choose to pay back those who hurt you with love and kindness and defeat and overcome evil with good.

Recently someone I care about corrected me in a harsh manner in front of an entire group of people. Although others believed it came out of her love for me and anger directed toward the enemy because of his lies, I judged her reaction as partly stemming from her own personal struggle with guilt and fear due to the uncontrollable situation in her own life. Justifying this situation helped me forgive and brought understanding, but it didn't remove the feelings of humiliation and hurt. God filled me with His love and gave me the strength to be gracious. She later called to straighten things out.

I would have preferred a more gentle approach. Albeit her method wasn't one of my choosing, perhaps a softer tone and alternative words may not have had the same altering affect. There was wisdom in her words that I needed to hear and apply to my life. Because I attained the right attitude, was obedient to the Lord, and accepted the truth, God used this situation to set me free from fear and unbelief.

With that said, God asks us to correct in gentleness out of love, not anger. We need to be patient with one another. When we put love into action, our faith has the power to perform. In other words, if we want our faith to work, we have to walk in love despite how others love or behave towards us. Making your mind up to forgive is very freeing. God blesses us when we choose to overlook an offence. We can love by letting go.

We must consistently choose to love to have a constant flow of God's miraculous power flowing in our lives. In other words, if you want a miracle to happen in your life, you need to purposely act out of love in everything you do! God asks us to edify and build each other up by speaking the truth. This may mean telling someone something what they need to hear rather than what they want to hear; spoken out of love, of course, in conjunction with the Word. Below is a wonderful Scripture I often use to pray for myself and others, to increase our love.

Dear Lord,

I pray that my love would abound more and more in depth and knowledge and insight so that I can become pure and blameless until the coming day of Jesus Christ our Lord, bearing fruits of righteousness for Your name's sake. May God Himself, the God of peace, sanctify me through and through. May my whole spirit, soul and body be kept blameless at the coming of our Lord Jesus Christ (1 Thessalonians 5:23). *In Jesus' name I pray. Amen.*

When Christ returns for His people, it is those who are full of His power that will rise with Him; people who walk in faith and love. To do this, we must put God first and observe His commandments of love in our lives.

Getting to Our Promised Land

"But my righteous one will live by faith. And if he shrinks back, I will not be pleased with him." (Hebrew 10:38)

After the great exodus of the Israelites from Egypt, they spent 40 years in the desert. After this time had passed, the Lord told Moses the people had camped around the mountain long enough. They were to break camp and advance into the mountains, foothills, and along the coasts of specific neighbouring villages as far as the great river of the Euphrates. The Lord gave specific direction as to what land the Israelites were to conquer and possess and which they were to leave. God directed the people where to go and helped defeat the enemy each step of the way.

"See, I have given you this land. Go in and take possession of the land that the Lord swore he would give to your fathers—to Abraham, Isaac and Jacob—and to their descendants after them." (Deuteronomy 1:8)

Their numbers had grown more than they were able to count, so Moses had the people choose one wise, respected man from each tribe to represent their group and sent them out to spy in the new land to get a better perspective before battle. Caleb and Joshua were the only two out of the 12 spies that returned with a positive report. Although the other 10 agreed the land was prosperous and brought back an amazing yield of fruit, they held an entirely opposite outlook because they were full of doubt and fear. They had forgotten the great miracles God had performed in the desert as they looked at the size and strength of the opposition and cities. They were focused on the appearance of the natural circumstances rather than on God's promise and ability. *"Then Caleb silenced the people before Moses and said, 'We should go up and take possession of the land, for we can certainly do it.' But the men who had gone up with him said, 'We can't attack those people; they are stronger than we are.'"* (Numbers 13: 30, 31)

Are you like the 10 remaining Israelite spies who were full of excuses? They had all the different reasons lined up about how they wouldn't or couldn't win. No one has ever accomplished their life dreams or goals by concentrating on all the underlying principles of why their circumstances won't work out! If you think that way you'll be defeated even before you start. I realize that facing new challenges, whether positive or negative, can be scary. Choose to think positive thoughts; it's much easier that way! Draw your strength from the Lord and decide to do things even if you're afraid. The author of Hebrews 10 encourages us to not throw away our confidence (vs.35). This is essential to attaining your goal and becoming all that you can be. Trust God; if He's called you to do something, He'll make a way when your motives are pure. Isaiah 30:21 says, *"Whether you turn to the right or to the left, your ears will hear a voice behind you, saying, "This is the way; walk in it."* Choose to step out with confidence. If you make the wrong choice, God will close the door and if it's the right one, He'll usher you through. He not only has your best interest in mind, He only calls you into things that are attainable (Deuteronomy 30:11). He wants you to succeed and provides help along the way. You may fall and get a few bumps and bruises along the way. The pain from these sores will act as a reminder of what mistakes not to repeat and give you greater determination to get up and remain steadfast until you reach your desired destination.

Is there doubt and fear holding you back from entering your promised land? When you focus on the obstacles, you give them the power to paralyze your mind, which brings defeat. However, when you believe God's promises, He will bless you with the strength and courage needed to overcome. Having a positive outlook is the first step towards victory!

The men who brought back a negative report spread rumours among the people and grumbled and complained before Moses and God, questioning God's motives for bringing them out of Egypt. Out of fear of the enemy, they longed to return to Egypt. They had forgotten the great miracles God had performed in the desert to get them to their present position. Because of this rebellion the people where forbidden to enter the Promised Land and Jacob and Caleb were the only two out of the original group that were able to enter. These were the two spies who brought back the positive report and believed with God's help they would be able to conquer the land. The others were held back by their unbelief that carried negative attitudes, mindsets, and rebellion (Numbers 14).

Even though the Israelites heard God speak, their hearts were hardened through unbelief and they were unable to enter the rest of God (Hebrews 3:7–13). The promise of God's rest remains only for those who believe through the eyes of faith.

Are you facing a crossroad in life, a pivotal place where you must make a decision either to retreat where it's comfortable and familiar or to press on toward your goal? Looking towards the opposition can be very intimidating and hard, but the reward in the end will be well worth it! Trust God to take you to your promised land, a land that is full of wonderful things for you to enjoy. If we argue, grumble, and complain we quench the Holy Spirit from helping us. The opposite can be said about being thankful, for when we worship the Lord, His presence is available to guide us.

As discussed in previous chapters, we no longer need a priest to make sacrifices for our sins or to come before God on our behalf. We can come boldly before the throne of God and cast our care on Him because Jesus sacrificed His life for us (*Hebrews 4:16*). His blood appeased God's anger caused by our sin. There is no longer the need for the shedding of animal blood to cover these sins or to gain righteousness through works. God's grace allows us to enjoy this rest every day!

"Come to me, all you who are weary and burdened, and I will give you rest. Take my yoke upon you and learn from me, for I am gentle and humble in heart, and you will find rest for your souls. For my yoke is easy and my burden is light." (Matthew 11:28)

Are there issues overwhelming you at the moment? Fear and worry will drag you down and hold you back, just as excuses will. The yoke placed on oxen helps balance their load so that they're able to carry even more. God is our yoke. Scripture says His yoke is easy. We're encouraged to take His yoke upon us by sharing our concerns. This takes the weight off our shoulders and creates stability in our lives to enable us to move forward. Jesus wants to take you to your destination. However, you must place your burdens at His feet and place your trust in Him. Put Him in control of your situation and follow His leading.

Crossing the Jordon

The Israelites wandered back out in the desert until the last of the original fighting men had died. Moses was forbidden to go into the Promised Land because he didn't uphold God's holiness and broke faith in the presence of the Israelites in the desert. This is a lesson for all. The Lord humbled them until they were ready to follow God's commandments and revealed His miraculous power that they might remember the Lord and not fall back into old patterns of destruction.

In Deuteronomy 8, the people were reminded to follow God's instructions and commands, so that they would prosper and increase in their promised land. They were reminded that it is God that gives the ability to prosper and increase and not to become inflated with pride. When people believe they've succeeded all on their own, it causes them to turn away from God. God amazes me. He promised to fulfill His covenant and swore an oath unto Himself, promising that even if someone turned away from Him, He wouldn't abandon or destroy them, but would bring them back into relationship with Him. That promise still stands today!

This next Scripture has profoundly impacted my life. Take a few minutes and meditate on it asking God to bring revelation.

"He humbled you, causing you to hunger and then feeding you with manna, which neither you nor your fathers had known, to teach you that man does not live on bread alone but on every word that comes from the mouth of the Lord" (Deuteronomy 8:3)

This verse gives us clear insight as to how life itself operates. There are two points I would like you to see, the latter being the most important.

First, God humbled the Israelites so that they would realize that God is the one that blesses and provides life. Without Him we would have and be nothing. God, with the power in His spoken word, brought forth food for them to eat. We know that God's words are powerful because He created the whole earth through His spoken word. Sending manna from the heavens simply confirmed God's power. My second point not only reemphasizes the first, it increases its significance. Let's take another look at the ending of the Scripture, it says we live...*"on every word that comes from the mouth of the Lord."* We need to eat food to live, but we live because God says so! Do you see what I mean? There's no devil or demon in hell that can snatch us out of God's hand. Our confessions do have an impact on our lives regarding what situations we go through, and often determine how long we stay in those situations, but it is "only" God that determines how long we live! You can breathe easy now and let go of all that fear. Trust God with your life. You're in good hands!

Nearing the time of Moses' death, God appointed Joshua to succeed Moses as leader. Moses imparted the spirit of wisdom into him and encouraged him in the Lord before climbing to the top of Mount Nebo where he could see the Promised Land with his own eyes. Although still strong in body, Moses died at the age of 120. The people gathered and buried him. After they grieved for 30 days, God spoke to Joshua and commanded him to get ready to cross the Jordan, for just on the other side was Canaan, the Promised Land.

"Be strong and courageous, because you will lead these people to inherit the land I swore to their forefathers to give them. Be strong and very courageous. Be careful to obey all the law my servant Moses gave you; do not turn from it to the right or to the left, that you may be successful wherever you go. Do not let this Book of the Law depart from your mouth; meditate on it day and night, so that you may be careful to do everything written in it. Then you will be prosperous and successful. Have I not commanded you? Be strong

and courageous. Do not be terrified; do not be discouraged, for the Lord your God will be with you wherever you go." (Joshua 1:6–9)

Joshua sent out two spies into the land before them to get a closer look. They went and stayed at the house of Rahab, the town prostitute. The king of Jericho got word and sent a message to Rahab to bring out the men because they were spies. She had heard the stories of how God had dried up the Red Sea and how He had helped them deliver the enemy into the Israelites' hands. The people were melting in fear because of them. She lied to the king's messengers and told them to go look for the men outside the city. She hid the spies on her roof under stalks of flax and made them swear that she and her family would be spared because of the kindness she showed them. The promise of safety was binding as long as she brought her family into her house and hung a scarlet cord in her window as a sign to the Israelites to pass over. The next morning she let the men down through her window that was part of the city wall so they could hide in the hills for a few days and return to their camp.

I love this story about Rahab because it represents how God chooses to use people from every walk of life. The world may look at her through eyes of disdain, but God saw Rahab's faith. God knew she wasn't perfect. In spite of her lifestyle, God gave her a chance. He redeemed her from her past and gave her a future, all because she believed. Do you believe? Your past doesn't have to dictate your future. God loves you. It doesn't matter where you've come from or what mistakes you've made, God's waiting to change your life. He wants to redeem it. Will you let him?

God had already promised the land east of the Jordan to the Reubenites, the Gadites, and the half-tribe of Manasseh. The women, children, and livestock were to remain in that land, but their fully armed fighting men were to go on ahead with the rest of the Israelites until they had taken possession of their land.

When it was time for the people to cross the Jordan, Joshua instructed them to consecrate themselves as the Lord was going to perform amazing miracles among them. God instructed Joshua to have the people follow the Ark of the Covenant when they saw the priests carrying it, so they'd know where to go. The moment the priests stood in the river, the water stopped flowing downstream and stood up in a heap even though it was flood time in that area. The priests remained in the middle of the dry river bed until every last woman and child had crossed. One man was chosen from each tribe to gather a stone from the centre of the river bed and carry it on their shoulders over to the other side. These stones were taken from the middle of the Jordan, to build an altar as a remembrance to the people and further generations regarding the amazing things the Lord had done!

It's in the dark times that we need to remember the goodness of God and the positive blessings that He has brought to our lives.[15] These are the stones of remembrance that will help carry you through to the other side to victory.[16] What are the stones of remembrance you can take from your past that will give you the needed perseverance in your situation?[17] Meditating on these areas will provide you with confidence.

As I take a reflective look back through the years of my life I can see the wonderful touch of God's hand, His strong yet gentle fingerprints marking the fragile crystal glass that represents my existence. There have been moments filled with abounding love and goodness alongside heart wrenching fear and turmoil. Challenges one believes they should never have to endure or face.

Although my family was abandoned by our father, God placed numerous individuals in our lives to encourage and help us along the way with all the different needs we encountered. Many believe God has abandoned them to face life struggles to cope and search for answers themselves. But I have learned through life's experience that God is just as present in the difficult times as He is in the good. He's always watching over us, waiting to reach out in our time of need. It's His love that sends a word of encouragement when you are feeling down, the delivery man who drops off milk when the fridge is empty or shows up with a meal when you're too sick to cook. Yes, God is always with us, lavishing us in His wonderful love! However, it's only through a grateful heart that we're able to see His loving gaze.

Due to circumstances, my grandparents were not very active in our lives. They lived in Montreal, so I only ever saw them a handful of times. Family friends (Sanger & Disheau) took us under their wings. Nanny Dee was more than happy to step in with lots of hugs and kisses, Aunt Carolyn cut our hair, and her brother Wally cut our grass. We enjoyed many gatherings where we were able to experience the connection of family even though they weren't our own.

God placed Mrs. Styles, (my grade three teacher) into my life to show me that I had potential and that all the lies spoken over me about being stupid were just that, lies! I can still picture her. She was a short, stocky lady that didn't tolerate any guff off the boys. She was always full of encouragement and demanded respect and integrity from each of her students.

I clearly recall the time she grabbed one of the boys by the ankles and hung him upside down. She told him she was going to shake him until his gizzard fell out on the floor if he ever misbehaved again. He was always as good as gold after that. Teachers would never get away with that now; nevertheless he certainly learned his lesson. God only knows what she saved him from in the end.

I've already shared the account about of how God provided a miracle for our family Christmas when I was nine because there wasn't enough money for food or gifts. Again, God also ordained my father's return which put an end to the sexual and physical abuse. My family no longer had to live in desperation and my father helped bring order to our house. Although my father struggled with anger, he cared about us and added some really positive experiences to my life. He put me in gymnastics to build my confidence, and wouldn't tolerate my siblings calling me names. He took us for toboggan rides with his tractor, sent us to camp, bought me nice things, took our family on a trip to Wonderland, and chased older boys away.

My mother led me to the Lord through her shining example and continued to draw me along the right path. I inherited her contagious gift of the gab, her smile, and her laugh. My mom knew how to have fun and tried to make life that way for others whenever she could. She always had a listening ear for others. Most of our friends called her mom because she always made them feel welcome. They practically lived at our house. My most cherished memories come from the hours she spent playing board games with us kids. Mom took us ice skating and camping even when her back was so sore that she could hardly walk. She even sat up with me until four in the morning eating chips and watching a movie instead of judging me when I was late and ditched the car.

Even though I ignored God's voice warning me to stay away from sugar, He continued to faithfully tap on the door of my heart and remained my savoir, healer and friend.

When life smacked me "upside the head" with the huge wake-up call, called cancer, it was God that wrapped His loving arms around me and covered me with an unexplainable warmth and peace whispering, "Be still and know that I am God." He revealed His loving heart to me and stood by me each step of the way! God anointed me in His presence and gripped me with an amazing strength while surrounding me with an incredible army of support.

The doctor's diagnosis may have been grim, but God's Word said something entirely different. Remember how we experienced the healing power of God firsthand when He healed our two boys from food allergies.

As I walked through this journey, God held my hand and revealed His true character to me, guiding me each step of the way. He reminded me that nothing could separate me from His love and that His plans were to prosper me, to give me hope and a future. Any misconceptions I believed about Him fell away as He gently washed me in the truth of His Word and engrained these facts within each experience. In Romans 8:28, God promises that He will always work everything out for the good for those who love Him. This can truly be said of my journey with cancer. He didn't allow these crushing circumstances to break me, only to polish me like a fine piece of crystal that has been brought out of the fire. He used the painful hurts of the past to bring healing and victory not only within my own life, but to others. A precision design only the Great Master could create Himself from the erupting lava and char. The places I once saw as flaws and defects, I can now see as intricate designs of His glory and grace. As you look back over your life, can you see the places God has had His hand on you?

Gilgal

The Israelites had finally stepped foot on the first part of the promise land. Gilgal was located just west of the Jordan River and it was there that they stopped to build an altar of remembrance with the 12 stones that were taken from the Jordan and renewed their covenant with God by circumcising the young men who were born out in the desert.[18] This was a symbol of cutting off the old nature with its disobedience and unbelief, marking themselves as different.[19] With this act, God rolled away the reproach of Egypt and rose up the sons of those who died in the desert keeping His promise.

The name Gilgal means "circle" which held great significance for the Israelites.[20] God had taken them from 430 years of slavery to deliverance, through times of testings and trials that were marked with failure, to establishing them with a solid foundation of belief and set their feet on Promised Land.[21] God brought them full circle.

They no longer had to carry the disgrace of unbelief and disobedience or the shame of Egypt, they were free to start over and put the past behind them. This was a fresh chance to start over and do things differently, to walk in faith rather than unbelief. They stayed at Gilgal until they had healed and celebrated the Passover with the produce from the land. When the manna stopped and they were able to eat the yield off the land this was the first significant sign from God that their lives had changed. News of God's mighty wonders had spread across the land and caused their enemies hearts to weaken with fear.

Are you still carrying shame and guilt from your past? Do you carry its stigma around with you everywhere you go? Every person on the face of this earth has made mistakes they're not proud of. Jesus was wounded for our transgressions and bruised for our iniquities; we don't need to hold onto them any longer. It's time to let it go and let Jesus be your redeemer, to put off the old self and put on the new robes of righteousness that He died to give you!

After being diagnosed with a life–threatening disease, my perspective has become extremely clear. The glasses I now wear to view life are no longer streaked with meaningless array, as I hold a heightened desire to thrive and experience life as never before. Again, it doesn't matter where you started in life or where you have come from along the way, it's how you finish that matters! You don't have to get sick to change your perspective. If you want to make a difference in the lives of others, now is your chance to do things differently and start afresh. And remember, even mistakes hold valuable lessons!

A New Action Plan

Believe God and take Him at His word, take care of yourself, enjoy life more by taking time for family and friends, value relationships more and material things less, talk less, listen more, be frivolous once in awhile, express your feelings, don't miss an opportunity to tell someone you love them, live each day as if it were your last and forgive!

God can take you from the pain of the past, through your tests, trials, and failures and bring you full circle to triumph. You can have your own Gilgal in a sense and begin again. The shame and reproach can be removed from long-ago by choosing to believe God. Let Him use your failures in a glorious way. Find the positive points in situations instead of staring at the negative ones. Reframe them with a positive twist.[22] Stay positive, hopeful, and continually connected with God, looking for His direction.

We all have things in our past that we regret. When we ask God to forgive us, He takes our sins and throws them into the sea of forgetfulness. What a God! He remembers His promises and forgets our sins for His benefit. Allow Him to take you full circle and redeem your life. You too cannot move from your Gilgal until your hurts are healed and your reproach is removed. God is asking us to circumcise ourselves from the stigmas of our past and our hearts from the junk of this world as a sign of our dedication to Him. He wants to know that you love Him more than anything or anyone else!

I pray that, *"The Lord your God will circumcise your hearts and the hearts of your descendants, so that you may love him with all your heart and with all your soul, and live."* (Deuteronomy 30:6)

The Fall of Jericho

On the way to Jericho, Joshua saw the commander of the Lord's army standing in front of him with a drawn sword. Joshua was commanded to take off his sandals because he was standing on holy ground. In reverence, he fell facedown. I absolutely love what the angel said next. Although the commander of the Lord gave Joshua specific instructions for the defeat of Jericho, he told Joshua that He was neither for Joshua nor for his enemy. I hope you get that! God shows no favourites. He loves each one of us equally.

By the time the Israelites arrived at Jericho, the news of their success had spread across the land. The people were terrified and had tightly barricaded the city. This was of no concern for the Israelites because God had shown them a unique plan. They carefully followed the Lord's instructions each day with the armed guard going before them. For six days they quietly preceded once around the city walls behind the Ark of the Covenant and then returned back to camp. One the seventh day they marched around the walls seven times as the priests made a loud racket with their horns in front of the Ark. During the seventh time around, after hearing the loud trumpet call, the people gave a loud "Shout." The walls of Jericho tumbled down as promised and they immediately seized the land!

If we are obedient to God's direction, we will be victorious even when our circumstances look impossible. God's ways of doing things are often the opposite of how the world operates. I've heard it described as the upside-down kingdom. People often have good intentions, but often don't understand and will try to discourage you from entering your Promised Land where God is calling you. When the walls or obstacles in life seem too high to climb, look for God's direction. He will give you the answers that will bring them tumbling down.

"So be careful to do what the Lord your God has commanded you; do not turn aside to the right or to the left. Walk in all the way that the Lord your God has commanded you, so that you may live and prosper and prolong your days in the land that you will possess." (Deuteronomy 5:32, 33)

"Observe the commands of the Lord your God, walking in his ways and revering him. For the Lord is bringing you into a good land." (Deuteronomy 8:6–7a)

As promised, the Lord helped the new generation of Israelites defeat the enemy everywhere they set their foot. They inhabited the Promised Land, enjoying their new found freedom. They defeated the Canaanites, Hittites, Perizzites, and all the other "ites". You, too, can defeat the enemy and enter your Promised Land if you are willing to obey the Lord's direction. Are you ready?

The Blessing

"If you pay attention to these laws and are careful to follow them, than the Lord your God will keep his covenant of love with you, as he swore to your forefathers. He will love you and bless you and increase your numbers. He will bless the fruit of your womb, the crops of your land—your grain, new wine and oil—the calves of your herds and the lambs of your flocks in the land that he swore to your forefathers to give you. You will be blessed more than any other people; none of your men or women will be childless, nor any of your livestock without young. The Lord will keep you free from every disease." (Deuteronomy 7:12–15a)

This passage describes the covenant blessing promised to Abraham and his descendants. God blessed Abraham so that he could be a blessing to others. When we have given our lives to Jesus, these promises also belong to us; however, we must follow through with our part of the conditions.

"If you belong to Christ, then you are Abraham's seed, and heirs according to the promise." (Galatians 3:29)

At numerous times, Abraham built altars and called on God for direction. God must have shared the principles of sowing and reaping with Abraham because he gave with a gracious heart. We, too, can be blessed by God if we have a giving heart rather than one that hoards and holds. When Abraham had finished defeating Kedorlaomer and the other kings associated with him, Melchizedek, the king of Sodom and also a priest of God, came to meet with him in the valley of Shaveh. They partook of bread and wine together as an act of covenant and Abraham gave him a tenth of everything he owned (Genesis 14:18–20). Abraham tithed even before God introduced it to the Israelites during Old Testament time.

"Abraham was now old and well advanced in years, and the Lord had blessed him in every way." (Genesis 24:1)

"The Lord has blessed my master abundantly, and he has become wealthy. He has given him sheep and cattle, silver and gold, menservants and maidservants, and camels and donkeys." (Genesis 24:35)

For those who are unfamiliar with tithing it is a way of sowing a blessing into our lives in every area by giving back a portion of what God gives you. This principle is based on the foundational laws of the universe, better known as the law of reaping and sowing. In Deuteronomy, God set before the people the laws that brought blessings and revealed the curses that would result because of disobedience. God told the people to choose His way. It was never His desire for anyone to reap the negative, but we're the ones that will reap from our choices because of the laws that were set in place from the beginning. We suffer as a result of our own free will!

The act of tithing puts the promise of healing, prosperity, salvation, and well-being for your family into action. It holds promise to prosper in every area of our lives. Even though Abraham was old, he was healthy in body and lacked nothing. God doesn't need our money because He owns everything to begin with. When we give, God will bless our remaining money to stretch even farther than what the full amount would have gone if we had kept it. God wants us to be good stewards of our money and asks us to be obedient in this area so He can bless us here on earth as well as in eternity. All in all, it is an act of obedience that keeps the devourer away.

"The Blessing of the Lord brings wealth, and he adds no trouble to it." (Proverbs 10:22)

"Bring the whole tithe into the storehouse, that there may be food in my house. Test me in this," says the Lord Almighty, "and see if I will not throw open the flood-gates of heaven and pour out so much blessing that you will not have room enough for it. I will prevent pests from devouring your crops, and the vines in your fields will not cast their fruit," says the Lord Almighty. "Then all the nations will call you blessed, for yours will be a delightful land," says the Lord Almighty." (Malachi 3:10–12)

There you have it. God is asking us to test Him in this area and witness His goodness as He opens Heaven's windows to pour out a blessing on you, one of great bounty. This is the only area in the whole Bible where the Lord asks us to test Him. If we allow God to get involved in our finances, we, too, will become blessed as richly as Abraham. God promises to meet all of our needs according to His riches in glory. Abraham was blessed because he believed and lived according to God's covenant. The Old Covenant Law required giving 10 percent of the first fruits of one's labour. The New Covenant of grace doesn't give us a specific amount.[23] However, it does say that our offering must be given willingly, not from compulsion or given grudgingly for all grace to abound to us (2 Corinthians 9:5, 7).[24] Some still give 10 percent as a base amount, while others believe it should be more because of what Christ has done for us. Either way, we are blessed. Jay Snell, author of "How to claim the Abrahamic Covenant," explains the meaning of the word "blessed" as "the beneficial enduement of God's power to produce well–being in every area of a person's life."[25] Tithing puts this blessing into effect. One must give out of a grateful, generous heart to receive its benefits. Our desire to give should stem from our love for God and longing to see His work continued and not seen as a means for gain or viewed as a loss.[26] God doesn't need our money. He asks us to tithe so we can be blessed. Some may have the mindset that God is taking from us when in fact He wants us to be obedient so He can give us a boun- tiful harvest. It's a means to continue the covenant blessing. God promises that when we give, He will bless the remainder to go further and meet all of our needs according to His riches in glory. When we give God our wallet, we're really giving Him our heart!

As we tithe, God rebukes the devourer (the devil) from stealing our earnings and belongings. Do you feel as if you can never get ahead? Is something always breaking down? It's natural to have normal wear and tear on our belongings but not continuously. If we stop tithing, it gives the devil legal right to start right where he left off before you started being a giver. He wants to steal your health, your wealth, your relationships, and everything near and dear to your heart.

The blessing begins with the principle of tithing. Think of tithing as the seed that produces your harvest. The amount you decide within your heart will bring back 30–, 60– or 100–fold in return (Mark 4:8). Picture a farmer for a moment. After a cash cropper has worked up the soil on his land, he takes his seed and plants it in the ground. Every farmer knows they must wait patiently because it takes time for the seed to sprout. They don't overturn the soil to check out what the seed is doing. No, they have the faith to know that at just the right time each seed will produce a plant that carries many more seeds within that will continue the cycle.

Just as the farmer, we, too, must possess the faith to believe our seed will reap a harvest. Again, watch what you say over your seed; if you're always talking about being broke, you will be; if you speak death over your relationships, you'll have disunity. You must believe that God rewards those who come to Him diligently and trust that you can have what you say, as described in Mark 11:24.

Again, God is sovereign, yet He chooses to work through His people. When we don't tithe, we're throwing away our seed. It is stolen by the destroyer, never to be planted and in the process we're challenged in every area.

"Do not be deceived: God cannot be mocked. A man reaps what he sows. The one who sows to please his sinful nature, from that nature will reap destruction; the one who sows to please the Spirit, from the Spirit will reap eternal life. Let us not become weary in doing good, for at the proper time we will reap a harvest if we do not give up." (Galatians 6:7–9)

We need to plant our seeds of blessing in rich soil from where you get spiritually fed and have faith knowing that God will bring about a bountiful harvest that will bring a blessing. God promises to bless your seed a hundred–fold. There are some in a position who are unable to tithe from their husband's earnings for various reasons. God knows your heart and if you are faithful with what He tells you to do, I believe God will allow grace to abound to you in your situation and put the law of the blessing in action on your behalf.

"And God is able to make all grace abound to you, so that in all things at all times, having all that you need, you will abound in every good work." (2 Corinthians 9:8)

"Remember this: Whoever sows sparingly will also reap sparingly, and whoever sows generously will also reap generously. Each man should give what he has decided in his heart to give, not reluctantly or under compulsion, for God loves a cheerful giver." (2 Corinthians 9:6–7)

God starts working with our seed the moment we put our faith in motion. This is the most critical time to be patient and remain in faith. Patience gives our faith the strength to stand while we are waiting for the desired outcome to manifest into existence![27] The waiting can be difficult. It's important to do whatever you can to keep hope. You can't afford to become weak. Make a list of hopes and dreams with Scripture to meditate on (see *Romans 15:4*). This will keep your promise and faith from being stolen! Keep your words in line with the promise and praise God for His goodness.

God wants us to have hope and offers it to us through His written Word. If you want to be encouraged, read Colossians 1:1–11 to see the faith and love that is available to us through Christ Jesus.

Patience Keeps Our Faith Strong!

It's imperative to practice patience when undesirable events happen. As Christians, we need to react in a way that is pleasing to God. Take a deep breath and ask yourself the famous question, "What would Jesus do in this situation?" or "How would God want me to react?" Give yourself a moment to think about it and then behave accordingly. When you exhale, let go of all the frustration and any other negative emotion felt. Applying this exercise will ground you with patience and self-control and aid in making wise decisions. The more you exercise your patience, the more natural this reaction will become. Patience is only developed through practice. Eventually this will become automatic and you'll be able to handle bigger challenges in the future more easily. God promises He will strengthen us with His glorious might, giving us great endurance and patience to run our race if we do not give up (Colossians 1:11).

God instructs us to take joy from our trials because through them we learn to press forward (*Romans 5:3–5*). This perseverance develops character within us which produces the hope we need to endure. What kind of character are you developing? Hope gives us the strength to carry us through. God's love fills our hearts with joy as He fills us with His Holy Spirit. This hope will never disappoint us! Those who know me are probably in shock right now. Knowing that I'm a diehard about never, saying never! However, I'm going to make an exception this time because God doesn't lie. If He promises that hope will never disappoint us, than it won't!

"Be completely humble and gentle; be patient bearing with one another in love. Make every effort to keep the unity of the Spirit through the bond of peace." (Ephesians 4:2, 3)

Peace brings unity. Keeping peace is a way of walking in God's love and brings strength to our lives and into our relationships. When we choose to walk in love with others at all times, we receive a complete understanding of wisdom, and knowledge of God's will, and are filled with steadfast faith (Colossians 2:2–5). When we put on peace, we put on the power to endure whatever happens and love binds everything together to strengthen us to endure.

"Therefore, as God's chosen people, holy and dearly loved, clothe yourselves with compassion, kindness, humility, gentleness and patience. Bear with each other and forgive whatever grievances you may have against one another. Forgive as the Lord forgave you. And over all these virtues put on love, which binds them all together in perfect unity." (Colossians 3:12–14)

Dear Heavenly Father,

You are so good! You're a wonderful Father, with good plans for His children. Please give this dear friend of mine the wisdom, guidance, and direction they need to attain their goal and the discernment to recognize Your path. May they walk in Your strength to persevere without shrinking back, so that they'll remain in Your will and receive what You've promised. Help them to place their confidence in Jesus and have peace in the process. In Jesus' name I pray, Amen.

---

[1] Osteen, Joel. *Your Best Life Now* (New York, NY: Faith Words, 2004).

[2] Bevere, John. *The Bait of Satan* DVD Video Lessons, John Bevere Ministries (Orchard Park, NY: Eastco Multi Media Solutions, 2002).

[3] Copeland, Kenneth & Gloria. *Healing & Wellness* (Fort Worth, TX: Kenneth Copeland Publications, 2008).

[4] "Paul and the Old Covenant." *Grace Communion International.* 18 Nov. 2010 (http://www.wcg.org/lit/law/otl/ot106.htm).

[5] Copeland, Kenneth. *The Force of Faith* (Fort Worth, TX: Kenneth Copeland Publications, 1983).

[6] Nelson. *Canadian Dictionary* (Scarborough, ON: ITP Nelson. A Division of Thomson Canada, Ltd., 1997), p. 1006.

[7] Copeland, Kenneth. *Faith and Patience; The Power Twins* (Fort Worth, TX: Kenneth Copeland Publications, 1992).

[8] Copeland, Kenneth. *The Force of Faith* (Fort Worth, TX: Kenneth Copeland Publications, 1983).

[9] "The Ten Commandments -Ten Commandment Scriptures." *The Ten Commandments.org.* 18 May 2009 (http://www.the-ten-commandments.org/tencommandsments.html).

[10] Ibid.

[11] Ibid.

[12] Ibid.

[13] Meyer, Joyce. *The Love Revolution* (New York, NY, Faith Words, Hachette Book Group, 2009).

[14] Chan, Francis. Yankoski, Danae. *Crazy Love* (Colorado Springs, CO: David C. Cook, 2008).

[15] Moore, Beth. *Believing God* (Nashville, TN: Life Way Press, 2004).

[16] Ibid.

[17] Ibid.

[18] Ibid.

[19] Ibid.

[20] Ibid.

[21] Ibid.

[22] Ibid.

[23] "Is Tithing Required in the New Covenant?" *Grace Communion International*. 18 Nov. 2010 (http://www.gci.org/law/tithing).

[24] Ibid.

[25] Snell, Jay. *How to claim the Abrahamic Covenant* (Livingston, TX: Jay Snell Evangelistic Association, 1995), p. 5.

[26] "Is Tithing Required in the New Covenant?" *Grace Communion International*. 18 Nov. 2010 (http://www.gci.org/law/tithing).

[27] Copeland, Kenneth. *The Force of Faith* (Fort Worth, TX: Kenneth Copeland Publications, 1983).

Chapter Thirteen
God's Will to Heal!

Jesus went throughout Galilee, teaching in their synagogues,
preaching the good news of the kingdom, and healing every disease
and sickness among the people.

Matthew 4:23

All through the New Testament, the Bible recounts the amazing and wonderful things Jesus did while He walked on the face of this earth. Everywhere He went, He was filled with compassion for the lost, sick, hurting, and needy. He healed all the sick and delivered all who were oppressed with evil spirits. Not one left without receiving the miracle they sought!

"When evening came, many who were demon-possessed were brought to him, and he drove out the spirits with a word and healed all the sick." (Matthew 8:16)

"Many followed him, and he healed all their sick." (Matthew 12:15b)

"Those troubled by evil spirits were cured, and the people all tried to touch him, because power was coming from him and healing them all." (Luke 6:18b, 19)

Did you hear that? Jesus healed them all!

"Jesus gave them this answer: "I tell you the truth, the Son can do nothing by himself; he can do only what he sees his Father doing, because whatever the Father does

the Son also does. For the Father loves the Son and shows him all he does. Yes, to your amazement he will show him even greater things than these." (John 5:19–20)

"For I have come down from heaven not to do my will but to do the will of him who sent me." (John 6:38)

"He sent forth his word and healed them; he rescued them from the grave." (Psalm 107:20)

The above verses truly reveal God's willingness to heal. Jesus always acted on what He saw the Father do, and healing was clearly in His will. Even the sacrifice of Jesus' life was in accordance with God's divine plan, for God's Word states; *"But he was pierced for our transgressions, he was crushed for our iniquities; the punishment that brought us peace was upon him, and by his wounds we are healed."*(Isaiah 53:5)

God loves each one of us so much that He sent Jesus, His only Son, to die on the cross to pay the penalty for our sins; and to break the curse of sin, poverty, sickness, pain, and death that we might have and enjoy life now and for eternity with Him. By His death and resurrection, Jesus defeated the enemy once and for all! When He died on the cross, His work was completed perfectly. This means there was and is nothing left to be done. To quote Jesus' last words in John 19:30, He said, "It is finished." Jesus had defeated the enemy and captured the prize, a reward offered to each one of us as a gift of grace. Jesus rose from the dead and is sitting on the throne of God, with the enemy under His feet.

Since sickness is from the enemy, that means cancer and every other rotten disease is under Jesus' feet too. All we need to do is receive this free gift with our faith, choosing to believe what God's Word says about our situation, and take our eyes off of our circumstances and onto Jesus, the one who has the answers to all our problems.

This explanation in itself should answer this perplexing question bothering so many people. To reinforce my point, let's look at another Scripture that gives additional proof of God's willingness to heal.

"A man with leprosy came to him and begged him on his knees, 'If you are willing, you can make me clean.' Filled with compassion, Jesus reached out his hand and touched the man. 'I am willing,' he said. 'Be clean!' Immediately the leprosy left him and he was cured." (Mark 1:40–42)

Jesus was willing and still is! Some sceptics may say that was then and this is now. Yes, over 2,000 years have passed in time, but the Bible clearly tells us that Jesus is the same, yesterday, today, and forever (Hebrews 13:8). He has not changed! He still wants to see people saved, healed, and set free.

Jesus got into a boat to cross to the other side of the lake. While still near shore, a ruler of the synagogue, named Jairus, came and fell at Jesus' feet, begging Him to come heal his little daughter who was dying. Jairus believed with all his heart that if Jesus just touched her, she would live. Jesus was sympathetic and immediately left for Jairus's house to heal the dying girl. When He arrived at the little girl's home, the mourners had already arrived! Jesus told Jairus not to be afraid but to believe. Our faith needs to be active to receive!

"When Jesus entered the ruler's house and saw the flute players and the noisy crowd, he said, "Go away. The girl is not dead but asleep." But they laughed at him. After the crowd had been put outside, he went in and took the girl by the hand, and she got up." (Matthew 9:23–25)

Again, Jesus reveals the Father's will to heal! News had travelled quickly about the miracles preformed by Jesus. A woman suffering from an issue of bleeding for 12 long years pressed through the crowd to touch the hem of His garment. This desperate woman had spent every cent she had on doctor bills and still continued to get worse! She also knew that if she managed to touch Him, she would be healed.

The moment she touched the hem of His garment, Jesus felt the power go out of His body and asked the disciples who had touched Him. The crowd was so large with people pressing all around Him that He was unable to see who had, yet He knew in His spirit someone had, because He felt the power flow out from Him (Matthew 9:18–22)!

"Jesus turned and saw her. 'Take heart, daughter,' he said, 'your faith has healed you.' And the woman was healed from that moment." (Matthew 9:22)

This woman had amazing faith and determination! She ignored the Judicial Law that wouldn't allow a woman to come out in her type of condition, which held serious consequences if caught, and likely had to crawl on her hands and knees to get to Him through the pressing crowd.[1] She believed Jesus was able to heal her and came expecting to receive a miracle.

"*As Jesus went on from there, two blind men followed him, calling out, 'Have mercy on us, Son of David!' When he had gone indoors, the blind men came to him, and he asked them, 'Do you believe that I am able to do this?'*

"'*Yes Lord,' they replied. Then he touched their eyes and said, 'According to your faith will it be done to you;' and their sight was restored.*" (Matthew 9:27–30a)

At a later date, after Jesus had finished teaching in the synagogue, He went with two of the disciples to Simon and Andrew's house. When they arrived, Simon's mother-in-law was in bed sick with a fever. Jesus immediately went to her. The moment He touched her hand she was healed. To show her gratitude, she got up and made them something to eat (Mark 1:29–31).

It is unmistakably God's will to heal. Jesus touched and healed everyone who ever came to Him!

"That evening after sunset the people brought to Jesus all the sick and demon possessed. The whole town gathered at the door, and Jesus healed many who had various diseases. He also drove out many demons." (Mark 1:32–34a)

"A few days later, when Jesus again entered Capernaum, the people heard that he had come home. So many gathered that there was no room left, not even outside the door, and he preached the word to them. Some men came, bringing to him a paralytic, carried by four of them. Since they could not get him to Jesus because of the crowd, they made an opening in the roof above Jesus and, after digging through it, lowered the mat the paralyzed man was lying on. When Jesus saw their faith, he said to the paralytic, 'Son, your sins are forgiven.' He said to the paralytic, 'I tell you, get up, take your mat and go home.' He got up, took his mat and walked out in full view of them all. This amazed everyone and they praised God, saying, 'We have never seen anything like this!'" (Mark 2:1–5, 10b–11)

Jesus doesn't have a list of requirements you must fill before receiving your healing. We don't have to be perfect. Jesus admired their faith that brought them seeking. He's not a respecter of persons, which means that what He's willing to do for one, He's willing to do for all. And that's exactly what He did! God doesn't show favouritism (Acts 10:34), contrary to some earthly fathers. We do, however, have a responsibility to look after ourselves and turn from our sin so we don't get sick again.

When we look at Jesus' life, we see a reflection of God's character. Jesus is made in the exact image of God and is perfect in every way. He was tempted in all things, yet He was without sin; the same remains today (Hebrews 4:14, 15). Therefore, if Jesus is the exact representation of the Father, this proves that God doesn't make mistakes. A perfect Father wants what's best for His children!

God Gives Good Gifts to His Children

"Every good and perfect gift is from above, coming down from the Father of the heavenly lights, who does not change like shifting shadows." (James 1:17)

God desires to bless His children with wonderful things to enjoy. This is revealed in 1 Timothy 6:17 which says; *"God richly provides us with everything for our enjoyment."* He is a good Father who wants His children to have good things and healing is definitely a good thing!

"Which of you, if his son asks for bread, will give him a stone? Or if he asks for a fish, will give him a snake? If you, then, though you are evil, know how to give good gifts to your children, how much more will your Father in heaven give good gifts to those who ask him!" (Matthew 7:9)

"Dear friend, I pray that you may enjoy good health and that all may go well with you, even as your soul is getting along well." (3 John 2)

It's God's desire for His children to prosper in every way. This includes divine health. He wants you to be whole in your body, mind and soul. 1 Peter 2:24 says, *"He himself bore our sins in his body on the tree, so that we might die to sins and live for righteousness; by His wounds you have been healed."* Jesus bore our sicknesses and diseases so we wouldn't have to. He already paid the price for our sins and healing. God's Word says by Jesus' stripes we have been healed. Your healing has already been accomplished. This goes beyond being a promise. God made it fact! It is a free gift, but you must receive it with your faith.

Sickness is oppression from Satan. God doesn't purposely make His kids sick so He can turn around and heal them. People often give God a bad rap for what the enemy has done! This is the work of the devil. John 10:10 tells us that Satan is the one who comes to steal, kill, and destroy, but Jesus came to give us life and life more abundantly. God is the Great Physician, not the inflictor. God sent Jesus to destroy the works of the devil and sickness is straight from the pit of hell! May

God open your eyes to see this! Mental sickness and disorders are also a work of the enemy. When he sees a weakness, he takes advantage where he can. He torments people's minds with evil spirits and robs their brains of chemicals. It's not just hereditary. It may be a weakness in the family line that Satan preys on, but from what God has shown me, I believe it's most likely rooted in spiritual issues. Jesus cured those who were troubled by these spirits. He is the answer for all types of ailments, large and small. Can you see? Jesus wants to heal you. He healed them all!

In addition, 3 John 2 also declares that God cares just as much about our physical body as He desires for you to be in spiritual health. Did you know that our physical health is relative to our spiritual health? Have you had a spiritual check-up lately? Scripture tells us to judge ourselves now so we won't be under judgment later. The way we judge ourselves is to come to God and inspect our hearts to see if there are sinful ways we need to change in our lives. When there is, ask God for forgiveness and then choose to change.

Some people receive their healing and then go right back to the same lifestyle they once had before and then wonder why they end up sick again. In John 5, Jesus healed a crippled man who was lame for 38 years. Then *Jesus said to him, "Get up! Pick up your mat and walk." At once the man was cured: he picked up his mat and walked. Later Jesus found him at the temple and said to him, "See, you are well again. Stop sinning or something worse may happen to you."* (John 5:8-9, 14)

Several years after Carter, our second son, was born, I had a procedure called an upper GI endoscopy performed by an Internal Specialist and was diagnosed with acid reflux syndrome, a common condition many people suffer from. The stomach produces too much acid due to stress, poor eating habits or from eating before bed. When lying down at night, the esophagus relaxes and allows the acid to travel up and eat away at the tissue in the esophagus and throat, making the throat and sometimes the mouth very red and raw. This also causes a decrease in appetite and often an upset stomach. The doctor recommended that I cut out all caffeine including chocolate and spicy, fatty, and highly acidic foods.

I followed the doctor's directions very closely for several years. After I finished nursing our third son, Spencer, I began drinking the odd cup of coffee on weekend mornings with my husband. And of course, who can live without chocolate? It didn't take long before the limited amount of coffee bothered my stomach and made me jittery. I felt that still-small voice within me, speaking to my heart about cutting out coffee completely. I finally kicked the habit, but wondered why other people could enjoy it and I couldn't! Eventually, I came to terms with the fact that the years of abusing my body as a teen by eating hot pickled peppers by the bowlful and drinking pickle juice had taken their toll. I needed to take responsibility and start pampering it. Just because someone is young doesn't mean they'll get away with poor eating habits. It will eventually catch up with them!

A year before I was diagnosed with cancer, I again felt the Lord prompting me to change my diet. This time it concerned my consumption of sugar. A concerned friend came to me with information about hyperglycaemia. She obviously recognized the signs. I was unaware that my body was even craving it as a way to keep up with my busy lifestyle. I was addicted, although I didn't want to admit it. I loved dessert! I ate it anywhere from three to six times a day and hefty servings, I might add. I was quite proud of how much I could pack back and stay the size I was. I did cut back a little, but not as much as I should have. I considered my diet healthy because I ate three balanced meals, as well as three snacks a day and didn't eat a lot of processed junk like chips, pop or fast food. God continued to send the message about eliminating sugar altogether from different avenues until I finally gave in. But I wasn't impressed at all! Matter of fact, I was downright resentful. After about a month, I began to reason my conviction away and convinced myself it would be all right to allow myself the pleasure of eating dessert once a week. It didn't take long before once turned into twice, and the next thing I knew, I was eating dessert once a day. I justified my decision by the fact that it was an improvement. It wasn't until after I was diagnosed with cancer that I gained wisdom through several naturopath doctors and from reading several of Dr. Don Colbert's books that cancer feeds off sugar.[2] I then realized God was only trying to protect me instead of taking away something I enjoyed. The "old Nancy" thought God wanted to punish her! I always knew that sugar lowers one's immune system, but I lived in denial thinking it would never happen to me. I repented for not taking proper care of my body and asked God to forgive me for my anger and resentment towards Him.

On January 26, 2006, I received the first of two intercellular blood tests by my naturopath doctor to determine possible deficiencies of certain vitamins and minerals within my blood. The lack of certain substances can cause sickness and disease within one's body. I learned from Dr. Colbert that *there are decreased vitamins and minerals in our food sources today because of the depleted minerals in our earth's soil; our food doesn't have the same nutritional value it did 50 years ago because of the use of pesticides and herbicides as well as the lack of rotating crops or letting the soil rest every seven years like in olden days. Poor eating habits may also contribute to sickness and disease as well as lack of exercise and toxins within our environment, food, and water supply.*[3] My body was lacking quite a number of different vitamins and minerals that aren't commonly known. Dr. Ken says sugar can also rob your body of essential vitamins and minerals.

The Bible says all things are permissible but not all things are beneficial (1 Corinthians 10:23). The Lord gave us guidelines in the Bible in Leviticus 11 as to how to eat. People have made food an addiction and the world is laden with disease because of it. We need to stop bowing down to our flesh, rise up, and take responsibility for our actions.

"The one who sows to please his sinful nature, from that nature will reap destruction; the one who sows to please the Spirit, from the Spirit will reap eternal life." (Galatians 6:8)

Our bodies aren't invincible; we will reap from what we sow. God never intended for us to eat food that is heavily laden with chemicals, preservatives, color dies, sugar, and salt; our bodies will break down and get sick if we abuse them.[4] If we drive our cars nonstop without putting in the proper gas or doing the necessary maintenance procedures, our cars will cease up. Our bodies are no different. It is God's desire for you to be healed and made whole in your body, mind, and spirit. However, you must take action and do the things you know you should do. Ask God for wisdom. I'm sure He will gladly show you. Keep up with what He tells you. You're not doing yourself any favours by reverting back to old habits. It's easy to regress when you feel good. I've learned this the hard way! But we need to remember the Lord's commands for our life and remain faithful.

The Lord sent down manna from Heaven for the Israelites to feed them during the Exodus from captivity. Each household was to collect a certain amount for each person. This food was nutrient packed with everything they needed and would rot by the next day. Each day a fresh provision would fall. Notice this food didn't have chemicals and preservatives. I don't know about you, but I don't really feel great about eating something that sometimes doesn't break down for years.[5] Go check out a few expiration dates on the boxes in the cereal aisle.[6] Perhaps you have never really given any thought to what those chemicals and preservatives could do to your body?[7] I know I didn't; I automatically put my trust in those companies.

"It is for freedom that Christ has set us free. Stand firm, then, and do not let yourselves be burdened again by a yoke of slavery… You, my brothers, were called to be free. But do not use your freedom to indulge the sinful nature." (Galatians 5:1, 13a)

During the late winter months of 2009, I again developed acid reflux. This time, my throat was raw and strained with canker sores. Even my tongue and mouth were burned from the acid and felt as if they were on fire, with my voice often sounding raspy. I was quite perplexed because I seemed to be eating all the right things and wasn't feeling stressed. My doctor swabbed my throat for strep and prescribed an antibiotic, along with some acid reflux medication. I experienced partial, short-term relief. By spring, lumps developed throughout my entire neck and the pain increased to the point that I couldn't lift my chin. My doctor changed my prescription and ordered an ultrasound. The medication again reduced my symptoms to a minimum, as long as I ate a bland diet. The ultrasound revealed that I had numerous cysts throughout my salivary glands, with one particularly large one. This was of concern because the mass was partially solid! My family doctor thought it best to send me to a specialist in internal medicine. After a thorough examination by her, she decided to advise a surgeon as to how to proceed with the biopsy. After collaborating, the doctors decided to send me for a CT scan early in July before proceeding. In the meantime, I received prayer at church. The CT scan revealed that the cysts were benign, yet chronic, due to the acid, and the solid mass had shrunk. The doctor put me on an even more limited diet to help achieve alkalinity in my body and told me to double the medication my family doctor prescribed and to keep praying because it was working. The lumps went down in my neck and the acid became tolerable. Shortly after, I discovered I had parasites in my stool and treated them with over-the-counter medication as directed by my doctor. Four doses were necessary for their elimination.

Around the same time as all the testing, I mentioned to my oncologist and internal specialist that I was experiencing the odd sharp twinge in my abdominal area near my liver and the top of my stomach. They both told me that everyone experiences the odd ache and pain and that it was probably my brain playing tricks on me! I understood that they didn't want to subject me to anymore radiation in case it wasn't anything. Yet, my intuition spoke different.

During our summer holidays, I woke up in the middle of the night in a cold, clammy sweat with terrible abdominal cramping. I stumbled to the washroom, barely making it without blacking out. As I sat on the toilet with my head against the wall, the room began to swirl. I felt nauseous, shaky, and weak. An audible voice said, "You're very ill, Nancy." Was God trying to warn me, or was the devil trying to fill me with fear? I immediately started to pray. Then Isaiah 30:21 came to mind. It says: *"Whether you turn to the right or to the left, your ears will hear a voice behind you, saying, "This is the way; walk in it."* After about half an hour had passed, I started to feel a bit better. I went back to bed, changed my soaking wet pajamas and continued to pray until I fell asleep. The next morning, I felt completely fine when I woke up. I thought maybe I had a reaction to the artificially flavoured crab I ate on my salad the evening before. I mentioned it to both my oncologist and internal specialist, but they both agreed that it was probably a virus. I still wasn't convinced! Regardless, I let the issue go and went on about life.

Still having problems with the acid reflux, my family doctor switched my medication again. With a four hundred dollar prescription for the month in hand, I finally found some relief. Not wanting to take medication all my life, I decided to return to Dr. Ken, my naturopath, to get to the root of the problem. The tests verified that I had (Elmeria stredae) parasites in my liver and in my intestinal track. Dr. Ken told me the acid reflux resulted from my system being so sensitive to the parasites. He gave me three different herbal supplements to take twice a day and recommended that I take probiotics because of the toxic bacteria they produce. My skin, especially my face, had a green tone.

One night, I dreamt I was invited to my friend Nancy Steele's house for supper. When we sat down she placed a huge bowl in the middle of the table with cooked carrots and asparagus. I looked at her as if to say, "Are you sure you invited me to supper?" Then she gave me a look back as if to say, "You know it, girl!"

I knew God was telling me to change my diet again. I believed it was only for a short time! For the next three days, all I ate was lots of vegetables, but especially cooked carrots and asparagus. I felt great! Both the pain and the acid reflux had disappeared. The next day, I ate meat with my supper in assumption that my timeline was up. Unfortunately, the abdominal pain returned with a vengeance. That night I dreamt that I was in a room with a girl with some destructive bad habits and a teacher from high school that practiced pagan religion (witchcraft). I stood, puzzled, holding two black roses, not knowing how I got them. Everyone else around me embraced vibrant flowers.

"Where is my bouquet?" I asked, turning to the nervous girl with bad habits. She pointed to a small wooden box on the floor buried in junk that resembled an infant's coffin. I then handed the teacher back the black roses and picked up my bouquet of vibrant peach-coloured roses, walked out under a covering to a cute silver car, put the flowers in the trunk and went on my way.

God showed me that the black roses represented death and the dying of old habits. Discarding unhealthy habits would bring about rebirth. One represented my first brush with death; the second concerned the issue with parasites. The fact that I gave the black roses back meant that I wasn't going to die. Yet, I was about to die (put an end) to the old habits that cause death, including toxic emotional reactions to issues, and I set out on a new journey where I would flourish (the new car represented a new journey; taking the living flowers with me meant I would flourish). I realized that I'd relaxed by making a few too many food allowances and wasn't paying proper attention to my fat intake. I needed to follow what the Lord initially asked me strictly, so that I'd receive the new beginning at life God had shown me. His promises were revealed through previous dreams; one symbolized by the infant and now the flowers.

The nervous girl in my dream represented bad habits and the person who needs to lean on the Lord instead of turning to other things for comfort. She also needed healing from the emotional issues from the past, where she, like I, felt less valued than others within her family. She also needed to give up some things to benefit her health. I learned from Mark Virkler that when we dream of other people, they represent the character within ourselves unless we are only an onlooker towards the dream.[8]

The teacher (authority figure) in my dream signified the pagan emblems, rituals and or belief systems that people accept into their lives that place them under demonic authority, whether they realize it or not. What on earth had I allowed into my life to open myself up to the demonic? I'll explain this at the end of this section, but until then, keep in mind that it is at the hand of Satan, not God, that sickness comes into effect.

The teacher in my dream used two products (hair dye and lipstick) that contain lead. There is a great amount of controversy over whether they contribute to the cause of cancer. At the time of the dream, I'd been contemplating getting highlights. When I awoke, I felt impressed by the Lord to start the cleanse. I felt Him wanting me to start during the summer but had been putting off because of the drastic dietary change. The alkaline cleanse completely healed my acid reflux problem after one week with absolutely no medication. I was then able to eat foods such as onions, garlic, peppers, tomatoes, etc. that doctors list as contributors to acid reflux. I learned from watching Dr. Oz on television that garlic and onions relax the esophagus which allow acid to rise. When the pH level is balanced in the body, there isn't any acid to rise. This isn't a ticket for people to start eating greasy, fatty food, but will allow them to get to the root of the problem so they can once again eat the healthy, healing foods that cleanse and restore health to the body in other ways!

The cleanse I used as a guideline came from a book called *The Complete Cancer Cleanse*. Completing each stage aids the body to help prevent and/or overcome cancer. It rids the body of unwanted chemicals, toxins, parasites, tumours, and kidney stones, etc. It also helps cleanse the body from toxic emotions that hinder healing and cause sickness. Our cells and tissues hold memory of these toxic negative emotions and trauma when not released. When these emotions or memories are triggered, it causes the brain to reproduce cancer cells. This is why it's so important to deal with our issues right away instead of stuffing our emotions![9]

Scripture indicates that for some healings to manifest, prayer and fasting must be involved. Denying yourself of food while you're sick isn't a good idea and I'm sure medical doctors wouldn't recommend it. However, Isaiah 58 talks of a different kind of fast. A true fast that rids oneself of strife and selfishness, to look past one's own fleshly desires, to honour the Sabbath and to meet the needs of the poor to experience the healing that breaks forth like the light at dawn. God is asking us to honour Him by eliminating sin from our lives and blessing those who are less fortunate. During my–cleanse, I considered this to be the same type of fasting because as I denied my body harmful things, I prayerfully allowed God to work and remove sin from my life. Giving to others comes naturally for me but God used eliminating certain foods as a means to deal with self-pity and resentment. Please remember, the only reason I needed to eliminate certain foods from my diet was because of the stress I'd put myself through, as well as the choices I made while younger. God only used the situation to teach me; He doesn't take pleasure in taking things away from us.

As I cleansed my body of the unwanted toxins, the Lord began to reveal to me the additional areas that needed purification in my life. This is where the dream of dying to old habits comes into play and how my life was opened to the demonic which can also cause sickness. The demonic can bother Christians and non–Christians alike where there is legal access through sin whether direct or indirect such as generational, through soul ties, or unconfessed sin past or present, including pride and especially fear.[10] Worrying was my biggest problem. The constant stress created from worrying made me sick. When we worry, fret, fear or doubt, we are not putting our trust in God! That means instead of walking in faith, we're really walking in sin! We often think of "sin" as the big stuff like lying, cheating, stealing, murder, etc. But in reality, anything against God's will is sin. There's no such thing as a little white lie in God's eyes. Sin is sin! Our sin can be as simple as harbouring little offenses! Don't forget, that's unforgiveness!

Our world is saturated with misleading ideas that cause confusion. The biggest areas are usually the topics that bring the most controversy. The Bible clearly maps out what is and isn't sin. Reading the Bible will give you clarity. When in doubt, read the Book. A year ago, I was given a gift certificate to buy an expensive article of clothing from what I thought was an athletic store. I felt extremely blessed that this individual regarded me to that degree. I could hardly wait to spend it, but found it difficult to find the time to get into the city. One day, while out for a walk with a friend, she mentioned how her daughter wanted to get a pair of pants from the same store where I had the certificate. She also informed me that I may not be comfortable with wearing such an article and proceeded to tell me about the store. Earlier in my relationship with her, I'd shared my concerns about yoga because I didn't want my children participating in yoga while over at her house. That's something they did on a regular basis. After you read the next chapter you'll understand why this was such a dilemma for me. Each day was filled with anxiety about what to do. I didn't want to offend the person who gave me such a thoughtful gift, yet I wanted to obey the Lord. I tried to ignore the problem but every time I saw this person, they'd ask me if I'd gone shopping yet. I had a check in my heart saying no, while my earthly desire said yes.

I decided to get advice from someone in spiritual leadership, even though I disagreed with a few of his basic beliefs. That should have been a red flag! He encouraged me to buy and wear the article of clothing out of love and respect for the individual. That was just what my flesh wanted to hear. That way I wouldn't offend the person that gave me the gift and I could have something nice and trendy to wear. I could hear God's voice quietly telling me to listen to Him and not others, but I ignored His voice. Instead, I reasoned my convictions aside with the words that said it's only an article of clothing, and it wasn't like you're actively taking part in yoga. I threw in an additional $65 and bought a hoody with the most discrete emblem on it I could find.

Ignoring God's voice was a bad idea! Every time I wore the coat, I was tormented in my mind by the words of my conviction. I felt as if I was advertising something that I knew had spiritual consequences and didn't want to be seen as a hypocrite by others who knew my position regarding yoga. I even contemplated sewing a patch over the emblem and cutting off the ties that also carried the symbol. Directly after I bought and started wearing the coat, the acid reflux and cysts developed in my throat. I decided to research the foundational beliefs behind the company and uncovered information that confirmed the check in my spirit. The entire foundational belief system of the company was rooted in the Hindu religion. I finally understood what God was protecting me from. Please note that I'm not prejudiced. God made all people equally in His image and we are to love everyone the same regardless of skin color, religion, wealth or lack thereof. However, it's the sin that we're to judge to protect ourselves from falling into it, not the people. That's the difference! I no longer wanted anything to do with this article even if it caused hard feelings. It wasn't until after I got rid of the item that I found relief within my body, mind, and spirit. Do yourself a huge favour and listen to the Lord the first time. You'll save yourself a lot of grief! If you have unconfessed sin in your life, it can become an open door for Satan to put sickness on you. It is God's desire for all to be saved, healed, and delivered. That was the main purpose of Jesus' ministry on the earth.

If you have been seeking God for healing and you are not getting a breakthrough, ask yourself these important questions: Am I walking in faith? Does my church believe in healing? If not, go where they do! Jesus' miracles were hindered by the people's unbelief in Nazareth (Mark 6:1–

69). Am I reading, meditating, and praying healing Scriptures? Do I speak positive confessions? This needs to be done consistently. It will build up your faith. Remember, God acts on His Word. Am I allowing Satan access into my life through sin? Sin inhibits God's grace from flowing into our lives. Even when you think you've forgiven or confessed everything, ask God to reveal any hidden sin. Do I continually walk in love with others? Is there a generational curse or stronghold of sin in my life that needs to be broken? Sickness can linger when a person needs deliverance of an evil spirit.[11]

As long as you have unconfessed sin in your life, Satan will continue to keep rights of access. Jesus came to save, heal, and deliver. The choice is yours. Do you want to be set free? If you don't deal with the root of the problem, the symptoms will continue to pop up like bad weeds. Family ties of freemasonry, witchcraft, and the occult need to be broken with prayer. If you've prayed the prayers in this book and are still having problems, go to a Christian counsellor that has the necessary material to renounce the actual vows and practices family members made, to break off the chains that bind you.

When we submit to any way that is against God's best for our lives, we open ourselves up to the demonic. For example, if we allow ungodly movies to be watched in the home, the spirit attached to such movies will be granted access in our lives. Horror movies allow the spirit of fear to lurk and torment, just as movies with sexual content invite a spirit of lust to temp and manipulate. Each one of Satan's demons has an assigned task to complete.[12] These demonic spirits will gain access anywhere they can to gain authority in your life. Often teenage girls will read horoscopes, play with Ouija boards, and go to fortune tellers for fun. What they don't realize is that this allows divination spirits to cause destruction in their lives, even down the road, until confessed, repented of, and renounced. We cannot serve both God and Satan. When we choose sin over God, it's the same as worshipping Satan. Can you see how careful we must be with what we allow into our homes and lives? Ask God to reveal to you the areas of sin and clean your homes of any artefacts tied to such things. Certain objects can hold satanic influence or presence. Confessing these sins and renouncing any further involvement will close the door on Satan and his demons. This removes his legal right in your life. Be on your guard! He'll try to gain access again if he can.

Do you need to get rid of any occult possessions? We must deal with all entry points so that they are unable to return. Ask God for the strength you need to be obedient. When we are, it brings us back under God's protective covering.

- Articles of witchcraft: Spell books, Ouija boards, tarot cards, horoscopes, palm reading, fortune telling, pentagram, hexagram, good luck charms, crystals, divining rod, amulet, etc.

- Video games: dungeons and dragons, and other dark games etc.

- Satanic music (heavy metal, punk, or gothic rock)

- Dark television programs, movies and even dark cartoons

- Masonic artefacts, jewellery, books etc.

- New Age Crystals, symbols, books, and jewellery etc.

- Idols (Ezekiel 14:6)[13]

"If my people, who are called by my name, will humble themselves and pray and seek my face and turn from their wicked ways, then will I hear from heaven and forgive their sin and will heal their land." (2 Chronicles 7:14)

Sin can be a direct result of sickness. It is the open door the devil uses to put sickness on people as a result of poor eating habits, abusing their bodies through addictions, unforgiveness, worshipping other gods, etc. You may think it is no big deal but sin is sin and Satan will hold any legal right he can. Many bad things that happen in this life are often the repercussion of our sins, the poor choices of man or the lack of wisdom. Not all cases of sickness are a result of sin! Regardless of the reason, God heals to reveal His glory and draws the lost to Him by His goodness.

"Praise the Lord, O my soul, and forget not all his benefits—who forgives all your sins and heals all your diseases, who redeems your life from the pit and crowns you with love and compassion, who satisfies your desires with good things, so that your youth is renewed like the eagle's. The Lord works righteousness and justice for all the oppressed." (Psalm 103:2–6)

The Lord reminds us to remember all the benefits He offers. It is His desire to forgive all our sins and heal all our sicknesses and diseases. It doesn't say He might, the Word says He does. For it says, *"He does not treat us as our sins deserve or repay us according to our iniquities. For as high as the heavens are above the earth, so great is his love for those who fear him."* (Psalm 103:10, 11)

Notice in Psalm 103:10 that Jesus didn't withhold healing because someone was wicked and He certainly didn't just heal those who were righteous. Jesus didn't come to call on the righteous, He came for us sinners (Mark 2:17). We don't have to have our act together to receive our healing, but we do need to accept responsibility and change our habits to keep it. This again puts the ball of free will back into our court. It's up to us how we're going to play. Unfortunately, our bodies suffer the consequences when we don't make the right choices. In reality, life isn't a game. Our decision will determine whether we win or lose a serious battle in the long run. Taking ownership and doing our part by handling the ball wisely will determine whether we have a successful outcome. Many people only concern themselves with the physical here and now. There will be a time when they won't be able to ignore the spiritual side of life which is of greater significance. Our bodies are only temporary while our souls experience afterlife for eternity. We're human and at times we'll make mistakes; there is no doubt about that. When we do mess up, it's important to keep short accounts with God asking Him to forgive us. He is gracious and will heal our lives (souls and bodies) as we humble ourselves and repent and pray.

God's Plans Are Always For Our Good

"For I know the plans I have for you," declares the Lord, "plans to prosper you and not to harm you, plans to give you hope and a future." (Jeremiah 29:11)

Some people think that it's God's will for them to be sick. There is no evil in God. It says He is the light of the world and there is no darkness in Him, so why on earth would God want something bad to happen to His children! He doesn't! God doesn't discipline His children with sickness or allow them to be sick to teach them a lesson. The words prosper; hope and future are all wonderful blessings God wants to give His children. Satan uses doubt and unbelief to confuse God's children so that they will walk in defeat instead of victory! We need to operate in active faith to receive. Jesus commissioned all believers to go out and deliver others from sickness and death as a means to continue the work of God. Satan wants to stop this from happening. Our body is God's temple which Jesus bought at a great price (1 Corinthians 6:19, 20). He wants us to be healthy.

Christians aren't able to effectively minister to others if they're sick or broken. One way he does this is to make them question God's will and heart. He wants people to think that it's God's will for them to be sick so that they will become passive and stagnant in their faith, which makes them ineffective in the kingdom of God. One Scripture that has caused confusion for Christians in this area is the story of Apostle Paul and the thorn in his flesh. When Paul asked God to remove this hindrance he was told by God that His grace was sufficient enough for him (2 Corinthians 12:9). Many Christians have assumed that the thorn in Paul's side was a type of sickness without studying the actual Greek meaning for this word. This misconception has caused people to question God's will to heal. The translation for the word "thorn" means "messenger of Satan." This means that the thorn in Paul's flesh was a messenger sent by Satan. Satan has always made it his goal to try and stop the good news of God's Word from spreading. God didn't say no to Paul about removing his sickness because there wasn't any sickness to remove! He would have been more than willing if there had been. Scripture proves it! Doubt of God's willingness to heal has robbed countless people of the faith they needed to receive their healing. God provided Paul with the grace and authority he needed to overcome every persecution he suffered (2 Timothy 3:11).[14]

God's grace is more than sufficient for us as well. We are not empty-handed. God has equipped us with the full armour of God to defeat the enemy, but we must use it. Even when we're weak, God is strong and it is then that He's at His strongest!

Sickness is of the devil and healing is from God. Jesus said there would be tribulation in the world. He also encourages us with the reminder to cheer up because He has overcome the world (John 16:33). In addition, God promises to use everything the devil throws at us for our good (Romans 8:28), but this suffering isn't from God's hand. We reap and sow from the repercussions of a fallen world and the "choices" of man. God is a gentleman and will not force Himself on anyone. Remember our God–given right of free will. As a result, we reap from the choices we make, whether they're wise or foolish. Yet God in His goodness brings good out of these situations because of His faithfulness.

In Deuteronomy, God explained all the blessings we could expect if we obey His laws and precepts and warned the people of the curses which would fall upon those who disobeyed. It was never God's intention for anyone to get sick. He clearly laid out the blessing that followed righteousness and the curses that would result from disobedience and told us to choose life and blessing. It is, without a doubt, His desire for mankind to choose His way, the right way of doing things. To settle this matter deep within your spirit, I'm going to repeat myself one last time. God doesn't punish His children with sickness. That's not a characteristic of a good parent. God is good all the time! Sickness is a result of poor choices made by ourselves and or others and the lack of wisdom and knowledge.

God's Word says His people perish for lack of knowledge (Hosea 4:6). This is because many people don't know the Word well enough to follow through with what it says to reap the blessings from it. The devil does whatever he can to keep people from learning God's will.

God is and always will be the supreme authority. Although God has the power to do whatever He wants, He continues to give us free will. It's our legal right! People fight for freedom of speech and the expression of their rights and then complain when they get what they've asked for. Don't you think it breaks God's heart to see His children making bad choices and suffering because of them? God is always there trying to guide us the right way. However, it's up to us to choose our path.

Some people have the belief system that God doesn't allow us any choice in life. They believe that everything that happens whether good or bad was dealt from His hand. I had a friend absolutely furious with me because she held this view and didn't understand the power in confessing God's Word. I hope and pray God has given her revelation in this area so that she can gain victory in her life!

At the beginning of my diagnosis, a friend had a vision of me lying in a casket. After that, every time she thought of me she would cry. It was because of the traditional teaching taught in her church about God's sovereignty that she struggled with this issue so much. I told her God can and will change the outcome of events if we pray. I believe God's plan was to put an overwhelming thought on her heart to draw her into intercession on my behalf. I'm forever grateful for her prayers. When you place the truth of God's Word over traditional beliefs, you'll never go wrong.

In the Old Testament days, King Hezekiah became ill to the point of death and was told through the prophet Isaiah to get his house in order because he was not going to recover. Hezekiah turned his face to the wall, weeping, and prayed to the Lord (Isaiah 38:1, 2). Isaiah 38:4, 5 says, *"Then the word of the Lord came to Isaiah: "Go and tell Hezekiah, 'This is what the Lord, the God of your father David, says: I have heard your prayer and seen your tears; I will add fifteen years to your life."* This is a sure example that prayer can change the outcome of our circumstances. We're not a bunch of puppets that God uses to hold absolute rule-ship over. He reveals and offers the way to a prosperous life, but we're not forced to accept. He always wants us to choose what's best out of His great love for us. Even so, the choice is ultimately ours.

"He himself bore our sins in his body on the tree, so that we might die to sins and live for righteousness; by his wounds you have been healed." (1 Peter 2:24)

It's God's desire for us to die to our sins and live for righteousness. In other words, we need to choose to stop sinning and live God's way. Jesus took the beating that justice demanded for our healing. He took our sicknesses upon Himself over 2000 years ago. It doesn't matter whether we need emotional, physical or spiritual healing, what needed

to be done was done. It was finished on the cross. We need to take this free gift, by faith, for it to manifest in the natural. God's Word says...
"That if you confess with your mouth, "Jesus is Lord," and believe in your heart that God raised him from the dead, you will be saved. For it is with your heart that you believe and are justified, and it is with your mouth that you confess and are saved. As the Scripture says, "Everyone who trusts in him will never be put to shame." For there is no difference between Jew and Gentile—the same Lord is Lord of all and richly blesses all who call on him, for, "Everyone who calls on the name of the Lord will be saved." (Romans 10:9–13)

It is by the confessions of our mouths that we are saved. Many years ago, when Ben had his life–threatening allergies, Joyce Meyer taught me that the Greek word used for "saved" in this passage is "*sozo*" which means wholeness. This one little word offers three great gifts all in one complete package. The word "*sozo*" is used interchangeably for the words healing, deliverance, and saved.[15] Jesus died so we could be healed physically, emotionally, and spiritually so that we could enjoy all blessings of prosperity.

God dearly loves you. It's His heart's desire for you to be healed and made whole. If you need healing, pray the prayer below and expect your healing to manifest. Many people notice an immediate change while others find their healing happens over a period of time. Remember the parable that Jesus told about the old widow who kept coming day after day before the judge with her request until she received what she asked for. There's nothing wrong with asking God daily for something until you receive it! He's waiting for you to ask!

Healing Prayer

Dear Heavenly Father,

I am grateful that You are a wonderful Father who desires good things for His children. I believe that You are the Great Physician and I ask that out of Your great mercy You would extend Your right hand and touch my body where there is sickness and infirmity. By the power and authority given me in Jesus' name, I command all sickness, disease, and pain to come out of my body right now. I command my body to be healed and made whole in Jesus' name. Your Word says when I am in trouble and call out to You, You will save me from my distress. Please send forth Your Word and heal me and rescue me from the grave (Psalm 107:19, 20). "O Lord my God, I cry out to You now, and ask You to completely heal me. Thank You Jesus, for being wounded for my transgressions and bruised for my iniquities; I am thankful that the chastisement for my peace was upon You, and that by Your stripes I am healed (Isaiah 53:5). Bless me with the wisdom I need and fill me with Your Holy Spirit that I may overcome. In Jesus' name I pray. Amen.

Once you've repented of your sins, don't forget to pray for those who have hurt you. When you release these people into God's hands, He will act on your behalf and bring justice. God will not allow others to mistreat you and get away with it. It may take awhile for you to see the result. If you don't forgive, you place yourself into the enemy's captivity, which hinders your ability to receive your healing. Remember to stay in the healing Scriptures so that your faith doesn't waver. Healing often weighs heavily on our expectation!

Healing Scriptures

"O Lord my God, I called to you for help and you healed me." (Psalm 30:2)

"He sent forth his word and healed them; he rescued them from the grave." (Psalm 107:20)

"He himself bore our sins in his body on the tree, so that we might die to sins and live for righteousness; by his wounds you have been healed." (1 Peter 2:24)

"I will not die but live, and will proclaim what the Lord has done." (Psalm 118:17)

"Heal me, O Lord, and I will be healed; save me and I will be saved, for you are the one I praise." (Jeremiah 17:14)

"Then your light will break forth like the dawn, and your healing will quickly appear; then your righteousness will go before you, and the glory of the Lord will be your rear guard." (Isaiah 58:8)

(See: Mark 16: 17, 18; James 5:14, 15; Psalm 103:2–5 & Isaiah 53:4–5.)

---

[1] Copeland, Kenneth & Gloria. *Healing & Wellness* (Fort Worth, TX: Kenneth Copeland Publications, 2008).

[2] Colbert, Don, MD. *The Seven Pillars of Health* (Lake Mary, Florida: Siloam, 2007).

[3] Ibid.

[4] Maccaro, Janet, PhD, CNC, *90 – Day Immune System Make Over* (Lake Mary, Florida: Siloam, 2006).

[5] Ibid.

[6] Ibid.

[7] Ibid.

[8] Virkler, Mark & Patti. *Hear God Through Your Dreams* (Elma, New York, USA: Communion With God Ministries, 2003).

[9] Calbom, Cherie, M.S., Calbom, John, M.A., Mahaffey, Michael, P.C. *The Complete Cancer Cleanse* (Nashville, Tennessee: Thomas Nelson, 2006)

[10] Horrobin, Peter. *Healing through Deliverance, The Foundation of Deliverance Ministry Vol#2* (Grand Rapids, MI: Chosen; A Division of Baker Book House Company, 2003).

[11] Ibid.

[12] Ibid.

[13] Ibid.

[14] Copeland, Kenneth & Gloria. *Healing & Wellness* (Fort Worth TX: Kenneth Copeland Publications, 2008).

[15] Ibid.

Chapter Fourteen
Jesus Our Great Shepherd!

The Lord is my shepherd, I shall not be in want. He makes me lie down in green pastures, he leads me beside quiet waters, he restores my soul. He guides me in paths of righteousness for his name's sake. Even though I walk through the valley of the shadow of death, I will fear no evil, for you are with me; your rod and your staff, they comfort me. You prepare a table before me in the presence of my enemies. You anoint my head with oil; my cup overflows. Surely goodness and love will follow me all the days of my life, and I will dwell in the house of the Lord forever.

Psalm 23

These are the famous words of David, a ruddy little shepherd boy who eventually became a King over Israel. Over the period of his existence, David became all too familiar with life's great valleys. As a youth, He lived in isolation and loneliness as he guarded his father's sheep along the rocky hills of Judea while his brothers fought at war. He often passed the time with singing and praying to the Lord. Herding could be quite dangerous with the threat of wild beasts. If danger lurked, a hired hand might run and leave the sheep but David, with God's help, killed both a lion and a bear to protect his family's livelihood. David also stood before a beast of human nature that threatened to kill him and place fellow countrymen into slavery. Imagine standing before a giant whose muscles protrude like rigid rocks bulging from a cliff wall and eyes that burn with hate. Just the thought would make you want to run and hide! That's what his brothers, along with the army, did every time this Philistine giant confronted them. Goliath threatened to pulverize David, feed him to the birds, and put all the people of the land into a life-time of captivity. Even though he was small and unable to bear the weight of armour, David went forward into battle with a few small stones and a sling. Despite the outward appearance of his meagre body, David took the gifts of inner strength, fortitude, and confidence that can only come from spending time with our Heavenly Father. Again, with God's help he defeated the Philistine giant and maintained freedom and peace in the land.

He was young when he was anointed by Samuel to be the successor over King Saul. David had a special musical ability that brought him into King Saul's kingdom and over time David married the King's daughter. David's popularity increased rapidly due to his success in battle and he had to flee for safety when his life became threatened by his own father-in-law, due to jealousy. David was forced to live on the run and hide in mountain caves for several years while Saul hunted him day and night.

Like many, David experienced great loss in his lifetime. While David was running for his life, King Saul gave his wife away to another man. Later, after he'd become King, David married Bathsheba after a scandalous affair and as a result his infant son died (2 Samuel 11, 12). Years later, his son Amnon raped David's daughter Tamar (his half sister). This forced the princess to live as a common girl and brought shame upon their family. Absalom, David's other son, caused division amongst his father's kingdom in anger over this situation. This eventually resulted in the death of all his sons (2 Samuel 13). Yes, David was no stranger to the valleys in life that reside at the base of the mountaintops. We all enjoy the exhilaration that comes from these mountaintop experiences, but we need to remember that there wouldn't be mountaintops without the valleys.[1] I've learned that it's in these valleys that God is always present to guide, bless, and comfort us. He always leads us to the places we can rest in His goodness and mercy even when things don't go the way we would like. It's here that life's lessons are learned. As we spend time with Jesus, He fills us with supernatural peace and joy that quiets and rejuvenates our weary souls.

In the Eastern lands, during Bible times, it was a common welcoming gesture for hosts to anoint their guests' heads with oil which bestowed a delightful fragrance.[2] Jesus invites and anoints us with the Holy Spirit to strengthen us and enable us to cope far beyond our natural ability and fills our hungry souls with gladness even when facing a situation of despair (Zechariah 4:1–6; Psalm 45:7).

Jesus is our good shepherd and never leaves us, especially when oppressed by the negative situations in life. It's human nature to feel anxious and overwhelmed; especially if you don't know what to do or where to turn. As we learn to communicate with Jesus, He'll show us what to do and give us peace along these thorny patches. We often think of death when we hear the 23rd Psalm because it's often read at funerals. Still it offers so much more, as a valley can refer to any type of negative experience.

It's a shepherd's job to take his sheep through the valleys, up over the mountaintops and over to the other side to graze on green pastures.[3] He uses his rod and staff to keep the sheep from getting into trouble. If he sees his sheep about to fall over the side of a cliff, he carefully hooks it with his rod and brings it closer to himself out of harm's way. Similarly, Jesus always remains by our sides to guide us throughout the ups and downs of life's experiences.

The Bible is the rod and staff our Good Shepherd uses to keep us from straying off into danger. It is a beacon of light for our lives to keep us from slipping or stumbling. Reading the New Testament is a wonderful way to get to know our Shepherd. Mature Christians will often tell new believers to start in John and then read Matthew, Mark and Luke and so on. It is filled with the wonderful accounts when Jesus walked on earth and reveals His heart of compassion for mankind. Reading Scripture is extremely important to help you recognize and learn the voice of the Good Shepherd so that you don't wander off and follow a false shepherd, one that will lead you off the side of a cliff.

Health Dangers

"Therefore, since we are surrounded by such a great cloud of witnesses, let us throw off everything that hinders and the sin that so easily entangles, and let us run with perseverance the race marked out for us. Let us fix our eyes on Jesus, the author and perfecter of our faith, who for the joy set before him endured the cross, scorning its shame, and sat down at the right hand of the throne of God." (Hebrews 12:1, 2)

The Lord has placed a very strong concern on my heart to inform you of some grave dangers. We have talked about some of the different methods the Lord uses to bring healing and how He's created our bodies to heal themselves with techniques such as Scripture meditation, prayer, natural foods, laughter, rest, and sleep. In the world, there are many other approaches that appear to be good and acceptable. Ways people assume are leading them on the right road to health and wholeness because they appear to bring about some positive results, or so they seem. People are desperately searching in all directions for answers that will bring the hope they need and desire.

Satan, the father of lies, knows this and has devised a very sneaky plan. The Bible warns us that he disguises himself as an angel of light. He takes truth and mixes it with deceptive lies to draw people down the wrong paths. There is enough truth on such paths to lead people into believing they've found the answer they've been looking for, yet these same paths are filled with deception that will lure them astray. I cringe when I hear people say that people should do whatever method works for them, knowing that some options give Satan doors of access to cause deception and harm. People that hold this frame of mind need our prayers. The enemy has deceived them into thinking that such options are okay. I would agree only in cases referring to those options that are acceptable with God. We are all called to walk different paths, although some are similar. Some methods are successful for some, while others are not. There are demonic powers able to heal; this is why some people are led astray. This was prophesied in the New Testament and is why God tells us for our protection to test the spirits to see where they are rooted. There is a fine line between science and false religion. Ask God for discernment. It's important to be aware of the practitioner's belief system behind their treatment and for what purpose they employ them. Some methods are completely of the devil. When you let Jesus the good shepherd guide you, you'll never go wrong.

Just as the serpent in the Garden of Eden tricked Adam and Eve into eating the forbidden fruit off the tree, which brought spiritual death upon all mankind, he's trying to deceive people into a similar trap by leading them down deceptive paths. These paths appear to be truth, but are twisted with misleading lies that lead to spiritual death.

"And the Lord God commanded the man, "You are free to eat from any tree in the garden; but you must not eat from the tree of the knowledge of good and evil, for when you eat of it you will surely die." (Genesis 2:16, 17)

Satan wanted to confuse Eve and cause her to doubt what God had said, knowing this would make it easier for her to believe his lies.

"Now the serpent was more crafty than any of the wild animals the Lord God had made. He said to the woman, 'Did God really say, 'You must not eat fruit from any tree in the garden'?"

"The woman said to the serpent, 'We may eat fruit from the trees in the garden, but God did say, 'You must not eat fruit from the tree that is in the middle of the garden, and you must not touch it, or you will die.'"

"'You will not surely die,' the serpent said to the woman, 'for God knows that when you eat of it your eyes will be opened, and you will be like God, knowing good and evil.'" (Genesis 3:1–5)

Adam and Eve forgot that they were already formed in the image of God (Genesis 1:27). The boundaries God had set out for them were placed for their own protection and benefit; not to withhold good from them! Not only did their disobedience cause our bodies to age and cause eventual death, this act of sin separated them and us from God and caused spiritual death for our souls. I urge you please be very careful about which avenues you seek healing from!

God is the true source of our healing and He has the answers that will lead you to life both spiritually and physically. There are different types of medicine and practices that are rooted in cultures that worship other gods. These false gods are demonic spirits. Their practices are not from the God of Love I know. I'm very careful about what I open myself up to spiritually because there are spiritual attachments to such customs. You may think that sounds a little far-fetched, but it's not. I've learned this the hard way! We often give our children advice hoping they'll learn from our mistakes rather than having to learn firsthand. So, as my spiritual child, can you please listen to what I'm saying and save yourself an immense amount of grief and pain!

Even when something appears to be beneficial on the surface and the results seem positive, it's important to do a background check to ensure all desired paths guide you to spiritually healthy avenues. I hope you will be careful about what you tap yourself into spiritually. Opening yourself to the ways of the occult will close your eyes off to truth, open your mind up for the deceptive lies of Satan, and place a barrier between you and God. *The word occult is taken from the Latin word "occultus" which means "hidden."*[4] This is to cause deception. Be aware and stay away from any methods or religions that lead you away from God and place the focus on centering yourself (making yourself an idol or god) or the universe. Just because something is spiritual doesn't mean it's godly or good. Please ask God to give you wisdom, knowledge, and clear discernment before doing anything. He will give you the wisdom to filter out those things whose foundations aren't of God, and are based on the schemes of Satan's deception.

"And no wonder, for Satan himself masquerades as an angel of light. It is not surprising, then, if his servants masquerade as servants of righteousness. Their end will be what their actions deserve." (2 Corinthians 11:14–15)

There is only one true God and He is jealous for your soul. He is not jealous of you, He's jealous for you. There is a difference. God loves you and wants you to prosper in every way including your spirit, soul (which is made up of your mind, will, and emotions), and body. When He created the entire universe, He knew what our needs would be and therefore made everything on the earth for our benefit and pleasure. He did not create the sun, moon, stars, trees, water, etc. for us to worship, nor did He intend for us to make our own religions out of them. He is asking us to serve Him and Him alone!

"You shall have no other gods before me. "You shall not make for yourself an idol in the form of anything in heaven above or on the earth beneath or in the waters below.

You shall not bow down to them or worship them; for I, the Lord your God, am a jealous God." (Exodus 20:3–5a)

Let's take a closer look at a few different ways people turn to for healing. But first, let's pray.

Dear Heavenly Father,

Please unveil my eyes and ears so that I would see and hear all the spiritual truths you have for me, including the discernment I need for the path I'm on. Protect and keep me from slipping down destructive paths and lead me to the way everlasting. In Jesus' name I pray. Amen.

Yoga

Yoga is a part of an Eastern religion that originated in India. Although they worship over 300 million deities, there are three main ones they recognize.[5] One is called "Brahman" which they believe to be the "creator," the second is Vishnu, whom they believe is the "preserver" and Shiva, the "destroyer" which is always seen around India in the common sitting stance, as seen in yoga advertisements.[6] Each position practiced during yoga is an actual worship position to their sun gods.[7] The word "yoga" comes from the ancient Sanskrit language word "Yuj" which means: to yoke, join or unite.[8] When a person practices yoga, they become yoked with the spirits worshipped in the Hindu religion and the chants or mantras are used to summon or welcome these spirits within.[9] There are eight different branches of yoga (derived from the 29th Sutra of the second book) which are primarily about the mental and spiritual aspects rather than physical actions and are still being taught in the core of practically all yoga variations.[10] Their belief is that when they attain a certain level (enlightenment) they will no longer be bound by chains of constant reincarnation and will reach ultimate freedom for their body, mind, and soul with the supreme. The supreme they are referring to is not God Almighty, our Creator of Heaven and earth. They believe the universe and everything in it is God, including self. Their objective of self–realization is to initiate one to look deeply within oneself and to ascertain or discover that the so–called "true self" or "higher self" is God.[11]   In other words, "you are the supreme!" We were made in God's image, but we are not God! When you were born, the earth was already in existence wasn't it? We as humans don't have the ability to create something out of nothing! Only God is able. Yogis' beliefs intertwine with Taoism which is interlocked with the evolution theory (the big bang theory), which rejects God as Creator.[12] It's Satan's goal to deceive people and remove any credit from God any way he can. The Hindu religion also denies Jesus Christ as Saviour and Lord. The core of yoga is Hinduism and is based on Hindi Scripture which was developed by Hindu sages.[13]

Johanna Michaelsen, author of *Like Lambs to the Slaughter* writes:

> "Hatha yoga is one of six acknowledged classifications of traditional or orthodox Hinduism. The term "*hatha*" comes from the verb "*hath*" which means "oppress." The practice of hatha yoga is designed to suppress the flow of the psychic energies through these channels (symbolic or psychic passages on either side of the spinal columns: thereby forcing the serpent power or the "kundalini" to rise through the central psychic channel in the spine (the sushumna) and up through the chakras, the supposed psychic centers of human personality and power. Westerners mistakenly believe that one can practice hatha–yoga apart from the philosophical and

religious beliefs that undergrid it. This is an absolutely false belief...

"You cannot separate the exercises from the philosophy... 'The movements themselves become a form of meditation.' The continued practice of the exercises will, whether you...intend it or not, eventually influence you toward an Eastern/mystical perspective. That is what it is meant to do!... There is, by definition, no such thing as 'neutral' Yoga."[14]

This type of yoga is the most difficult and the most potentially spiritually dangerous." In other words, when someone practises this branch of Yoga they're inviting the serpent's (Satan's) power to travel up their spine and to rise up within their body, mind, soul, and spirit.

Now, after everything I've shared with you in this book, can you see the danger of inviting an evil spirit within your body to dwell? Do you still feel comfortable about participating in a practice that bases their foundational beliefs on such a thing? Do you want to partake in something that rejects your healer, Saviour, and friend as just another religion?

Some people feel that as long as they're only participating in yoga for exercise purposes without repeating chants or prayers, that it has nothing to do with the religion and isn't spiritually dangerous. However, I beg to differ! During an interview, Sannyasin Arumugaswani, Managing Editor of Hinduism Today stated, "...*Hinduism is the soul of yoga 'based as it is on Hindu Scripture and developed by Hindu sages. Yoga opens up new and more refined states of mind, and to understand them one needs to believe in and understand the Hindu way of looking at God...A Christian trying to adapt these practices will likely disrupt their own Christian beliefs...*"[15]

Dr. John Ankerberg, author of "Innocent Yoga?" also writes, "When Westerners employ yoga techniques as a means to improve their health, they should understand that they can also be producing subtle changes within themselves which will have dramatic spiritual consequences that will not be for the better. Regardless of the school or spiritual tradition, yoga practice tends to alter a person's consciousness in an occult direction."[16]

Simply being present has spiritual consequences. I've heard of someone being thrown clearly across the room when they tried to worship Jesus in one of these classes. Don't confuse this with the power of God! It was clearly the devil!

From all the research I've done, I strongly believe that it is truly a misconception that a person can practice yoga without altering their philosophical and religious beliefs. Meditation is incorporated with each position and will eventually cause a person to undertake and be influenced by the aspects of the Eastern, mystical perspectives that are connected with this false religion. Even the special breathing is used to invite the Kundalini spirit within.[17] Yoga textbooks will confirm this.[18] Doing yoga opens oneself up to the demonic and will cause spiritual consequences. As a person executes these worship moves, they're submitting themselves under the authority of the Kundalini spirit. The Kundalini spirit is then able to influence that person's life in any negative way it can, whether through sickness, relationship failure, financial trouble, etc.; wherever it can find weaknesses. In the same respect, a person who visits a foreign country and takes off their shoes to go into a temple that worships other gods, surrenders and shows submission to that temple god. This happens even when an individual does so out of respect for others' beliefs and traditions. This creates a spiritual tie or connection with that false god, which is Satan himself. Therefore it's wise for a Christian not to enter such places. The same connection is formed when a person gets involved in martial arts. Each type of art is rooted in the same occult philosophy. For example: Kung Fu holds Buddhist philosophical roots that are rooted in forms of divination, and Tao te ching is based on the belief that salvation comes by observing nature.[19] Martial arts were formed through transcendental meditation, a very dangerous practice used to open the mind and allow what they believe to be the universal spirit to flow.[20] The *"enlightenment"* they receive is actually from evil spirits. This is also practiced in yoga. *In Revelation 16:14 it says, "They are spirits of demons performing miraculous signs, and they go out to the kings of the whole world, to gather them for the battle on the great day of God Almighty."* Have you forgotten about the empowered rebellious angels that were thrown down from above? Satan is the ruler of the air according to 2 Corinthians 4:4, and Luke 4:6–7 confirms this authority. A person involved in martial arts opens themselves up to the spirits attached to such a practice. Their devotion and act of bowing down to their Sensei (meaning Master) affirms this submission. This kind of devotion and honour should only be given to God! The Bible clearly states that we can only have one Master!

As Christians, God is to be our authority. Mankind needs a shepherd to function and carry out God's purposed will properly. God Himself is a God of order even within Himself. First there is God the Father, then God the Son (Jesus, God in the flesh) and third, God the Holy Spirit. All are equally God; yet each One has a very distinct role. God created order as a means to bring structure and success within our countries, churches, and homes. He commands us in His Word to submit only to the authority that He places over us. We are to honour and respect those in government, police, pastors, elders, teachers, etc., to receive the covenant of God's blessing. God has placed them in their ordained position for a purpose. However, when this authority is abusive or asks us to go against God's will, for instance by breaking the law, we aren't obligated to submit. God always gets the final say!

I'm not comfortable with doing yoga in any form and I refuse to put my boys in martial arts because of this. As a matter of fact, when I found out my son's fourth grade teacher was teaching yoga in her physical education class, I went to her to share my concerns. Keep in mind that this conversation wasn't confrontational in the least. She assured me that they were only stretching and posing and they weren't doing chants or any other practices which related to this eastern religion. Knowing that I was still uncomfortable, she offered to lend me the video tape to view at home the next time she brought it in. I prayed and asked God that if what the class was doing displeased Him, He would stop them from practicing this at school. Before she had a chance to bring the tape in for me to view, she lost it. And that was the end of the yoga! Some people may think that was a coincidence; I call that an answer to prayer!

I realize stretching and deep breathing is beneficial for the body. There's nothing wrong with doing stretching or breathing exercises that are NOT related to yoga. Many people, including Christians, are participating in yoga, unaware of its background and its spiritual effects. They merely trust its ability to calm, de-stress, focus, and bring about the physical benefits they desire.

When it comes right down to the bottom line, yoga has roots in the sin of idolatry. There is no getting around it. You can't dabble with something that worships "self" or other gods and expect God to be Kosher with it. It mixes about as well as oil and water with God and is as flammable as gasoline with a lit match. Sin is sin! There is no getting around it. God loves the sinner, but hates sin. God is holy! He is completely pure, without blemish. That's why sin and God don't mix; they can't. We need to keep our lives pure because it's the pure in heart that will see God. Please remember that God is merciful and will forgive you if you truly repent and turn away from this sin.

The Dark Side of Reiki

One day while out for a walk with a friend, she shared that she'd seen a Reiki practitioner hoping to find relief for her arm. Even though I didn't know much about Reiki at the time, I felt extremely unsettled in my spirit. I shared what I knew and encouraged her to turn to God for her healing. She mentioned she'd initially thought the experience was helpful, but began experiencing weird outbursts of anger. Over time her arm got worse and the problem spread to other areas. This compelled me to research Reiki more in depth. The more information I learned, the more clear her situation became too me. This is what I learned: Reiki is another deceptive path the enemy uses where people seek healing. Reiki is a form of the New Age belief system. According to the large Reiki organization, Reiki can be defined as a non-physical healing energy made up of life force energy that is guided by the Higher Intelligence, or spiritually-guided life force energy."[21]

A Reiki practitioner depends on a spirit guide connection to bring healing.[22] This life force energy they're referring to is not God. An individual going to a Reiki to receive a healing touch may be unaware that the energy force the Reiki practitioner is drawing from is actually an evil spirit.[23] Reiki practitioners themselves have divulged this dark secret and brought them to the light after turning to the church in desperation, hoping to seek true healing from God after their own lives have fallen apart from mental and physical illnesses, financial trouble, and broken marriages.[24]

How does a Reiki attain the energy by such a spirit, you may ask? A Reiki opens the doorway to these spirits through their own words and actions. Do you recall the power that our words possess for either God or Satan to use in our situations? The Reiki prays to dead Reiki masters, welcoming and accepting their energy life force through a worship ritual as they sit in front of a homemade altar set up with candles, incense, and photos of dead Reiki masters.[25]

The secret initiation symbol the Reiki master embraces as holy is called "Dia ko mio."[26] When a Reiki calls on this spirit, he acts as a channel and connects the person receiving Reiki to Phoenix, the demon who claims to have risen from the ashes.[27] After the Reiki has performed healing on a client, they then return to their shrine to pay gratitude to the dead Reiki master and these spirits.[28] This is not only worshipping false gods, it's a form of witchcraft!

People need to know the truth. Many times people don't want to hear the truth. They fear it and would rather avoid it. Regardless, God has asked me to share these facts because He loves you and wants you to be free. If you've opened yourself up spiritually to such darkness there's still hope! There's a deliverance prayer below that will lead you to spiritual freedom in Christ.

Acupuncture

Most people are familiar with the practice of using needles to numb nerves, called acupuncture. But did you know that it is rooted in a false religion? Asians used this ancient art to implement and endorse their faith. Like yoga, it can open spiritual doors of deception. Unaware of this controversial issue, I agreed to have acupuncture performed on my back after having herniated disks, even though I felt a little uneasy about it. Afterwards even though I couldn't put my finger on it, something seemed different in my spirit. I felt as if I'd fallen into a slump with God, like there was some type of barrier between us. God began to send the message through books and people that I needed to go to prayer counselling. One day, after hearing Dr. Carolyn Leaf speak on television about the connection between sickness and unresolved emotional matters, I decided I'd waited long enough. I'd worked my way through many issues over the years, yet knew I must have been missing something because I was still struggling with health problems.

When I met with Diane, the prayer counsellor in my church, she shared how God had already given her a dream to show her where my issues lay, which was amazing because she knew very little about me. God is so amazing. She went through deliverance prayers with me to cut off all spiritual ties with this practice and others. Some I'd naively practiced as a child and others I'd been inadvertently been exposed to. Repentance is such a wonderful thing. The joy that rushes through your soul is so invigorating. It is the true feeling of freedom. My peace returned and I immediately felt the barrier come down. It was wonderful to clearly hear God's voice again.

The next time I went to physiotherapy, I asked her to treat me using a different method. As an alternative, she effectively used traction and stretching. Since then, I've found an excellent massage therapist working in the medical field that has helped me retain even longer-lasting results.

Some people believe that receiving acupuncture is acceptable under certain conditions. They feel that as long as the practitioner's frame of mind and intentions are for scientific reasons and they aren't performing this procedure as an act of worship to release or transfer "blocked energy", then it is okay. To my therapist, acupuncture was all about the science. She trained in the medical field and strictly performed this treatment for medical purposes. She never used any jargon referring to "transferring of energy," or used smoke and mirrors so, with this in mind, I must disagree after what I've experienced.

At times we tend to rely on the opinions of others to make our decisions because of our own lack of confidence. There are many intelligent, knowledgeable people in the world. If you are going to them for direction you need to find out what their source of knowledge is. There is no one who is as all-knowing and all-wise as God. Best of all, He's unable to be deceived. He is God! I'm not saying we're unable to get good, godly counselling when we're stuck, but ultimately we need to depend on God. When we pray and ask God for guidance He'll never steer us in the wrong direction.

Why waste your time asking around when you can go straight to the true source of knowledge. Ask God what you should do! Then go directly to the Word for confirmation. It is the unchanging standard from which we must live by.

Are you making decisions based on other people's opinions? I'm amazed at what people will try or do without researching first. All because their neighbour's friend may have tried a certain method that worked for them! Just because they thought it was all right, doesn't make it all right. It's not their approval you need, it is God's. He's the Good Shepherd that will never lead you down the wrong path. There is wisdom in multitudes. Therefore ask God to give you confirmation through two or three godly people who are well grounded in the Word. Well-meaning, good Christian and non-Christian people alike can make mistakes. We're all human! People's intentions may be admirable, but it's God's direction you need. He will give you the correct answers you need!

Massage Therapy

Massage therapy can be a wonderful way to combat stress and also boost your immune system. But this is another avenue in which you should carefully seek direction. A few summers ago, I won a trip to the spa for a day while participating in a cancer walk. I was thrilled! I had recently finished nine months of Herceptin treatments and felt completely worn down at the time. Have you ever experienced the sensation that you've been hit by a Mac truck? Well, that's how I felt.

I welcomed every moment of the sticky seaweed mud body wrap, facial, Jacuzzi jet massage soak, manicure and pedicure, and hair and makeup makeover. The girls even served me a lovely lunch part way through the day. I truly felt like I was in Heaven until I was led into a small, dimly lit room and told to remove my fluffy white robe. I was then directed to lie face down into a very precise position on the mattress with a thin white sheet draped over me by the female masseuse. Every ounce of divine emotion I felt earlier dissipated as I lay in this seductive atmosphere. The room seemed to hold an uncomfortable presence.

As she began working my weary muscles, I began praying in my head for protection and discernment. Almost immediately she stopped and left the room. Since my eyes had adjusted to the lack of light by then, I propped myself up on my elbows to get a clearer view around the room. My eyes automatically were drawn to a picture of a deceased Buddha Master hung on the wall straight across from where I was lying. It was then that I realized she had me in a prostrate position of serenity and was worshiping and paying respect to this deceased Buddha master with acts of service. I need not fear! God's spirit lives within me and is greater than any evil spirit in that room. God protected me from any negative spiritual transference. However, I still wouldn't purposely place myself in this type of situation again. Be careful about what situations you allow yourself to be in. Above all, please remember that we're to love all people. They aren't the enemy, some are just deceived.

There are scientific facts that prove there are several physical benefits to massage. I'm not knocking that, but it's important to have some background knowledge regarding the practitioners we use. There are parlours around the nation that use methods of false religions while treating you and may transfer ungodly spiritual energy over while they lay their hands on you, without you even being aware. Again, what are the intentions of the practitioner? This is a very important question you need to ask yourself. Wives beware! There are also places that give massage that are discretely offering sexual services as well! If your husband's got a bad back it might be in your best interest to do a little homework before sending him out for a backrub. Even better, maybe you should rub it for him!

Don't be afraid to ask questions. Sometimes it may feel a little uncomfortable or even intimidating, but you'll be better off in the long run. Take your matters to the Lord in prayer. Sometimes situations may be blatantly obvious while others are sketchy. We need to be careful. My passion is to help others because I love people and want to lead them in the way of truth by sharing what I have learned and hopefully stop them from repeating any mistakes that I've made.

Sometimes things that emerge our way may appear to be blessings on the surface. We automatically assume they're from God because they appear to be good. However, I've learned that at times the enemy will dangle baited hooks in front of our noses with deceptive morsels on them. We naively think that everything that passes our way is from God.

Although every good gift is from God, we need to pray to ensure that the gift given is actually from Him. Regardless, I believe God used this situation to reveal truth to me to expose the darkness, so that others may see. We can overcome the trickery of the enemy by putting on the armour of God, staying prayerful and standing our guard.

A bank teller learns to identify counterfeit money by handling the real thing day after day. We learn to decipher the Lord's voice by spending time with Him daily as we read His Word and wait in His presence. In the same manner, we too can learn to identify what's false by reading the truth in God's Word.

Always ask the Lord for clear direction about everything. He always leads everyone to the path of everlasting truth. Let peace be your guide. If you start out in a certain direction and you lose your peace, turn back, pray again, and go where God leads you. Don't be afraid to follow your gut instinct. God's the One who put it there! Be careful not to reason yourself out of what God shows you. Remember, Satan is the author of confusion. He'll try to bring it. Prayer, praise, and worship are the best ways to fight this. The spirit that brings confusion isn't able to stay in God's presence.

Meditation

God encourages us to reflect and meditate on Scripture daily to renew our minds (Joshua 1:8; Psalm 119:9–11). When His Word becomes part of us, we're able to make righteous decisions when needed, even in the most difficult circumstances. It's when we act in obedience that we're promised long life and prosperity. There are other forms of meditation that aren't only dangerous, but counterfeit. When a person empties their mind completely, it alters their state of consciousness and allows demons to come in and take control of their psyche. The enemy seeks to kill and destroy by disguising himself in ways that seem harmless, like a wolf in lamb's clothing. Mind control, mantra meditation, transcendental meditation, and hypnosis should also be avoided for the same reasons.

Arts Formed By Practices Rooted in False Religions:

- Acupuncture[29]

- Astrology/horoscopes: is the study of the positions of the Moon, Sun, and other planets in the belief that their motions affect human beings.[30]

- Mantra Meditation: Stilling the mind (thoughtless, empty, silent) to shift and alter consciousness.[31]

- Martial Arts: All types of martial arts hold underlying occult philosophies.[32]

- Past Life Therapy[33]

- Qi gong: A Chinese method of physical and mental training for health, martial arts, and self–enlightenment.

- New Age: believes God is an impersonal source and that the universe and everything within it is God. They also believe in reincarnation and in karma. Karma is a Hinduism and Buddhism belief. They think a person's destiny is determined by their successive phases in a person's existence.[34]

- Crystal therapy: New age belief used to contact the divine within themselves with meditation. They think it magnifies a person's energy by focusing and connecting themselves with universal powers (form of witchcraft, divination, and idolatry). Also used in sound therapy.[35]

- Good luck charms and superstitions: Looking to objects to bring luck or good fortune rather than putting trust and faith in God? This seems innocent, but what isn't done in faith is considered sin (Romans 14:23).

- Homeopathy[36]

- Feng Shui: Chinese superstition belief of placing certain objects in a particular placement to promote health.

- Reiki or radiance technique: a non-physical healing energy made up of life-force energy that is guided by the Higher Intelligence, or spiritually guided life-force energy."[37]

- Self-Hypnosis/hypnosis[38]

- Transcendental meditation[39]

- Psychic Healing/Psychic surgery[40]

- Freemasonry

- Universalism/Unitarianism

- Yoga

- Witchcraft (spells, divination, Ouija boards, etc.)

These are a few of many. If you have been involved with any of these occult ways or others not listed, don't be discouraged; there is hope, you can renounce these things and walk in spiritual freedom with God by breaking off these strongholds with prayer. God is your redeemer and wants you to come to Him with a humble heart of repentance so He can forgive you. As you repent and renounce all evil practices, you'll be set free from the spiritual bondage. Just pray the following prayers with a sincere heart and you can enjoy your new life of freedom (1 John 1:9).

Prayer to Renounce Any Ungodly Practices:

Dear Heavenly Father,

I am thankful that You created the universe and everything in it for my benefit. Please protect me from the lies of the enemy and guide me in the way of truth. Open my eyes that I may see those paths that lead to spiritual death and guide me in ways that bring spiritual and physical health and wellness. Break all curses or spiritual ties that I have opened myself up to. Provide me with Your wisdom, knowledge, and understanding and may I recognize Your path and walk in it.

I acknowledge You as God Almighty, Creator of heaven and earth and Lord of all. I confess that I have sinned against You and Your Word. Please forgive me for my involvement in the sin of idolatry and honouring false gods. I repent and renounce my sins and all occult involvements of _____ (Yoga, Reiki, etc). Bring to my mind any sin involvement that is either known or unknown that I may confess, repent of, and renounce that I may be set free. Lord, I ask You to cut off all ungodly ties that connect me to any ungodly experiences and restore Your godliness back to my soul. I place the cross of Jesus between these sins and myself and plead the blood of Jesus over my life. Thank You for the freedom and liberty You died to give me. I choose to forgive and release those who were also involved in these sins and receive Your forgiveness, grace, and mercy. In Jesus' name I pray. Amen.

Blood Transfusions/Organ Recipients

Sometimes it's necessary for an individual to receive a blood transfusions and/or organ transplant for survival purposes. There are stories of countless people who have received one of these procedures and then acquired new-found cravings and habits. Heart transplant survivors have even reported dreams of situations from the deceased donor's life and have helped solve police cases. Contrary to this, I've heard of others who have struggled with new-fangled emotions such as fear, anxiety, and anger afterwards. I believe the answer behind these phenomena results from "the life" that's in the blood. If you've received either treatment, it's important to pray and ask God to cut the soul tie off between yourself and the donor. This prayer can also be prayed for anyone connected through blood pacts as well.

Dear Heavenly Father,

Thank You for the gift of life that You have given me. I ask You to cut the soul tie created between myself and the donor in the name of Jesus and eliminate anything sinful that may have come into me through that soul tie and re–establish me the way You designed me to be. In Jesus' name I pray. Amen.

"Blessed are those who wash their robes, that they may have the right to the tree of life and may go through the gates into the city. Outside are the dogs, those who practice magic arts, the sexually immoral, the murders, the idolaters, and everyone who loves and practices falsehood." (Revelation 22:14, 15)

God wants us to be blessed. That's why He established covenant with us through Abraham in the beginning. He desires salvation for every man, woman, and child alike and for each one to come to a knowledge of the truth (1 Timothy 2:4). He doesn't want anyone to perish. Let's look at the word blessed for a minute. Blessed means to be set apart; it's something that is sanctified, consecrated, approved, and made holy and brings God's favour!

God is merciful. In His great mercy He gave us the commandments to reveal what sin was, and then instructed us to abide by them. Why? Parents who love their children set boundaries for their benefit. This type of parent wants their child to succeed and do well by informing them of the approach they should take and the repercussions of failing to follow these guidelines. The Israelites knew the penalty for their sins would be death if they didn't abide! (Deuteronomy 28:15) When God created our universe He set it up on a foundation of absolutes; laws of reaping and sowing that excluded no one. Gravity affects us whether we believe it exists or not. God revealed the blessings and the curses (which Satan brings) before the people and told them to choose life. He wanted them to prosper. And He still does!

God has come to our rescue because it's impossible for man to fulfill the Law completely. He sent Jesus, His only son, to pay the debt for our sins. His love and compassion for us is that immense! He gave us the most precious thing He had that we might choose to be in a relationship with Him. We can receive this gift of mercy and salvation by making Jesus the Lord of our lives. God wants us to choose His way, so we can be blessed. He wants to wash away your sin and place a robe of righteousness upon you, that you may inherit the kingdom of God.

"Jesus answered, "I am the way and the truth and the life. No one comes to the Father except through me." (John 14:6)

"Enter through the narrow gate. For wide is the gate and broad is the road that leads to destruction, and many enter through it. But small is the gate and narrow the road that leads to life, and only a few find it." (Matthew 7:13, 14)

Jesus is the narrow gate (John 10:7). Many in the world believe there are many ways to get to Heaven. This is the broad road, which the above Scripture talks about, leading to destruction. Jesus is the only way! Ciphering through all the lies in the world can be comparable to finding a needle in a haystack because there are huge amounts of chaff to wade through. The way to God is clearly marked out for us in Scripture. When you find this amazing treasure, you'll find life beyond compare.

Scripture declares that Christ will return for His church at the end of the age. At that point, all born again believers will rise up with Christ; first the spirits of those who have already passed away and then those remaining on the earth. Christ is looking for people who are pure in heart. On the "day of judgment" we will all stand before Him. But not everyone who comes before Jesus will enter God's kingdom. For His Word says:

"Not everyone who says to me, 'Lord, Lord,' will enter the kingdom of heaven, but only he who does the will of my Father who is in heaven. Many will say to me on that day, 'Lord, Lord, did we not prophesy in your name, and in your name drive out demons and perform many miracles?' Then I will tell them plainly, 'I never knew you. Away from me, you evildoers!'" (Matthew 7:21–23)

God knows each one of us personally. However, we need to know Him intimately. There is a huge difference between "knowing God' and "knowing of" or "about God." The above verse clearly states that it is those who do the Father's will that will enter His gates. True followers of Christ will remain connected with Him. Because of this, they will retain the needed knowledge of what He desires, and follow through with His plan.

"I am the true vine, and my Father is the gardener. He cuts off every branch in me that bears no fruit, while every branch that does bear fruit he prunes so that it will be even more fruitful..."I am the vine; you are the branches. If a man remains in me and I in him, he will bear much fruit; apart from me you can do nothing. If anyone does not remain in me, he is like a branch that is thrown away and withers; such branches are picked up, thrown into the fire and burned." (John 15:1, 2, 5, 6)

We stay connected with God through prayer and by reading His Word. He wants to have an intimate relationship with you, which includes speaking to you, so learn to listen for His voice. As I taught previously: get where it's quiet, praise and worship Him, read your Bible, then stay quiet and listen for what comes to mind. Journal everything; because you hear your own voice inside your head, it's common to

Jesus Our Great Shepherd! 371

think what you've heard is all your own thoughts. Questioning thoughts, phrases, pictures or feelings that come into your spirit is natural and is encouraged.[41] In 1 Thessalonians 5:21, Paul encourages us to test everything and to hold onto what's good. The Holy Spirit always speaks truth, and reveals only those things that will bring glory unto the Father (John 16:13, 14).[42] Ask yourself this simple question: Would Jesus Himself say or do what I think He's asking me to say or do?[43] If your answer is no, then you can be sure it wasn't Him! In the same respect, Satan is not going to encourage you or make you feel good about yourself. If what you've pictured or heard weakens your faith and fills you with condemnation, it's the enemy. God draws us into repentance to draw us closer to Him, not to make us feel bad. Compare everything with Scripture. If it isn't in harmony with the Word, then discard it.

The book of Revelation declares, Christ and His army will defeat the enemy and he will be thrown into the lake of fire with his followers. I don't know about you, but I certainly don't want this for myself! *"There will be weeping there, and gnashing of teeth."* (Luke 13:24a)

False Prophets

"This is how you can recognize the Spirit of God: Every spirit that acknowledges that Jesus Christ has come in the flesh is from God, but every spirit that does not acknowledge Jesus is not from God. This is the spirit of the antichrist, which you have heard is coming and even now is already in the world." (1 John 4:2, 3)

Jesus warns us in His Word that there will be many false prophets in the world that will try to deceive us (Matthew 24:11). The good news is that He also tells us how to differentiate between the good and the bad. Jesus warns us to test the spirits in 1 John 4:1. The antichrist is anyone who is against Jesus.

Idolatry and Worshipping Other Gods

"You shall not bow down to them or worship them; for I, the Lord your God, am a jealous God, punishing the children for the sin of the fathers to the third and fourth generation of those who hate me, but showing love to a thousand generations of those who love me and keep my commandments." (Deuteronomy 5:9)

Although some things we value are very important and should be placed in a position of honour, we must be careful not to put anyone or anything before God or worship them. Some people worship the ground their spouse, children, friend, a favourite performer, singer, or actor walks on. In some cases people worship themselves! We can make a god out of just about anything. Perhaps you worship a sport, your place of status, your earthly possessions or money. The list could be endless. To what or whom are you giving precedence in your life? Every god aside from the One true God, is counterfeit! I'm not going to get into the history or principles of what each religion believes; however, I will say this:

Only our Heavenly Father was able to create the entire universe with the spoken Word. He created you out of an expression of His love and filled the world with wonderful things for your enjoyment. All religions (other than relationship with Jesus, which really isn't a religion), are based on a person having to earn their salvation. Some religions demand sacrifice and punishment. God offers us the free gift of eternal pardon and redemption through Jesus. Out of all the beliefs in the world, Jesus is the only one who claimed to be God. He said He would die and would come back to life. He sacrificially laid down His life for our sins and took His life back up again! There were over 500 witnesses that saw Him after He rose from the grave. He proved He was God by fulfilling His own prophecy. Everything He said He would do, He did!

What I've Seen and Experienced!

I've experienced the personal touch of God many times firsthand. When I've called out to Him, He has always been there! I know He is the way, the truth, and the life. He is my absolute! He is the One and only true foundation on which we can stand. Unfortunately, many people have misinterpreted religion for having a relationship with God. It's not about following a bunch of rules so that we don't get our fingers rapped. God loves each one of us and wants to have a relationship with us. The choice is up to you! The reason God wants us to uphold the Law is so that we'll prosper and do well. It doesn't earn our salvation. Living according to man-made religion will cause failure, but a relationship won't, not with Jesus.

All Religions Do Not Lead to God!

All paths present themselves as truth. However, God's Word, which cannot be compromised, says: He is the One and only God.

My heart ached for the young mother who I used to meet at my son's bus stop. She practiced paganism and had no qualms about performing witchcraft. She was quite proud of it really. Her life was in such a mess, yet even after sharing the gospel with her she refused to believe its truth. I watched her as she slipped into depression, suffered from migraine headaches and seizures. She continued to see her pagan priest who advised her about spells and sorts. Her health continued to decline and her marriage fell apart. She eventually moved back home with her mother who also practiced this religion and took her two young boys with her. It makes me sad to think that the world is full of dying people who don't know Jesus.

Where Will You Spend Eternity?

Like all good shepherds who find a place for their sheep to rest, Jesus has promised to prepare a home in paradise for each one of His followers for when their time is finished on this earth. If you have accepted Jesus as your Lord and Saviour, you don't need to worry about where you'll spend eternity! I truly believe the length of our days is marked out for us. It's much more than fate (Ecclesiastes 3:1)! Our time to leave this earth may be tomorrow, it could be 30 or 40 years from now, or more. Only the Lord knows the answer to that question. But until that time, God is preparing an amazing dwelling place for you in Heaven where you'll be eternally secure if you accept Him as Your Lord and Saviour.

"Do not let your hearts be troubled. Trust in God; trust also in me. In my Father's house are many rooms; if it were not so, I would have told you. I am going there to prepare a place for you. And if I go and prepare a place for you, I will come back and take you to be with me that you also may be where I am. You know the way to the place where I am going." (John 14:1–3)

God planned our lives before He even created the world and all that is in it. Even before God spoke the actual words that placed your soul into your mother's womb (Ephesians 2:10). God is the Alpha and the Omega, the beginning and the end. He is the author of our lives from start to finish (Hebrews 12:2). Although Satan tries to destroy humankind (John 10:10), Jesus is right there rewriting the script of our lives to work everything out for good. He won't abandon you or your loved ones!

"In him we were also chosen, having been predestined according to the plan of him who works out everything in conformity with the purpose of his will." (Ephesians 1:11)

"And we know that in all things God works for the good of those who love him, who have been called according to his purpose." (Romans 8:28)

You can have peace knowing that whenever it's your time to go from this earth, God will be there to receive your soul and will remain faithful to watch over your family. God is larger than any problem they may face. Need I remind you that He measured out the water in His hands? He's a big God! When a mother gives birth to her newborn child she quickly discovers her heart opening wider than she could have ever imagined. The love she feels must be expressed, she finds herself wanting to do whatever possible to comfort and protect the fragile life of her baby. This nurturing quality comes from God Himself and it's with that same love that God will continue to love them. His Word says He fathers the fatherless and defends the widows (Psalms 68:5). Since God is no respecter of persons, He's not about to pick favourites. Men and women are equal in God's eyes. He delights in both and will therefore do the same for the motherless.

Quite a few friends of my friends only have boys in their family; we joke and say we belong to the "The Boys' Club". But there is one particular family who felt it was time to graduate from the all boys club and add a little pink to the mix for a change! Three wasn't enough. Eldon and Shelly Horner have an amazing story about how they came to adopt a little girl from Russia whose mother used narcotic substances while pregnant with her. God took this fragile, underweight girl from an orphanage, where she spent most of her time in a crib and placed her in a thriving home where she is loved and cared for as their very own. Katie has been given all the love and nurturing a little girl could ever want and is growing up to be a beautiful, bright, little girl who loves Jesus.

God's specialty is taking unfortunate situations and working things out for good! God wants to fill the voids in our lives with His presence. And He does it even in ways we don't realize. He's so good! If you take a good look back over the years of your life you should be able to see God's handprint in your life! Times where He has placed just the right person at the right time to encourage you or help you in a situation. We may not have always taken their advice or appreciated the guidance, but God has always been there trying to protect and point us in the right direction. God is not about to give up on your loved ones either. They were His children first!

For God's children, things always have a way of turning out, even in the worst situations. God promises He will work everything out according to His will for our good. Even when you can't see the evidence, you can have an assurance that He is working behind the scenes. God promises to continue the good work that He has started and will continue until Jesus comes back to rescue His church (Philippians 1:6). He knows what's best for us even though we don't always understand.

Do you have an assurance about where you'll spend eternity? Most people believe Heaven exists and many want to pretend that hell doesn't. Some even think hell is what you experience on earth! The truth cannot be ignored! Eventually it will affect everyone one way or another. The world has many ideas about how to get to heaven. Some believe they can get there by being a good person, whether by way of righteous works, acts of discipline or through self-glorification, while others believe religion is the key. These are all avenues in which a person must strive to achieve. You can't get to Heaven by following tradition or rules, they will only burden you. Rules are necessary in life. They help us differentiate between right and wrong and are put in place to keep us safe, but living by them is not what gets us to Heaven.

"For we maintain that a man is justified by faith apart from observing the law. Do we, then, nullify the law by this faith? Not at all! Rather we uphold the law." (Romans 3:28, 31)

We can only get to Heaven by our faith in Jesus Christ. That's it! That is how we're justified, all because of what Christ did for us. Jesus fulfilled the Law by what He did on the cross, making it possible for us to have a relationship with God the Father. When we come into a relationship with

God, He changes us on the inside by giving us a deep desire in our hearts to do what's right. This is how we're able to show God our love and appreciation in return for what He has done for us.

The Lord says: "These people come near to me with their mouth and honour me with their lips, but their hearts are far from me. Their worship of me is made up only of rules taught by men." (Isaiah 29:13)

It saddens my heart to think of how many people may be lost because they don't have hearts that honour God. Wonderful people, who believe they are on their way to Heaven because they go to church on Sunday, sing in the choir, and put money in the offering plate. We can do all the right things, but unless we have hearts that honour God in spirit and in truth, it means absolutely nothing. All the lip service in the world won't do us any good unless our hearts are involved.

"For it is by grace you have been saved, through faith—and this not from yourselves, it is the gift of God—not by works, so that no one can boast." (Ephesians 2:8)

God has given us a purpose and has planned good things for us to do while we're here on this planet (Romans 2:10). But the road to Heaven is not paved with good deeds and it certainly doesn't put us into a relationship with God. Salvation is a free gift we attain by believing. It is a wonderful gift of unmerited favour. Not one person will ever be able to boast in Heaven of the great things they have done to receive eternal salvation. Not one!

What does your family lineage look like? Do you come from a godly heritage? Are you hoping to get in by the grace of another family member? There is not one person on earth able to swing their way up to Heaven by their mama's apron strings (Ezekiel 14:12–23). Righteousness comes by our faith alone. Each one of us needs to make our own personal decision.

"This is good, and pleases God our Savior, who wants all men to be saved and to come to a knowledge of the truth." (1 Timothy 2: 3, 4)

"But God demonstrates his own love for us in this: While we were still sinners, Christ died for us." (Romans 5:8)

Our Heavenly Father Himself has made the way by reaching down to mankind by making the sacrifice for us. We don't have to be perfect, perform, strive for perfection or work our fingers to the bone. We just have to receive and accept this free gift by opening ourselves up to God and receive Him into our hearts by faith and live for Him. Jesus did it all!

"Here I am! I stand at the door and knock. If anyone hears my voice and opens the door, I will come in and eat with him, and he with me." (Revelation 3:20)

God wants and desires to have a personal relationship with every person on earth. He loves us so much that He gave His only son to die for our sins. Even if you were the only person on earth, Jesus would still have laid His life down for you because you mean that much to Him. It's His desire for you to come to know Him as your Heavenly Father. He wants to lead you into the way of everlasting life to spend eternity with Him. The description of Heaven in the Bible is amazing. There is no crying or pain, just peace and joy in God's presence. By sincerely opening your life up to God and making Him your Lord you can have the blessed assurance that even if you don't receive your healing on this earth the way you hoped for, you will experience it in eternity with Jesus.

"For to me, to live is Christ and to die is gain." (Philippians 1:21)

Prayer of Salvation

If you would like to ask the Lord into your heart and make Him the Lord and Saviour of your life, say the following prayer out loud.

Dear Heavenly Father,

I accept Your invitation to be in a relationship with You. Thank You for sending Jesus to die in my place that I may live more abundantly. I believe and act on Your Word that says if I confess with my mouth, "Jesus is Lord," and believe in my heart that God raised Him from the dead, I will be saved. For it is with my heart that I believe and am justified, and it is with my mouth that I confess and am saved (Romans 10:9, 10). Please forgive me for my sins and come into my heart and life. Fill me with Your Holy Spirit that I may live now and forevermore. In Jesus' name I pray. Amen.

If you sincerely prayed this prayer you have just begun your journey with our Heavenly Father. Welcome to the family of God! All the angels in Glory are rejoicing over your salvation for your name has been written in the Lambs' Book of Life. God has removed your sin from you as far as the east is from the west. God's Word promises that when *we confess our sins, He is faithful and just to forgive us our sins, and to cleanse us from all unrighteousness* (1 John 1:9).

Some Parting Wisdom...

When we accept Jesus as our Saviour, the seeds of God's character traits are placed within us. The Bible says, *"Therefore, if anyone is in Christ, he is a new creation; the old has gone, the new has come!"* As you read God's Word and allow His Spirit to work within you, those seeds will begin to grow and flourish. As they do, God changes you from the inside out to become all that you can be and helps you receive the desired life you were always meant to live. This doesn't mean that life will always be easy. I'm sure you'll still have your share of ups and downs. You will, however, have God's help, along with the reassurance of never being alone! Keep seeking God with all your heart. Don't rely on your own ability to understand life's situations. Instead acknowledge God in everything. Make

Him the Lord over your actions, motives and decisions and He will guide and direct you in everything with peace (Proverbs 3:5). Keep short accounts with God. When you sense in your heart that you've done something wrong quickly ask for forgiveness. It's as simple as that. It's important to feed your spirit with the Word of God, so that you can learn to discern God's voice. Find a good, Spirit-filled, Bible-believing church where you can feed your spirit and grow in the Lord. God has placed the seeds of righteousness within your heart, but it's up to you to nurture them. God is pleased with you! Rejoice and celebrate. Tell a friend about the wonderful choice you have made. You no longer live in condemnation! Take comfort in knowing that God's Holy Spirit is with you to guide your every step.

"And I will ask the Father, and he will give you another Counselor to be with you forever—the Spirit of truth. The world cannot accept him, because it neither sees him nor knows him. But you know him, for he lives with you and will be in you." (John 14:16, 17)

"Arise, shine, for your light has come, and the glory of the Lord rises upon you." (Isaiah 60:1)

I learned many valuable lessons through this experience. It is my hope and prayer that I will always hold onto the wisdom, knowledge, and understanding I've gained through this journey and stand firm on the ground I've attained in my battle. May God also grant you this same request.

The time has come to say goodbye! Thank you for spending time with me and allowing me to openly share my heart and life with you. I hope and pray this book has brought the spiritual, emotional, and physical healing needed in your life. Above all else, seek the great Healer, over and above your healing! Ultimately, having a relationship with God is what really matters in the end! God Bless!

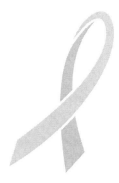

[1] "In Touch With Dr. Charles Stanley - Episode Guide /Locate TV" *Locate TV*, (Season 1 Episode 190, Good Shepherd) 16 Nov. 2010 (www.locatetv.com/tv/in-touch-with...charlesstanley/.../eposodeguide).

[2] Ibid.

[3] Ibid.

[4] Nelson. *ITP Nelson Canadian Dictionary of the English language. An Encyclopedic Reference* (Scarborough, ON: International Thompson Publishing, Nelson; A division of Thompson Canada Limited, 1997), p. 947.

[5] Rallo, Dr. Vito. *Shocking Secrets Behind Martial Arts & Yoga* (Riverview, FL: Free Indeed Ministries of Tampa Bay, 2009), pp. 6-7.

[6] Ibid, pp. 7, 23, 24.

[7] Ibid, p. 24.

[8] "Yoga." *Wikipedia.* 25 June 2010 (http://en.wikipedia.org/wiki/Yoga). Source: Flood, "*An introduction to Hinduism*" (Cambridge University Press, Cambridge, 1996), p. 94.

[9] Rallo, Dr. Vito. *Shocking Secrets Behind Martial Arts & Yoga* (Riverview, FL: Free Indeed Ministries of Tampa Bay, 2009), p. 24.

[10] "Yoga."*Wikipedia*. 25 June 2010 (http://en.wikipedia.org/wiki/Yoga). Source: Phillips, Stephen H., *"Classical Indian Metaphysics: Refutations of Realism and the Emergence of "New Logic."* (Open Court Publishing, 1995), pp. 12-13.

[11] "Yoga – Just Exercise or a Hindu Religion?" Let Us Reason Ministries, Oppenheimer, Mike. *Lighthouse Trails Research Project- Exposing Contemplative Spirituality*. 15 May 2010 (http://www.lighthousetrailresearch.com/yoga.htm).

[12] Rallo, Dr. Vito, *Shocking Secrets Behind Martial Arts & Yoga* (Riverview, FL: Free Indeed Ministries of Tampa Bay, 2009), pp. 19-20, 29.

[13] "There is no Christian Yoga?" Prem,Yogi Baba. *Lighthouse Trails Research Project- Exposing Contemplative Spirituality*. 15 May 2010 (http://www.lighthousetrailresearch.com/yoga.htm).

[14] "Can We Separate Exercise from the Philosophy?" Michaelsen, Johanna. *Lighthouse Trails Research Project- Exposing Contemplative Spirituality*. 15 May 2010. Exert from: *"Like Lambs to the Slaughter."* Harvest House Publishing, 1998), pp. 93-95, (http://www.lighthousetrailresearch.com/yoga.htm).

[15] "East and West, The Two Shall Never Meet, Can Yogic Practices Be Integrated With The Christian Faith?" DeBruyn, Pastor Larry, *Lighthouse Trails Research Project- Exposing Contemplative Spirituality*. 15 May 2010 (http://www.lighthousetrailresearch.com/yoga.htm). Also linked at:

(http://www.frbaptist.org/bin/view/Ptp/PtpTopic20060522141106)
Owens, Darryl E., "'Christian yoga' strikes a new
pose,"*DenverPost.com*, 18 May 2006
(http://www.denverpost.com/lifestyleles/ci_3819655).
[16] "Innocent Yoga?" Ankerberg, Dr. John. Weldon, Dr. John.
Lighthouse Trails Research Project- Exposing Contemplative Spirituality. 15
May 2010 (http://www.lighthousetrailresearch.com/yoga.htm).
Also linked at: (http://www.ankerberg.com/Articles/new-
age/NA1101W1.htm), Ankerberg, Dr. John, Weldon, Dr. John. *The
Coming Darkness: Confronting Occult Deception*, Eugene, OR: Harvest
House Publishers, 1993.
[17] Rallo, Dr. Vito. *Shocking Secrets Behind Martial Arts & Yoga*
(Riverview, FL: Free Indeed Ministries of Tampa Bay, 2009), p. 25.
[18] Ibid.
[19] "Wake up the Church, Get Biblical - The Spiritual Danger of
Martial Arts!" Larson, Bob. *Sound An Alarm Christian Faith Assembly*. 15
May 2010. (http://www.soundanalarm.com/wakeup/Martial
Arts.htm).
[20] Rallo, Dr. Vito, *Shocking Secrets Behind Martial Arts & Yoga*
(Riverview, FL: Free Indeed Ministries of Tampa Bay, 2009), p. 4, 7.
[21] "Reiki Energy, What is it? What does it heal?" Rand, William
Lee. *Lighthouse Trails Research Project- Exposing Contemplative Spirituality*.
15 May 2010 (http://www.lighthousetrailresearch.com/yoga.htm).
Link: Reiki News Articles; *The International Centre for Reiki Training*,
1990-2010 (http://www.reiki.org/reikinews/whaislg.html).
[22] "The Truth About Reiki, A Dangerous and Occultic Practice;
Jesus loves you," Editors at Lighthouse Trails Research Project,
Lighthouse Trails Research Project- Exposing Contemplative Spirituality. 15

May 2010 (http://www.lighthousetrailresearch.com/yoga.htm).
Link: (http://www.reikidangers.eu/spirit.htm).

[23] Ibid, 15 May 2010. Link: "Reiki Dangers-Testimonies."

[24] Ibid.

[25] "The Truth About Reiki, A Dangerous and Occultic Practice;
Jesus loves you," Editors at Lighthouse Trails Research Project,
Lighthouse Trails Research Project- Exposing Contemplative Spirituality. 15
May 2010 (http://www.lighthousetrailresearch.com/yoga.htm).
Link: (http://www.reikidangers.eu/spirit.htm).

[26] Ibid.

[27] Ibid.

[28] Ibid.

[29] Horrobin, Peter. *Healing through Deliverance, The Foundation of
Deliverance Ministry Vol#2* (Grand Rapids, MI: Chosen; A Division of
Baker Book House Company, 2003), p. 275.

[30] "*ITP Nelson Canadian Dictionary of the English language, An Encyclopaedic
Reference*", International Thompson Publishing, Nelson; A division of
Thompson Canada Limited, 1997, p. 84. Additional Resource:
"*Britannica Junior, (Vol. #2)*; An Encyclopaedia for Boys and Girls",
Published by Encyclopaedia Britannica, Inc., Chicago, Canada, Ltd.,
Toronto and Ltd., London, 1943), p. 276.

[31] Horrobin, p. 281.

[32] "Wake up the Church, Get Biblical – The Spiritual Danger of
Martial Arts!" Tardo, Dr. Russell. *Sound An Alarm, Christian Faith
Assembly*. 15 May 2010 (Faithful Word Publications, Arabi, LA.
(http://www.soundanalarm.com/wakeup/MartialArts.htm).

[33] Horrobin, p. 282.

[34] Ibid, 286.

[35] Ibid, p. 278.

[36] Ibid, p. 285;
(http//www.thenarrowwayministries.org/Articles.asp?Action=Article&intArticleID=21).

[37] "Reiki Energy, What is it? What does it heal?" Rand, William
Lee. *Lighthouse Trails Research Project- Exposing Contemplative Spirituality.*
15 May 2010 (http://www.lighthousetrailresearch.com/yoga.htm).
Link: Reiki News Articles; *The International Centre for Reiki Training,*
1990-2010.

[38] Horrobin, p. 280.

[39] Ibid, p. 287.

[40] Ibid, p. 290.

[41] Foy Savelle, Terry. *Make your Dreams Bigger Than Your Memories*
(Ventura, California, USA: Regal, 2010), p. 58.

[42] Ibid.

[43] Ibid.